Acute Medicine

A practical guide to the management
of medical emergencies

David C. Sprigings

Consultant Physician
Northampton General Hospital
Northampton, UK

John B. Chambers

Reader, Guy's and St Thomas' Hospitals
London, UK
and Consultant Cardiologist
Maidstone Hospital
Kent, UK

THIRD EDITION

Blackwell
Science

© 1990, 1995, 2001 by
Blackwell Science Ltd
Editorial Offices:
Osney Mead, Oxford OX2 0EL
25 John Street, London WC1N 2BS
23 Ainslie Place, Edinburgh EH3 6AJ
350 Main Street, Malden
  MA 02148-5018, USA
54 University Street, Carlton
  Victoria 3053, Australia
10, rue Casimir Delavigne
  75006 Paris, France

Other Editorial Offices:
Blackwell Wissenschafts-Verlag GmbH
Kurfürstendamm 57
10707 Berlin, Germany

Blackwell Science KK
MG Kodenmacho Building
7–10 Kodenmacho Nihombashi
Chuo-ku, Tokyo 104, Japan

Iowa State University Press
A Blackwell Science Company
2121 S. State Avenue
Ames, Iowa 50014-8300, USA

First published 1990
Reprinted 1991, 1992, 1993, 1994
Second edition 1995
Reprinted 1996 (twice), 1997, 1999
Third edition 2001

Set by Best-set Typesetter Ltd.,
Hong Kong
Printed and bound in Great Britain by
MPG Books, Bodmin, Cornwall

DISTRIBUTORS

Marston Book Services Ltd
PO Box 269
Abingdon, Oxon OX14 4YN
(*Orders*: Tel: 01235 465500
        Fax: 01235 465555)

USA
Blackwell Science, Inc.
Commerce Place
350 Main Street
Malden, MA 02148-5018
(*Orders*: Tel: 800 759 6102
          781 388 8250
        Fax: 781 388 8255)

Canada
Login Brothers Book Company
324 Saulteaux Crescent
Winnipeg, Manitoba R3J 3T2
(*Orders*: Tel: 204 837 2987)

Australia
Blackwell Science Pty Ltd
54 University Street
Carlton, Victoria 3053
(*Orders*: Tel: 3 9347 0300
        Fax: 3 9347 5001)

A catalogue record for this title
is available from the British Library

ISBN 0-632-05455-7

Library of Congress
Cataloging-in-publication Data

Sprigings, David.
    Acute medicine : a practical guide to
  the management of medical emergencies
  / David C. Sprigings, John B. Chambers.
  — 3rd ed.
      p.; cm.
    Includes bibliographical references
  and index.
    ISBN 0-632-05455-7
      1. Medical emergencies—
    Handbooks, manuals,
    etc.   I. Chambers, John,
    MD.   II. Title.
    [DNLM: 1. Emergencies—Handbooks.
  WB 39 S769a 2001]
  RC86.8 .S68 2001
  616.02′5—dc21   00-045449

For further information on
Blackwell Science, visit our website:
www.blackwell-science.com

Contents

Preface to the third edition, viii
Acknowledgements, ix

Section 1: Common Presentations

1 Cardiac arrest, 3
2 Cardiac arrhythmias, 10
3 Hypotension, 36
4 Acute chest pain, 46
5 Acute breathlessness, 57
6 The unconscious patient, 64
7 Transient loss of consciousness, 74
8 Acute confusional state, 84
9 Headache, 92
10 Sepsis syndrome, 100
11 Poisoning, 106
12 The critically ill patient, 127

Section 2: Specific Problems

Cardiovascular
13 Acute myocardial infarction, 137
14 Unstable angina, 151
15 Aortic dissection, 156
16 Severe hypertension, 160
17 Pulmonary oedema, 165
18 Pericarditis, 172
19 Cardiac tamponade, 175
20 Deep vein thrombosis, 178
21 Pulmonary embolism, 183

Respiratory

22 Acute asthma, 193

23 Acute exacerbation of chronic obstructive pulmonary disease, 198

24 Pneumonia, 206

25 Pneumothorax, 217

26 Haemoptysis, 221

Neurological

27 Stroke, 227

28 Transient ischaemic attack, 237

29 Subarachnoid haemorrhage, 242

30 Bacterial meningitis, 247

31 Spinal cord compression, 254

32 Guillain–Barré syndrome, 256

33 Epilepsy, 261

Gastrointestinal/Liver/Renal

34 Acute upper gastrointestinal haemorrhage, 273

35 Acute diarrhoea, 281

36 Acute abdominal pain, 288

37 Acute liver failure, 295

38 Acute renal failure, 302

Endocrine/Metabolic

39 Overview of diabetes, 319

40 Diabetic ketoacidosis, 328

41 Hyperosmolar non-ketotic hyperglycaemia, 335

42 Electrolyte disorders, 336

43 Acid–base disorders and arterial blood gases, 353

44 Acute adrenal insufficiency, 364

45 Thyrotoxic crisis, 369

46 Hypothermia (including myxoedema coma), 373

Infectious Diseases

47 Acute medical problems in the patient with HIV/AIDS, 381

48 Septic arthritis, 387

49 Fever on return from abroad, 392

Haematological

50 Management of anticoagulation, 403

51 Sickle cell crisis, 409

52 Anaphylaxis and anaphylactic shock, 414

Section 3: Procedures

53 Central vein cannulation, 419

54 Pulmonary artery catheterization, 429

55 Temporary cardiac pacing, 438

56 Pericardial aspiration, 447

57 DC cardioversion, 451

58 Insertion of a chest drain, 455

59 Lumbar puncture, 461

60 Peritoneal dialysis, 467

61 Insertion of a Sengstaken–Blakemore tube, 472

Appendices

62 Drug infusions, 479

63 Respiratory function tests, 486

64 Peripheral nervous system, 491

Further reading, 496

Index, 509

Preface to the third edition

The need for an easily portable practical guide to the management of medical emergencies has not diminished over the past five years. For this edition we have updated every chapter in line with current evidence and guidelines, and have added new chapters on the critically ill patient, acute diarrhoea, abdominal pain, electrolyte derangements and acid–base disorders. The layout has been improved to make key information even more accessible.

DCS
JBC
Northampton, May 2000

Acknowledgements

We are indebted to the following colleagues for expert criticism of sections of the manuscript of the third edition:

Christopher Blauth, Mac Cochrane, Paul Davies, Jules Dussek, David Goldsmith, Professor John Henry, Richard Heppell, Anne Kilvert, Bridget MacDonald, Iheanyi Okpala, Michael Polkey, John Rees, Anthony Rudd, Udi Shmueli, David Treacher and Mark Wilkinson. We thank Maureen Hyde for the electrocardiograms.

Section 1
Common Presentations

1 Cardiac arrest

- Cardiac arrest is defined as the sudden loss of consciousness with absent femoral or carotid pulses. The commonest cause is ventricular fibrillation (VF) or pulseless ventricular tachycardia (VT) (Table 1.1).
- Effective basic life support and early defibrillation are the key elements in successful resuscitation.
- Whenever possible, patients and their relatives should be involved in the decision whether to resuscitate in the event of cardiac arrest. The reasons for a decision not to resuscitate should be recorded in the casenotes, and the decision reviewed if the patient's condition changes.

Basic life support

- In witnessed ventricular fibrillation or pulseless ventricular tachycardia, basic life support should be preceded by a single precordial thump, followed by defibrillation if the thump does not restore an effective rhythm.

Figure 1.1 shows the algorithm for single rescuer basic life support in adults.

- The recommended rate of chest compression is 100/min, with 2 rescue breaths given after 15 compressions.

Advanced life support

Figure 1.2 shows the algorithm for advanced life support in adults.

1 Airway maintenance and ventilation
- Start with a bag-valve-mask device (Ambubag), which allows ventilation with 100% oxygen.

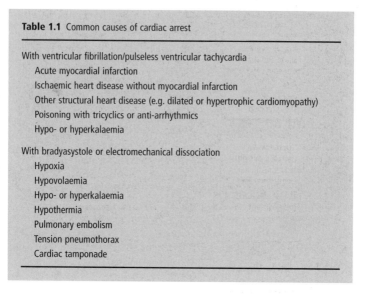

Table 1.1 Common causes of cardiac arrest

With ventricular fibrillation/pulseless ventricular tachycardia
   Acute myocardial infarction
   Ischaemic heart disease without myocardial infarction
   Other structural heart disease (e.g. dilated or hypertrophic cardiomyopathy)
   Poisoning with tricyclics or anti-arrhythmics
   Hypo- or hyperkalaemia

With bradyasystole or electromechanical dissociation
   Hypoxia
   Hypovolaemia
   Hypo- or hyperkalaemia
   Hypothermia
   Pulmonary embolism
   Tension pneumothorax
   Cardiac tamponade

• Aim for a tidal volume of 400–600 ml (enough to make the chest rise). This is adequate and less likely to cause gastric insufflation than larger volumes.
• Endotracheal intubation should be done as soon as possible by an anaesthetist or other person trained in the procedure.

2 Chest compression
• With two rescuers, the recommended ratio of chest compressions to ventilations is 5:1 (i.e. chest compression 100/min and ventilation 20/min).

3 Defibrillation for VF/VT
• Defibrillation is given in groups of 3 shocks. The initial sequence is 200 J, 200 J and 360 J. Subsequent shocks, if needed, are at 360 J.
• Defibrillation must be done safely. The first shock should be charged either on the patient's chest or in the machine, and not in the air. The paddles should then be kept on the chest for subsequent shocks as

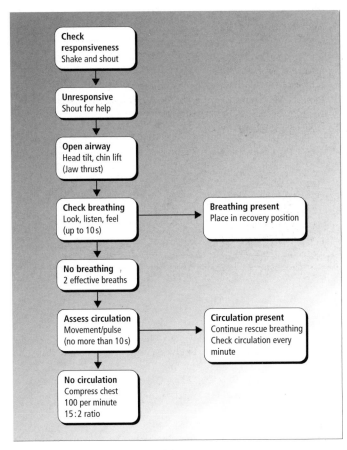

Fig. 1.1 Algorithm for adult basic life support.

required. If the defibrillator is charged but then not needed, it should be discharged with the paddles back in the machine. The operator should call to all staff that the defibrillator is being charged and again before delivering the shock, and should look to make sure that no one is in contact directly or indirectly with the patient before the shock is delivered.

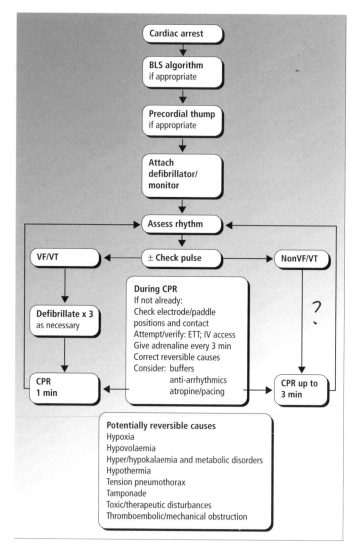

Fig. 1.2 Algorithm for adult advanced life support. Note that each successive step is based on the assumption that the one before has been unsuccessful.

• Only check the pulse between shocks if the ECG waveform changes to one compatible with a spontaneous output.

• Gel pads should be changed every 3 shocks, and strong pressure should be applied to the chest wall with the paddles to prevent the shock from arcing and to reduce transthoracic impedance.

4 Drug delivery

• If a central venous line is not already in place, put as large a bore cannula as possible (e.g. grey Venflon) in a large peripheral vein. Use a flush of 20 ml of normal saline after drug administration.

• If venous access cannot be established, adrenaline and atropine can be given via an endotracheal tube: give twice the dose used IV, diluted with isotonic saline to a volume of 10 ml.

5 Specific drug therapy

• **Adrenaline** (1 mg IV) should be given in each cycle (i.e. roughly every 3 min) to enhance basic life support irrespective of cardiac rhythm, except in cardiac arrest related to solvent abuse, cocaine or other sympathomimetic drugs, when it should not be used.

• **Atropine** (3 mg IV) should be given if arrest is due to bradyasystole.

• **Anti-arrhythmic drugs** may be given after 4 cycles of advanced life support (12 shocks) to patients with refractory ventricular fibrillation/ventricular tachycardia (Table 1.2).

• **Buffers** Sodium bicarbonate (50 ml of 8.4% solution (50 mmol)) should only be given if there is severe acidosis (arterial pH < 7.1) or in

Table 1.2 Drug therapy of refractory ventricular fibrillation/ventricular tachycardia

Lignocaine	100 mg (5 mL of 2% solution) IV over 30 s
Procainamide	100 mg by slow IV injection every 5 min up to a total dose of 1 g
Amiodarone	150–300 mg IV over 1–2 min
Bretylium	5–10 mg/kg IV over 15–30 min

the event of cardiac arrest due to hyperkalaemia (p. 344) or tricyclic poisoning.

6 Non-VF/VT rhythms

• Check electrode or paddle positions and contacts before concluding the rhythm is not VF/VT.

• Consider the treatable causes of cardiac arrest with bradyasystole or electromechanical dissociation (Table 1.1).

• Give atropine 3 mg IV if there is bradyasystole.

• Temporary pacing is indicated if the patient has severe bradycardia (<40/min) or ventricular asystole with visible P waves. While transvenous pacing is being arranged, use an external pacing system. If this is not available, external cardiac percussion ('thump' pacing, at a rate of 100/min) may generate an effective cardiac output.

• Reassess the rhythm after 3 min of resuscitation. If this is now VF/VT, manage accordingly with defibrillation. If not, continue resuscitation for as long as it is appropriate (see **7**).

7 When to stop resuscitation

• There is no universally applicable rule, but in most cases resuscitation should be stopped after 30 min if there is refractory asystole or electromechanical dissociation. Other rhythms may imply a potentially salvageable heart.

• Where cardiac arrest is due to hypothermia or poisoning, patients have survived neurologically intact after even longer resuscitation attempts.

• In patients without myocardial disease, do not stop resuscitation unless arterial pH and potassium are normal and core temperature is >36°C.

• Adrenaline causes dilatation of pupils and this sign should not be used as evidence of irreversible neurological damage during or immediately after resuscitation.

After successful resuscitation

1 The patient should be transferred to the CCU or ITU, with ECG monitoring during transfer. The airway should be protected until the patient is fully conscious. Mechanical ventilation should be continued if:

Table 1.3 Urgent investigation after successful resuscitation

ECG (? acute myocardial infarction, long QT interval)
Chest X-ray (? pulmonary oedema, pneumothorax, rib fracture)
Arterial blood gases and pH
Plasma potassium
Blood glucose

- the patient is comatose (Glasgow Coma Scale 8 or less (p. 72));
- there is severe pulmonary oedema;
- arterial Po_2 is < 9 kPa (70 mmHg) (breathing 60% oxygen) or Pco_2 is > 6.5 kPa (50 mmHg).

2 Decide why the arrest occurred (Table 1.3) and take action to deal with the underlying causes.

- Correct low or high potassium, low or high blood glucose, hypoxia and severe acidosis.
- Consider prophylactic anti-arrhythmic therapy in patients in whom arrest was due to VF/VT (p. 25), bearing in mind that these drugs have a negative inotropic effect.
- Place a transvenous pacing wire (p. 438) if arrest was due to bradyasystole.
- Arterial blood pressure should be maintained using inotropic/vasopressor agents if necessary (p. 42).

3 Intravenous lines inserted without sterile technique during the resuscitation should be changed.

2 Cardiac arrhythmias

Treatment should begin without a definitive electrical diagnosis if there is significant haemodynamic compromise (Fig. 2.1).

Priorities

If there is imminent cardiac arrest:
- Call the arrest team and manage along standard lines (see Chapter 1).

If there is a reduced level of consciousness, severe pulmonary oedema, or systolic BP is < 80 mmHg:
- Record a 12-lead ECG (if possible) for later analysis.
- **If the heart rate is >150/min:** call an anaesthetist in preparation for DC cardioversion starting at 200 J (p. 45).
- **If the heart rate is <50/min:** give atropine 0.6–1.2 mg IV, with further doses at 5-min intervals up to a total dose of 3 mg if the heart rate remains below 60/min. If the bradycardia is unresponsive or recurs, put in a transvenous pacing wire (see p. 438). If necessary, whilst transferring the patient to the screening room either start an isoprenaline infusion (Table 2.1) or use an external cardiac pacing system.

If the patient is haemodynamically stable:
- There is time to make a working diagnosis and plan management.
- Record a 12-lead electrocardiogram and a long rhythm strip.

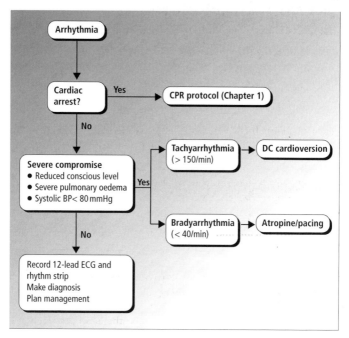

Fig. 2.1 Emergency treatment of cardiac arrhythmias.

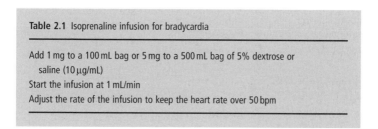

Table 2.1 Isoprenaline infusion for bradycardia

Add 1 mg to a 100 mL bag or 5 mg to a 500 mL bag of 5% dextrose or
   saline (10 μg/mL)
Start the infusion at 1 mL/min
Adjust the rate of the infusion to keep the heart rate over 50 bpm

Diagnosis of arrhythmias

Diagnosis of tachyarrhythmias (rate >120/min)

The diagnosis depends on the QRS width (normal or broader than 120 ms) and whether the rhythm is regular or irregular.

Broad and regular (Fig. 2.2)
• The diagnosis is usually ventricular tachycardia (VT) (Fig. 2.3). Haemodynamic stability does not exclude VT.
• If there is ischaemic heart disease or cardiomyopathy, the diagnosis is virtually always VT.
• Suspect diagnoses other than VT in young patients (age <40 years), or with known Wolff–Parkinson–White or bundle branch block. Assess the effect of adenosine (Table 2.2 and Fig. 2.2).
• Do not give verapamil as this may cause fatal hypotension in patients with VT.

Broad and irregular
• This is likely to be atrial fibrillation with bundle branch block or, less commonly, pre-excited atrial fibrillation (Fig. 2.4). The difference between the maximum and minimum instantaneous heart rates calculated from the shortest and longest RR intervals is usually >30/bpm.
• The differential diagnosis is torsade de pointes, an uncommon form of VT in which the QRS complexes are of variable size and shape and seem to revolve around the baseline, at a rate of 180–250/bpm.
• Torsade de pointes is usually due to therapy with anti-arrhythmic and other drugs which prolong the QT interval (e.g. quinidine, disopyramide, procainamide, amiodarone, sotalol), especially in patients with hypokalaemia or hypomagnesaemia.

Narrow and regular
• The differential diagnosis is given in Table 2.3.
• Vagotonic manoeuvres increase AV block and may reveal atrial activity. Try the Valsalva manoeuvre and carotid sinus massage (p. 81). If atrial waves outnumber QRS complexes, the diagnosis is atrial fibrillation, flutter or tachycardia.
• If vagotonic manoeuvres are unsuccessful, give adenosine (Table 2.2).
• Suspect atrial flutter with 2:1 AV conduction rather than sinus tachycardia if the rate is around 150/bpm (Fig. 2.5).

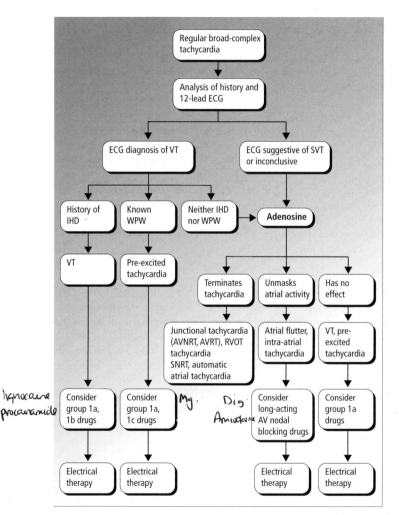

Fig. 2.2 Diagnosis and management of regular broad-complex tachycardia. AVNRT, atrioventricular nodal re-entrant tachycardia; AVRT, atrioventricular re-entrant tachycardia using an accessory pathway; RVOT, right ventricular outflow tract; SNRT, sinus node re-entrant tachycardia. From Camm A.J., Garratt C.J. *New England Journal of Medicine* 1991; **325**, 1621–9.

Cardiac arrhythmias

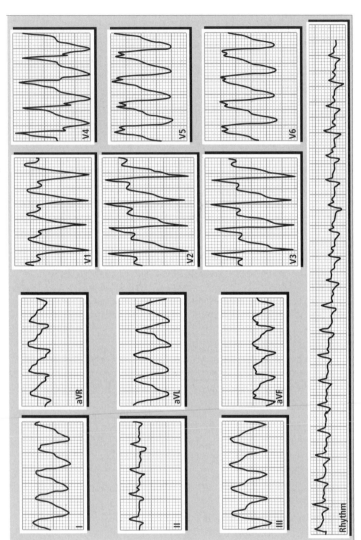

Table 2.2 Adenosine

Give as a rapid bolus into a large vein followed by a saline flush monitoring the
    ECG continuously
Start with 3 mg
If no response after 2 min give 6 mg
If still no response give 12 mg

Adverse effects
Transient chest discomfort, breathlessness, flushing and headache

Drug interactions
Antagonized by theophylline
Potentiated by dipyridamole (give half dose of adenosine)

- Suspect atrial tachycardia (Fig. 2.6) or nodal tachycardia if digoxin toxicity is possible. Digoxin toxicity is likely if plasma digoxin level is >3.0 ng/ml (>3.8 nmol/l), especially if there is hypokalaemia (<3.5 mmol/L), hypomagnesaemia or hypercalcaemia. Systemic features include nausea, vomiting, diarrhoea and confusional state.

Narrow and irregular (Table 2.3)
- The diagnosis is usually atrial fibrillation (AF) (Fig. 2.8).
- Other possibilities are sinus rhythm with frequent supraventricular extrasystoles or multifocal atrial tachycardia (the rhythm looks halfway between sinus and AF).

Fig. 2.3 (*Opposite.*) Ventricular tachycardia. The pathognomic feature of ventricular tachycardia is dissociation of atrial and ventricular electrical activity as shown by:
- P waves 'marching' in and out at a variable distance from the QRS complex and
- Capture or fusion beats (which are rare)
Other features suggesting VT are:
- Positive concordance (QRS predominantly positive in chest leads)
- Marked left axis deviation
- Rsr' complex if there is a positive QRS in V1
- QS in V6 if there is a negative QRS in V1.

Cardiac arrhythmias

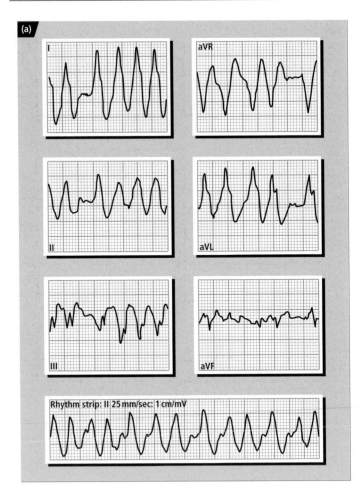

Fig. 2.4 Pre-excited atrial fibrillation (WPW). (a) There is marked variability of rate and QRS width. The difference between maximum and minimum instantaneous heart rates calculated from the minimum and maximum RR intervals is usually > 30 bpm.

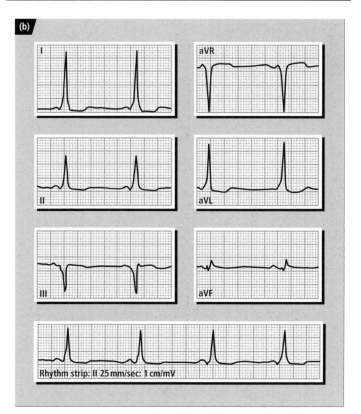

Cardiac arrhythmias

Fig. 2.4 (Continued) (b) After resolution of the tachycardia there is a short PR interval (always measure the minimum interval) and delta wave.

Diagnosis of bradyarrhythmias (rate < 60/min)

• Look carefully at the PR interval and the relationship between the P wave and QRS complex (Table 2.4).

• A regular ventricular rate <50/min in a patient with atrial fibrillation indicates complete heart block (not 'slow AF') (Fig. 2.8): always consider digoxin toxicity.

Cardiac arrhythmias

Table 2.3 Differential diagnosis of narrow-complex tachycardia

Arrhythmia	QRS rate (per min)	Atrial rate (per min)	Regular QRS?	Atrial activity	Effect of vagotonic manoeuvres or adenosine
Sinus tachycardia	100–200	100–200	Y	P wave precedes QRS	−
SVT	150–250	150–250	Y	Usually not seen or inverted P after QRS	++
Atrial tachycardia	100–200	120–250	Y	Abnormal shaped P wave May outnumber QRS	+
Atrial flutter	75–175	250–350	Y	'Saw-tooth' in the inferior leads/V1	+
Atrial fibrillation	<200	350–600	N	Chaotic (f waves)	+
MAT	100–130	100–130	N	P waves of three or more morphologies, irregular PP interval	−

SVT, Supraventricular tachycardia (re-entrant tachycardia involving the AV node or an accessory pathway); MAT, multifocal atrial tachycardia; − no effect or slight slowing; + slowing of ventricular rate; ++ may terminate tachycardia.

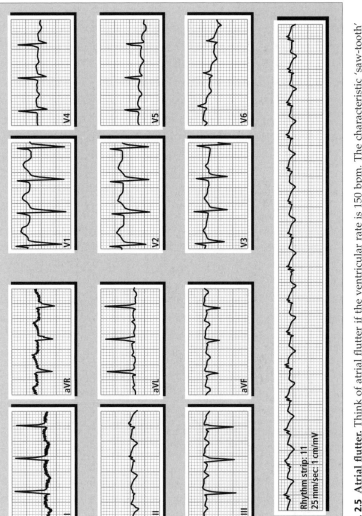

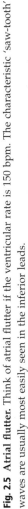

Rhythm strip: 11
25 mm/sec: 1 cm/mV

Fig. 2.5 Atrial flutter. Think of atrial flutter if the ventricular rate is 150 bpm. The characteristic 'saw-tooth' waves are usually most easily seen in the inferior leads.

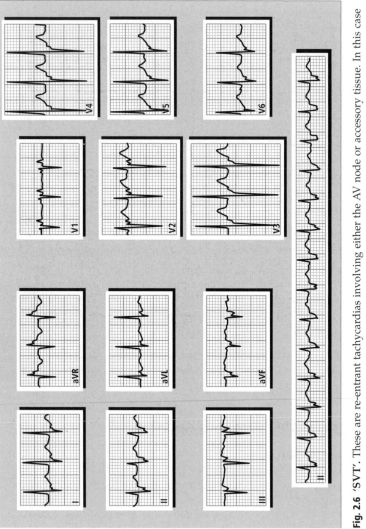

Fig. 2.6 'SVT'. These are re-entrant tachycardias involving either the AV node or accessory tissue. In this case the patient had WPW syndrome.

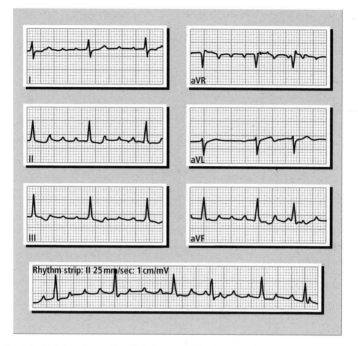

Fig. 2.7 Atrial tachycardia. This is caused by increased automaticity of the sinus or an ectopic atrial focus. In older subjects, it is often a sign of digoxin toxicity.

Management of individual arrhythmias

Ventricular tachycardia

To restore sinus rhythm

• If cardiac arrest or severely compromised haemodynamic state ('pulseless' VT): DC shock.

• If the patient is haemodynamically stable, give lignocaine 100 mg (5 mL of 2% solution) IV over 30 s. If this fails to restore sinus rhythm, give procainamide 200 mg IV over 1 min. If VT persists, use synchronized DC countershock. This is preferable to giving further anti-arrhythmic drugs.

Table 2.4 Diagnosis of bradycardia and atrioventricular block

Diagnosis	ECG features
Sinus bradycardia	Constant PR interval < 200 ms QRS regular
Junctional bradycardia	P wave absent or position constant either after, immediately before or hidden in the QRS complex
First-degree block	Constant PR interval > 200 ms
Second-degree block *Mobitz type I* (Wenckebach)	Progressively lengthening PR interval followed by dropped beat
Mobitz type II	Constant PR interval with dropped beats
Third-degree block (Complete heart block)	Relationship of P wave to QRS varies randomly P–P and R–R intervals constant but different

After correction of VT

• Establish the cause from the clinical assessment and investigation (Table 2.5).

• Correct hypokalaemia (p. 346).

• Correct hypoxia (Pao_2 should be kept > 9 kPa).

• Correct persistent severe metabolic acidosis: if arterial pH < 7.1 after restoration of spontaneous output, give sodium bicarbonate 50 mmol (50 ml of 8.4% solution) IV.

• Maintenance anti-arrhythmic therapy will usually be indicated (Table 2.6).

• Ask for specialist cardiological advice unless the VT occurred in the setting of a self-limiting condition (e.g. first 24 h after acute myocardial infarction, or metabolic disturbance).

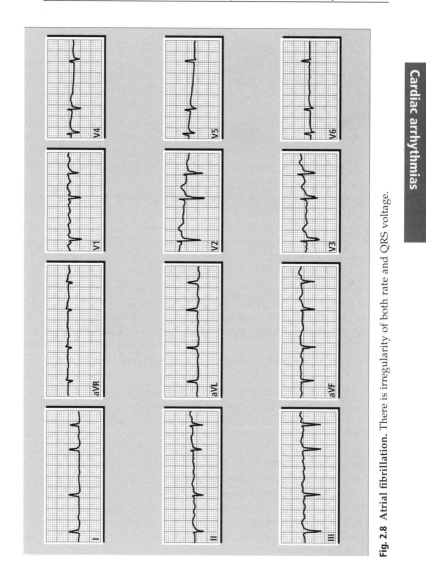

Fig. 2.8 Atrial fibrillation. There is irregularity of both rate and QRS voltage.

Cardiac arrhythmias

Table 2.5 Investigation after resolution of VT

ECG–? myocardial infarction, long QT interval

Chest X-ray–? pulmonary oedema, cardiomegaly

Plasma potassium should be kept in the range 4–5 mmol/L

Plasma magnesium (if taking diuretics)

Cardiac enzymes (for later analysis)

Arterial blood gases (if there is pulmonary oedema, a reduced conscious level or evidence of sepsis)

Echocardiography (to assess LV function and exclude other structural heart disease)

Torsade de pointes
• Give magnesium sulphate 2 g IV bolus over 2–3 min, repeated if necessary, and followed by an infusion of 2–8 mg/min.
• Use temporary pacing at 90/min (see p. 438) if this is ineffective.
• Stop drugs known to prolong the QT interval and check the electrolytes.
• In hereditary long QT syndromes consider a beta-blocker.

Atrial fibrillation
The aims of treatment are control of the ventricular rate, the restoration and maintenance of sinus rhythm where possible, and the prevention of systemic embolism.

Management (Fig. 2.13)
This depends on several factors including:
1 Duration of atrial fibrillation
   • Is the atrial fibrillation paroxysmal; if continuous, is it acute (<2 days' duration) or chronic?
2 Associated heart disease
Coronary and all forms of structural heart disease are relevant because they:
   • May cause atrial fibrillation.
   • Influence the risk of thromboembolism.

Table 2.6 Maintenance treatment of VT

In the first 24 h after acute myocardial infarction
Lignocaine
Loading dose (if not already given)
    100 mg (5 mL of 2% solution) IV over 30 s

Maintenance IV infusion (reduce by half if there is heart failure or cirrhosis)
4 mg/min for 30 min
2 mg/min for 2 h
1 mg/min for 12–24 h

If VT recurs give a further bolus of 50 mg and increase the infusion rate by
    1–2 mg/min

If VT still recurs add amiodarone (Table 2.7)

If VT does not recur during this period
Further anti-arrhythmic therapy is not required
If there are no signs of heart failure, start a beta-blocker
If there is heart failure, start an ACE inhibitor

24 h after myocardial infarction or due to other myocardial disease
Lignocaine by infusion
Start oral amiodarone (Table 2.7) if left ventricular function is poor or the patient
    has hypertrophic cardiomyopathy; otherwise start sotalol (80–160 mg 12 h PO)

Cardiac arrhythmias

- Affect the likelihood of cardioversion being successful.
3 Associated systemic disorder
- Atrial fibrillation is a common complication of acute illness (e.g. pneumonia, acute alcohol consumption), especially in the elderly.
- Thyrotoxicosis is a rare cause, but must not be forgotten because it radically affects treatment

Acute atrial fibrillation complicating intercurrent illness or surgery
- Rate control (Table 2.7) is usually needed if the ventricular rate is >120 bpm.
- Anticoagulation by SC heparin unless the risk of thromboembolism is high (thyrotoxicosis, mitral valve disease, previous event), when IV

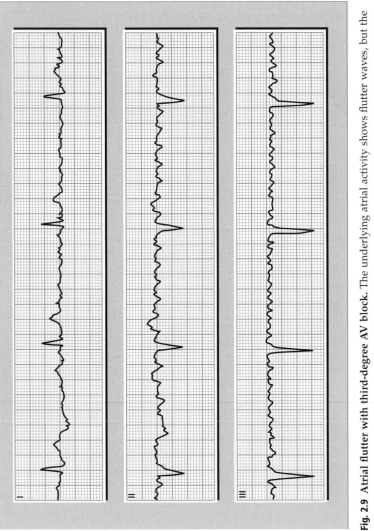

Fig. 2.9 **Atrial flutter with third-degree AV block.** The underlying atrial activity shows flutter waves, but the ventricular response is slow and regular.

Table 2.7 Drug doses in acute atrial fibrillation or flutter

Digoxin
Loading dose

IV: Give 0.75–1.0 mg digoxin in 50 mL of dextrose 5% or normal saline IV over
 2 h
PO: Give 0.5 mg 12-hly for two doses, followed by 0.25 mg 12-hly for 2 days

Maintenance dose
0.0625–0.25 mg/day. Take into account age, renal function and drug interactions

Verapamil
IV: Give 5 mg IV over 2 min. If no response after 5 min, give further doses of 5 mg
 every 5 min to a total dose of 20 mg (10 mg in patients with ischaemic heart
 disease or aged > 60 years)
PO: 40–120 mg 8-hly

Beta-blocker
IV: Atenolol 5–10 mg by slow IV injection; sotalol 20–60 mg by slow IV injection
PO: Atenolol 25–100 mg daily; sotalol 80–160 mg 12-hly

Amiodarone
Loading dose
IV: 300 mg (5 mg/kg) in dextrose 5% by IV infusion over 20–120 min, followed by
 900 mg over 24 h
PO: 200 mg 8-hly for 1 week (started concurrently with IV loading), followed by
 200 mg 12-hly for 1 week

Maintenance dose
PO: 100–200 mg once daily
Flecainide: see Table 2.8

heparin should be started. If atrial fibrillation is still present after 2 days, anticoagulate with warfarin.

• Cardioversion should be considered if still in atrial fibrillation after 4–6 weeks, unless there is thyrotoxicosis, in which case defer DC cardioversion until euthyroid for 6 weeks.

Acute onset (<48 h), no intercurrent illness
• Many attacks will resolve spontaneously. Consider modifying current therapy if known paroxysmal atrial fibrillation.

• Request echocardiography looking for structural heart disease (impaired LV systolic function, LVH, large left atrium or mitral valve thickening).

• If the heart is structurally normal, treatment options include:
Chemical cardioversion with flecainide (Table 2.8);
DC cardioversion without anticoagulation.

• If there is structural heart disease, treatment options include:
Transoesophageal echocardiography to exclude thrombus, then DC cardioversion;
Rate control, oral anticoagulation and outpatient review in 3–4 weeks to consider DC cardioversion.

Table 2.8 Chemical cardioversion with flecainide

Intravenously
As a slow intravenous injection at 2 mg/kg (to a maximum of 150 mg) over 10–30 min
then if necessary as an infusion at 1.5 mg/kg over 1 h
then if necessary as an infusion at 100–250 µg/kg/h over 24 h
Maximum dose in 24 h 600 mg

Orally
Initially 50 mg 12 h increasing to 100 mg 12 h

Atrial fibrillation for longer than 2 days or duration uncertain
• Start oral anticoagulation unless contraindicated (e.g. active bleeding, tendency to fall, high and variable alcohol consumption) or DC cardioversion not planned and thromboembolic risk low (e.g. age <60 years and normal heart).
• Treatment options include:
  • rate control alone (Table 2.7), or
  • start amiodarone for both rate control and possible chemical cardioversion. Plan DC cardioversion at 3–4 weeks if chemical cardioversion has not occurred and the chance of maintaining sinus rhythm is high (no significant structural abnormality, duration <3 months).

Atrial flutter
• Treatment is as for atrial fibrillation although flutter is less responsive to drugs (Fig. 2.13 and Table 2.7).
• DC cardioversion should be preceded by anticoagulation as for atrial fibrillation.

'SVT' (AV nodal re-entrant tachycardia/AV re-entrant tachycardia)
• This is a common arrhythmia associated with a structurally normal heart.
• Treatment options are given in Fig. 2.14. Doses are given in Table 2.9.

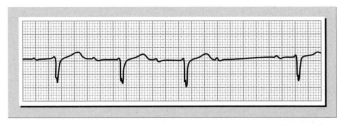

Fig. 2.10 Mobitz type I (Wenkebach) second-degree AV block. There is progressive lengthening of the PR interval followed by a dropped beat.

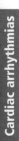

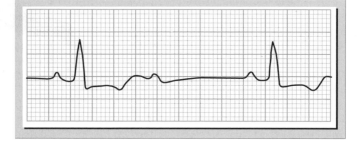

Fig. 2.11 2:1 second-degree AV block. There is a regular 'dropped' QRS complex every other beat.

Table 2.9 Drug doses in supraventricular tachycardia

Verapamil
Start with 5 mg IV over 2 min
If no response after 5 min, give further doses of 5 mg every 5 min to a total dose
    of 20 mg (10 mg in patients with ischaemic heart disease or aged >60 years)
Adenosine (see Table 2.2, p. 15)
Start with 3 mg IV bolus
If no response after 2 min, give 6 mg; if still no response, give 12 mg

Beta-blocker
Atenolol 5 mg IV or sotalol 20–60 mg IV

• Obtain a 12-lead ECG after sinus rhythm has been restored and check that it does not show features of Wolff–Parkinson–White syndrome (short PR interval and delta wave) (Fig. 2.4b).

Atrial tachycardia

This is an uncommon arrhythmia, but may be due to digoxin toxicity.
• Withdraw digoxin.
• Check the plasma potassium and maintain at 4–5 mmol/L.

• If the arrythmia does not resolve spontaneously and digoxin toxicity is likely, treatment is with phenytoin (5 mg/kg IV over 5 min) or beta-blockers (Table 2.9).

• If the patient is not taking digoxin and the tachycardia does not resolve spontaneously, sinus rhythm can be restored by synchronized DC countershock or a Class Ia anti-arrhythmic (quinidine, procainamide or disopyramide).

Multifocal atrial tachycardia
• Most commonly seen in COPD.

• Treatment is directed at the underlying disease and correction of hypoxia and hypercapnia.

• Consider verapamil if the ventricular rate is consistently > 110/min. DC cardioversion is ineffective.

Sinus or junctional bradycardia
Related to acute myocardial infarction (MI)

• This is common after inferior MI but only needs treatment if causing hypotension, low cardiac output or ventricular escape rhythms, in which case:

• Give atropine 0.6–1.2 mg IV, with further doses at 5-min intervals up to a total dose of 3 mg if the heart rate remains below 60/bpm.

• If there is little response to atropine, or frequent doses are needed, put in a temporary pacing wire.

• If a side-effect of beta-blockade, see Table 2.10.

Unrelated to myocardial infarction

• This is usually due to drugs (most commonly beta-blockers) or sinoatrial disease ('sick sinus syndrome'). Exclude hypothyroidism.

• No action is necessary if the patient is asymptomatic and the rate is > 40/bpm.

• If symptomatic (syncope/presyncope) or ventricular rate < 40/min, stop any drugs that may be contributing (if safe to do so), put in a temporary pacing wire and discuss permanent pacing with a cardiologist.

First-degree AV block (PR interval > 200 ms)
• This never needs treatment as an isolated finding.

• If associated with RBBB in acute myocardial infarction a temporary pacing electrode should be inserted.

Cardiac arrhythmias

Table 2.10 Reversal of beta-blockade

Beta-blockade must be reversed if contributing to pulmonary oedema,
hypotension or low cardiac output
• Give atropine and isoprenaline (dosage, see text) until the heart rate is over
60/min
• If the blood pressure remains low, start a dobutamine infusion at 10 μg/kg/min,
increasing the dose as required
• Glucagon can be combined with isoprenaline or dobutamine. Give an IV bolus of
50 μg/kg followed by an infusion of 1–5 mg/h

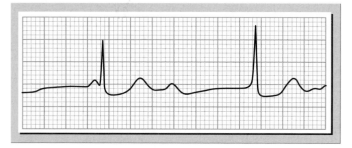

Fig. 2.12 Third-degree (complete) AV block. There is no regular
relationship between atrial and ventricular activity. Observation over
many cycles shows variability of the PR interval.

• It influences the decision to pace in a patient with syncope and
bundle branch block.
• It may indicate septal abscess formation in aortic valve endocarditis and should stimulate discussion of transoesophageal echocardiography with a cardiologist.

Second- and third-degree AV block (Figs 2.11–2.12)
Related to acute myocardial infarction (MI)
Put in a temporary pacing wire in patients with:
• Mobitz type I second-degree AV block if there is hypotension unre-
sponsive to atropine;

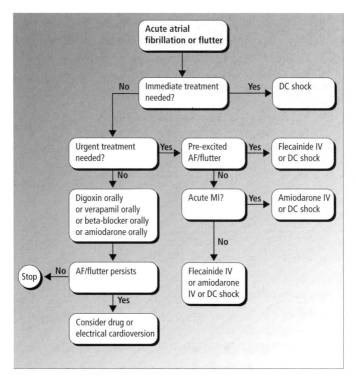

Fig. 2.13 Management of acute atrial fibrillation or flutter.

- Mobitz type II second-degree AV block;
- third-degree (complete) AV block.

Second-degree block unrelated to myocardial infarction
- Exclude digoxin toxicity or beta-blockade.
- If the patient has experienced syncope or presyncope, put in a temporary pacing wire, and arrange permanent pacing.
- If asymptomatic, record a 24-h ECG and discuss with a cardiologist whether permanent pacing is indicated.

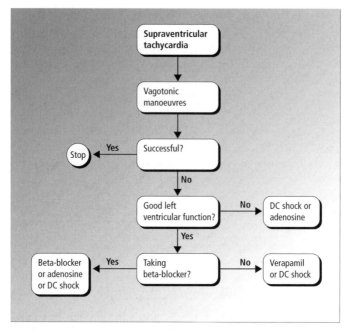

Fig. 2.14 Management of supraventricular tachycardia.

Third-degree AV block unrelated to myocardial infarction
• Even in asymptomatic patients, this carries a risk of sudden death.
• Put in a temporary pacing wire if the patient has experienced syncope or presyncope, or the ventricular rate is <40/min.
• Arrange permanent pacing.

Appendix

Suspected malfunction of permanent pacemaker (Table 2.11)
1 Check the details of the pacemaker: is it a single- or dual-chamber system, and what is the pacing mode? Contact the hospital where the system was implanted to obtain further details.

Table 2.11 Diagnosis of pacemaker malfunction

Feature	Causes
No spikes*	Normal sensing
	Malfunction of pulse generator
	Spike buried in QRS complex
	Electromagnetic interference
Spikes without capture (failure to capture)	High threshold:
	• lead fracture
	• lead displacement
	• myocardial fibrosis
	• myocardial perforation
	Lead not properly connected to pulse generator
	Depletion of battery of pulse generator
	Spike in ventricular refractory period
Spikes without sensing (failure to sense)	Lead displacement
	Low intrinsic QRS current (i.e. not at sensing threshold)

*Placing a magnet over the pulse generator converts nearly all units to fixed-rate pacing.

Cardiac arrhythmias

2 Obtain a 12-lead ECG, a long rhythm strip (with and without a magnet over the pulse generator) and a penetrated chest X-ray for the position of the leads.

3 If these show no abnormality:
- Record a 24-h ECG.
- Consider other causes of syncope or presyncope (Table 7.4, p. 83).

3 Hypotension

Hypotension needs urgent correction if:
• systolic BP is <80mmHg; or
• systolic BP has fallen >40mmHg and there are signs of low cardiac output: confusion or drowsiness; cold skin; oliguria; metabolic acidosis.

There are three groups of causes: hypovolaemia, cardiac pump failure and vasodilatation (Table 3.1). Initial management is summarized in Fig. 3.1.

Priorities

1 If hypovolaemia or vasodilatation is likely, lay the patient flat and elevate the foot of the bed.
2 Give oxygen. Put in a peripheral IV cannula. Attach an ECG monitor. Check oxygen saturation.
3 Make a rapid clinical assessment, with examination of the chest and abdomen. Check that breath sounds are heard over both lungs. Look carefully at the JVP, which may give a clue to the diagnosis (Table 3.2).
Questions to ask yourself include:
• Is there obvious haemorrhage from the gastrointestinal tract (p. 273) or other site (e.g. abdominal aortic aneurysm)?
• Is there a **major arrhythmia** (see *Further management*)?
• Is there pulmonary oedema (p. 165), i.e. the problem is **cardiogenic shock**?
• Is there fever, or other features pointing to **sepsis** (p. 100)?
• Is the patient at risk of **pulmonary embolism** (p. 183)? Hypotension and hypoxaemia without pulmonary oedema suggest pulmonary embolism or sepsis; in this setting, a raised JVP would favour pulmonary embolism and a low JVP sepsis.

Table 3.1 Causes of hypotension

Hypovolaemia
Haemorrhage
Urinary loss
Gastrointestinal fluid loss
Cutaneous loss (e.g. burns)
Third-space sequestration (e.g. acute pancreatitis)

Cardiac pump failure
Acute myocardial infarction (usually associated with pulmonary oedema, except
    when due to right ventricular infarction)
Acute myocardial ischaemia (usually associated with pulmonary oedema)
Arrhythmia (especially when associated with valve disorder, e.g. severe aortic
    stenosis, or impaired left ventricular function, in which case usually associated
    with pulmonary oedema)
Acute aortic or mitral regurgitation (due to endocarditis, aortic dissection, papillary
    muscle or chordal rupture) (always associated with pulmonary oedema)
Ventricular septal ruputure complicating myocardial infarction (often associated
    with pulmonary oedema)
Pulmonary embolism
Cardiac tamponade
Tension pneumothorax

Vasodilatation
Sepsis
Drugs and poisons
Anaphylaxis
Acute adrenal insufficiency (Addisonian crisis)

Hypotension

• Is **tension pneumothorax** a possibility (e.g. recent central vein cannulation)?
• Could this be **anaphylaxis** (p. 414)? If the patient has recently been exposed to a potential allergen, and has urticaria, erythema, angio-oedema or wheeze, treat as anaphylaxis and give adrenaline

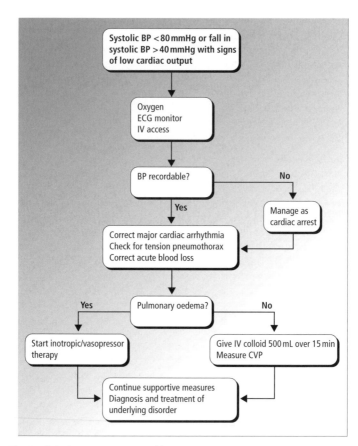

Fig. 3.1 Priority management of hypotension.

0.5–1 mg IM (0.5–1 ml of 1 in 1000 solution). Further management is detailed on p. 414.

4 Investigations needed urgently are given in Table 3.3. If hypotension does not respond promptly, put in a urinary catheter so that urine output can be monitored. The urine output is a rough guide to renal blood flow and cardiac output; the target is > 30 ml/h.

Table 3.2 The JVP in hypotension

Hypotension with a high JVP
Biventricular failure
Pulmonary embolism
Right ventricular infarction
Cardiac tamponade
Tension pneumothorax

Hypotension with a normal or low JVP
Hypovolaemia
Sepsis
Drugs or poisons
Left ventricular failure

5 If there is obvious haemorrhage:
• Get help from a gastroenterologist (if you are dealing with suspected upper gastrointestinal haemorrhage) or a surgeon.
• Put in a second large-bore IV cannula (e.g. grey Venflon).
• Rapidly transfuse colloid until the systolic BP is around 100 mmHg. Start transfusing blood as soon as it is available. If systolic BP is still <90 mmHg despite 1000 ml of colloid, and cross-matched blood is not yet available, use grouped but not cross-matched blood and save a sample of the transfused blood for a retrospective cross-match.
• Aim for a haemoglobin concentration of 10 g/dL.
• Correct clotting abnormalities. If the prothrombin time is >1.5 × control, give vitamin K 10 mg IV and 2 units of fresh frozen plasma. If the platelet count is <50 × 10^{12}/L, give platelet concentrate. Recheck the platelet count if >4 units of blood have been transfused.

6 If there is cardiogenic shock (hypotension with pulmonary oedema):
• Correct major arrhythmias (see *Further management*, pp. 42–4).

Table 3.3 Urgent investigation in hypotension

ECG
Chest X-ray
Creatinine, sodium and potassium
Blood glucose
Full blood count
Arterial blood gases and pH
Group and save (cross-match 6 units if haemorrhage suspected)
Clotting screen if low platelet count, suspected coagulation disorder, jaundice or
    purpura
Culture blood and urine
Echocardiography if suspected cardiac tamponade; suspected surgically
    correctable lesion (e.g. ventricular septal rupture after myocardial infarction
    (p. 147), acute aortic or mitral regurgitation); or diagnosis unclear

- If there is ECG evidence of acute myocardial infarction, consider thrombolysis (p. 138) or primary angioplasty if feasible.
- Increase the inspired oxygen aiming for an oxygen saturation of >90%/arterial Po_2 >8 kPa. If these targets are not met despite an inspired oxygen concentration of 60%, use a continuous positive airways pressure system if available.
- Start inotropic/vasopressor therapy (Tables 3.4 and 3.5).
- Arrange urgent echocardiography to assess left ventricular function and to exclude ventricular septal rupture and acute aortic or mitral regurgitation.
- Diuretics are relatively ineffective in patients with cardiogenic shock, but can be used once the cardiac output has increased (as shown by improvement in the patient's mental state and skin perfusion): if renal function is normal, give frusemide 40 mg IV.
- Providing the systolic BP has increased to at least 100 mmHg, start a nitrate infusion, initially at low dose (e.g. isosorbide dinitrate 2 mg/h).

Table 3.4 Guide to inotropic/vasopressor therapy—choice of therapy

Cause of hypotension	Choice of therapy
Left ventricular failure	Dobutamine if systolic BP is > 90 mmHg
Right ventricular infarction (p. 144)	Dopamine if systolic BP is 80–90 mmHg
Pulmonary embolism (p. 183)	Noradrenaline if systolic BP is < 80 mmHg
Cardiac tamponade (p. 175), while awaiting pericardiocentesis	Noradrenaline
Septic shock	Noradrenaline
	Dobutamine should be added if cardiac output is low
Anaphylactic shock	Adrenaline

Hypotension

• If the patient is not improving, consider placing a pulmonary artery catheter to allow more accurate titration of therapy. Adjust the doses of inotrope/vasopressor and nitrate, aiming for a PA diastolic or wedge pressure of 15–20 mmHg with a systolic BP of > 100 mmHg.

• Discuss management with a cardiologist if you suspect a surgically correctable cause (e.g. papillary muscle rupture) or there is evidence of acute myocardial ischaemia without infarction (unstable angina; p. 151).

Further management

The key points in the management of hypotension are to:
• Make a diagnosis and give specific treatment.
• Correct cardiac arrhythmias.
• Correct hypovolaemia.
• Correct hypoxia and biochemical abnormalities.
• Use inotropic/vasopressor therapy if there is refractory hypotension.

Table 3.5 Guide to inotropic/vasopressor therapy—dosages

Drug	Dosage (µg/kg/min)	Effect
Adrenaline	0.05	Beta-1 inotropism and beta-2 vasodilatation
	0.05–5	Beta-1 inotropism and alpha-1 vasoconstriction
Dobutamine	5–40	Beta-1 inotropism and beta-2 vasodilatation
Dopamine	5–10	Beta-1 inotropism
	10–40	Alpha-1 vasoconstriction
Noradrenaline	0.05–5	Alpha-1 vasoconstriction and beta-1 inotropism

For calculation of infusion rates, see pp. 481–5.

1 Make a diagnosis and give specific treatment
• Consider the causes in Table 3.1.
• Echocardiography is indicated if the diagnosis remains unclear.
• Give hydrocortisone 200 mg IV if the patient has been on previous long-term steroid treatment (prednisolone >7.5 mg daily) or you suspect acute adrenal insufficiency (p. 364).

2 Correct cardiac arrhythmias
• **Ventricular tachycardia** or **supraventricular tachycardia** with a ventricular rate >150/bpm should be treated with cardioversion (p. 451).
• **Acute atrial fibrillation**: **Consider DC cardioversion** if the ventricular rate is >140/bpm, after correction of hypoxia and electrolyte disorders. Otherwise give **amiodarone IV** (via a central line; 300 mg in dextrose 5% over 60 min, followed by 900 mg over 24 h). Most drugs used to control the ventricular rate in atrial fibrillation (p. 27) are con-

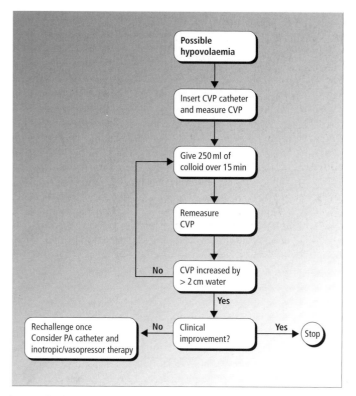

Fig. 3.2 Fluid challenge, with monitoring of the CVP.
The absolute value of the CVP is a poor guide to hydration as peripheral vasoconstriction will maintain this wherever possible. Patients with sepsis may require much higher circulating volumes than normal.

traindicated in hypotension. Digoxin is largely ineffective when sympathetic drive is high.
• If there is severe bradycardia (heart rate < 40/bpm), give atropine 0.6–1.2 mg IV, with further doses at 5-min intervals up to a total dose of 3 mg if the heart rate remains below 60/bpm. If there is little

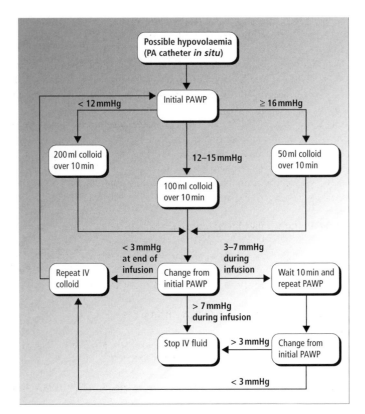

Fig. 3.3 Fluid challenge, with monitoring of the pulmonary artery wedge pressure. From Bossnert LL *et al. Drugs* 1991; **41**: 857–74.

response to atropine, use an external transcutaneous pacing system or put in temporary pacing wire (p. 438).

3 Correct hypovolaemia
• If there is obvious hypovolaemia (appropriate clinical setting; low JVP with flat neck veins), give IV fluid (blood, colloid or saline as

appropriate to the cause). A CVP line may be helpful (to avoid over-replacement of fluid), but the patient should be resuscitated first before this is placed.

• If the evidence for hypovolaemia is less certain, but there are no clinical signs of fluid overload, give a fluid challenge (Faigs 3.2 and 3.3), ideally with monitoring of the CVP, especially if the JVP is difficult to assess.

• The target range of CVP is 5–10 cm water, measured from a mid-axillary line zero reference point.

• If systolic BP remains <90 mmHg despite correction or exclusion of hypovolaemia, search for and treat other causes of hypotension, of which sepsis is the most likely (p. 100). If BP remains low, inotropic–vasopressor therapy will be needed.

4 Correct hypoxia and biochemical abnormalities

• Maintain Pao >8 kPa (60 mmHg), arterial saturation >90%.

• Severe metabolic acidosis may contribute to hypotension. Causes of metabolic acidosis are given on p. 359. If arterial pH is <7.1, give 50 ml of 8.4% sodium bicarbonate. Recheck pHa after 30 min.

5 Use inotropic/vasopressor therapy if there is refractory hypotension

• If systolic BP remains <90 mmHg despite adequate fluid therapy (CVP +10 cm water, PA wedge pressure 18 mmHg), start inotropic/vasopressor therapy.

• Choice of therapy and dosages are summarized in Tables 3.4 and 3.5. For calculation of infusion rates, see pp. 481–5.

4 Acute chest pain

- Consider the potentially lethal causes in all patients: acute coronary syndromes (acute myocardial infarction or unstable angina), pulmonary embolism and aortic dissection (Figs 4.1, 4.2 and Appendix).
- The initial management of acute chest pain is summarized in Fig. 4.3.
- If you cannot make a confident diagnosis of a minor and self-limiting disorder, admit the patient for observation and further investigation.

Priorities

1 Check the pulse and blood pressure, listen over the lungs and:
  - attach an ECG monitor and record an ECG;
  - give oxygen if the patient has severe pain, is breathless, or if oxygen saturation by pulse oximetry is <90%;
  - put in an IV cannula;
  - relieve severe pain with diamorphine 2.5–5 mg (or morphine 5–10 mg IV) plus an antiemetic, e.g. prochlorperazine 12.5 mg IV.

2 Correct major arrhythmias (p. 10) or hypotension (p. 36).

3 Take a preliminary history of the chest pain while recording a 12-lead ECG: Is it consistent with myocardial infarction? Are there any features suggesting aortic dissection (instantaneous onset, associated neurological symptoms)?

4 Look carefully at the ECG, and compare it with previous ECGs if available.
  - If there is ST elevation in 2 or more adjacent leads, or left bundle branch block, not known to be old, and the chest pain is consistent

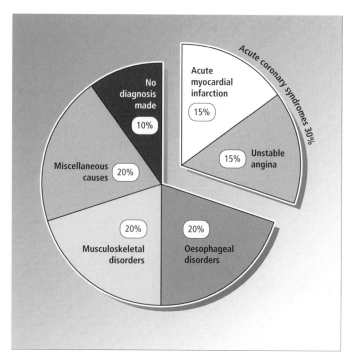

Fig. 4.1 Causes of acute chest pain presenting to the emergency department.

with myocardial ischaemia and has lasted >20 min, the working diagnosis is acute myocardial infarction. Give thrombolysis without delay, unless contraindicated (p. 141), or arrange primary angioplasty.

• Consider other causes of ST elevation (Table 4.1) if the history is not typical of acute myocardial infarction, and ask advice before giving thrombolysis.

5 If the clinical picture and ECG are not diagnostic of acute myocardial infarction, you need to adopt a systematic approach based on a

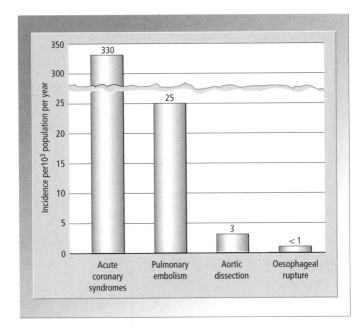

Fig. 4.2 Incidence of major disorders which may present with acute chest pain.

full history and examination, chest X-ray and, if the time interval is appropriate, measurement of plasma markers of myocardial necrosis (Table 4.2).

Points to cover in the history
Past history
• Is the patient known to have coronary disease?
• Has there been a previous myocardial infarction with similar pain?

Precipitation
• Previous similar chest pain brought on by effort and relieved by rest (within 10 min), i.e. exertional angina?

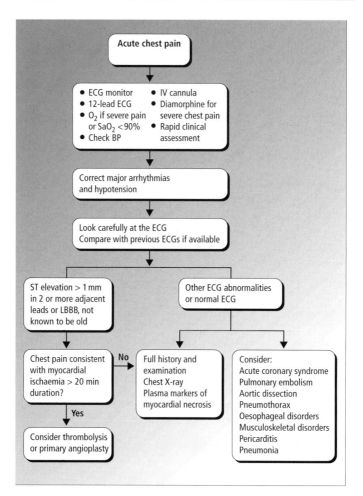

Fig. 4.3 Initial management of acute chest pain.

Table 4.1 Comparison of ECG features of acute myocardial infarction, early repolarization and pericarditis

ECG feature	Myocardial infarction	Early repolarization	Pericarditis
ST segment morphology	Convex upwards	Convex upwards	Concave upwards
Typical magnitude of ST elevation	1–10 mm	1–2 mm	1–5 mm
Distribution of ST elevation	Inferior, anterior and lateral patterns	Commonly septal, rarely limb leads	Both limb and chest leads
ST depression in V1	In posterior infarction	Rare	Common
ST elevation in V6	In infero- or anterolateral infarction	Uncommon	Common
ST/T wave evolution	Uniform in all involved leads	Does not occur	Various stages occur concurrently
Pathological Q waves	Commonly develop	Never develop	Never develop
Rhythm disturbances	May occur	Do not occur	Supraventricular tachyarrhythmias may occur

Table 4.2 Chest X-ray abnormalities which may be seen in pulmonary embolism, aortic dissection and oesophageal rupture

Diagnosis	Possible abnormalities (on PA and lateral films)
Pulmonary embolism	Focal infiltrate
	Segmental collapse
	Raised hemidiaphragm
	Pleural effusion
Aortic dissection	Widening or double lumen to aortic knuckle
	Irregular aortic contour
	Discrepancy in diameter of ascending and descending thoracic aorta
	Pleural effusion
	Mediastinal widening
	Displacement of calcified intima
Oesophageal rupture	Mediastinal and subcutaneous emphysema
	Paraspinal mass
	Pleural effusion
	Pneumothorax

Acute chest pain

• Did the pain follow oesophageal instrumentation (suspect perforation) or insertion of a central line (suspect pneumothorax)?
• If chest pain followed vomiting, suspect spontaneous oesophageal rupture.

Risk factors
• Ischaemic heart disease (cigarette smoking, hypertension, hyperlipidaemia, diabetes, family history of early coronary disease).
• Venous thromboembolism (p. 180).
• Aortic dissection (hypertension, Marfan syndrome, pregnancy).

Characteristics of the pain
• Instantaneous onset suggests dissection. In infarction, the pain usually peaks over many seconds.
• Radiation along the course of the aorta or its major branches (to neck, ear, back or abdomen) suggests dissection. Radiation to the back alone is a non-specific feature which also occurs in myocardial infarction, oesophageal pain and musculoskeletal causes including osteoarthritis.

Associated features
• Neurological symptoms, even minor transient blurring of vision, suggest dissection.
• Haemoptysis suggests pulmonary embolism.
• Purulent sputum.

Exacerbating or relieving factors
• Ask specifically about swallowing (oesophageal motility disorders), deep breathing (pleurisy or pericarditis) and movement of the trunk and arms (musculoskeletal).

Points to note on examination
• Blood pressure in both arms (>15 mmHg difference in systolic pressure is abnormal), and the presence and symmetry of major pulses (if abnormal, consider aortic dissection).
• Jugular venous pressure (if raised, consider pulmonary embolism or pericardial effusion with tamponade).
• Murmur (if you hear the early diastolic murmur of aortic regurgitation, aortic dissection must be excluded).
• Pericardial or pleural rub.
• Signs of pneumothorax, consolidation or pleural effusion.
• Localized chest wall or spinal tenderness (significant only if pressure exactly reproduces the spontaneous pain).
• Subcutaneous emphysema around the neck (which may occur with oesophageal rupture and pneumothorax).
• Are there any gross neurological abnormalities (suggesting dissection or vertebral crush fracture)?

Table 4.3 Plasma markers of myocardial necrosis

Marker	Rises after:	Peaks at:	Returns to normal:
Myoglobin	1–4 h	6–7 h	24 h
Troponin-I	3–12 h	24 h	5–10 days
Troponin-T	3–12 h	12–48 h	5–14 days
Creatine kinase	4–8 h	12–24 h	3–4 days
CK-MB	4–8 h	12–20 h	2–3 days

Points to check for on the chest X-ray
• Abnormalities suggesting pulmonary embolism, aortic dissection and oesophageal rupture are shown in Table 4.2.

Plasma markers of myocardial necrosis
• Plasma markers of myocardial necrosis (Table 4.3) should be measured if an acute coronary syndrome is suspected or cannot be excluded.
• Cardiac troponins T and I are specific markers of myocardial necrosis. Elevated levels of troponin T or I in a plasma sample taken 12 h or more after the onset of chest pain indicate acute myocardial infarction or high-risk unstable angina (p. 152).

Further management

If the diagnosis is still not obvious, you should ask yourself how closely the clinical picture matches the profile of any of the potentially lethal causes.

Could you be missing an acute coronary syndrome?
• Remember that the pain of myocardial ischaemia and oesophageal pain (due to acid reflux or spasm) may be indistinguishable. Both may radiate to the back or arms, and both may be burning or gripping in

Acute chest pain

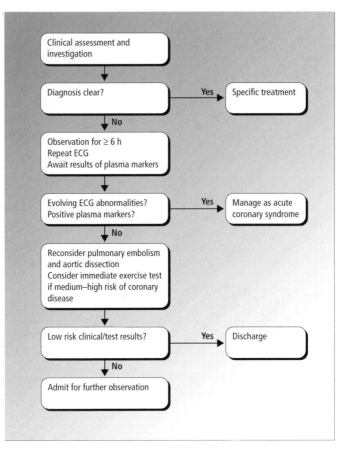

Fig. 4.4 Further management of acute chest pain.

quality. Both may be relieved transiently by belching. Angina may occur after meals, but usually during exercise after meals.
• The presence of ST segment depression or T wave inversion strongly favours an acute coronary syndrome rather than oesophageal pain. A normal ECG does not exclude unstable angina.

• The first sign of acute myocardial infarction may be hyperacute peaking of the T wave, which is often overlooked. If present, give aspirin and nitrate, and repeat the ECG in 20–30 min.
• If the history is compatible with myocardial ischaemia, or the patient is at moderate or high risk of ischaemic heart disease, admit for observation. Repeat the ECG initially after 1 h. Further management is shown in Fig. 4.4.

Could you be missing aortic dissection?

Aortic dissection must be excluded if:
• the chest pain was instantaneous in onset;
• there are associated neurological abnormalities;
• the patient has Marfan syndrome, known dilated aortic root or bicuspid aortic valve, or is pregnant.

Remember that the pulses and chest X-ray are normal in at least 50% of patients with aortic dissection. If you suspect aortic dissection, seek urgent advice on further management from a cardiologist.

Could you be missing pulmonary embolism?

• One or more risk factors for venous thromboembolism (p. 180) are found in 80–90% of patients with pulmonary embolism. In the absence of these, pleuritic chest pain is more likely to be caused by pneumonia or pleurisy.

Could you be missing a pneumothorax?

• Look again at the chest X-ray. It is easy to miss a small apical pneumothorax.

Could you be missing oesophageal rupture?

• Spontaneous rupture is very rare. Typically the pain follows vomiting (while, in acute myocardial infarction, vomiting follows pain).
• Check the chest X-ray for mediastinal gas (a crescentic radiolucent zone, which may be retrocardiac or along the right cardiac border), a pleural effusion or a widened mediastinum.
• If you suspect oesophageal rupture, put the patient nil by mouth and start antibiotic therapy with coamoxiclav and metronidazole. Discuss further management with a gastroenterologist or surgeon.

Acute chest pain

Appendix

Table 4.4 Causes of acute chest pain

	Common	Less common or rare
Coronary	Acute coronary syndrome	Angina due to tachyarrhythmia
Other cardiovascular	Pulmonary embolism	Aortic dissection
		Pericarditis
Oesophageal	Gastro-oesophageal reflux	Infective oesophagitis
	Oesophageal motility disorder	Oesophageal rupture
Pulmonary and pleural	Pneumonia	Pneumothorax
	Pleurisy	Pneumomediastinum
Musculoskeletal	Pain arising from costochondral or chondrosternal joints	Crush fracture of thoracic vertebra
	Rib fractures	
	Pain arising in intercostal or shoulder girdle muscles	
Others		Biliary tract disease
		Acute pancreatitis
		Perforated peptic ulcer
		Herpes zoster
		Vaso-occlusive crisis of sickle cell disease

5 Acute breathlessness

• The initial management of acute breathlessness is summarized in Fig. 5.1.

Priorities

1 Check the pulse and blood pressure, listen over the lungs, and:
   • attach an ECG monitor;
   • give oxygen 35%;
   • check oxygen saturation by pulse oximetry, and increase the inspired oxygen concentration if oxygen saturation is <90%;
   • put in an IV cannula.

2 If there are signs of a **tension pneumothorax** with impending cardiorespiratory arrest, insert a large-bore needle into the second intercostal space in the mid-clavicular line.

3 If there is **wheeze**, give nebulized salbutamol, 1 mg of nebulizer solution diluted in 2 ml of normal saline.
   • If the patient is hypoxic (oxygen saturation <90%), but does not have chronic obstructive pulmonary disease (COPD), the nebulizer should be driven with oxygen: check the necessary flow rate on the nebulizer packaging.
   • If the patient has COPD with known or potential CO_2 retention, use air as the driving gas.

4 If there is **severe pulmonary oedema** (the patient is exhaling froth):
   • correct major arrhythmias;
   • give:
   (i) diamorphine 2.5–5.0 mg (or morphine 5.0–10.0 mg) by slow IV injection;
   (ii) frusemide 40–80 mg IV; and if systolic BP is >100 mmHg;
   (iii) nitrate by IV infusion (e.g. isosorbide dinitrate 2 mg/h, increasing by 2 mg/h every 15–30 min until breathlessness is relieved or sys-

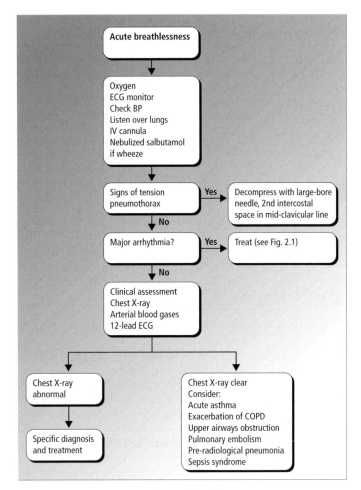

Fig. 5.1 Priority management of acute breathlessness.

tolic blood pressure falls below 100 mmHg or to a maximum of
10 mg/h) or buccal administration (glyceryl trinitrate buccal tablet,
5 mg).
5 Investigations required urgently are given in Table 5.1.

Table 5.1 Urgent investigations in acute breathlessness

Chest X-ray
Arterial blood gases and pH if oxygen saturation is < 90% or diagnosis is unclear
ECG (except in patients under 40 with pneumothorax or acute asthma)
Full blood count
Creatinine, sodium, potassium and glucose
Echocardiogram if:
   (a) suspected cardiac tamponade
   (b) suspected surgically correctable cause of pulmonary oedema

Further management

1 Complete your history and examination, including the following points:
- Known cardiac or respiratory disease?
- Associated chest pain (pleuritic or non-pleuritic)?
- Associated cough, with purulent sputum or haemoptysis?
- Change in sputum volume or purulence if chronic productive cough?
- Risk factors for venous thromboembolism (p. 180)?
- Usual exercise capacity and any recent change?
- Temperature, pulse, blood pressure, JVP, respiratory rate.
- Stridor or wheeze?
- Signs of heart failure?
- Focal lung crackles.
- Peak expiratory flow rate, related to predicted normal (p. 487).

2 The clinical assessment and investigation results should enable you to make a working diagnosis (Table 5.2). Further management of specific disorders is given in Section 2.

Acute breathlessness

Table 5.2 Features pointing to a diagnosis in the breathless patient

Diagnosis	Features
Acute asthma (p. 193)	Wheeze with reduced peak flow rate Previous similar episodes responding to bronchodilator therapy Diurnal and seasonal variation in symptoms Symptoms provoked by allergen exposure or exercise Sleep disturbance by breathlessness and wheeze
Pulmonary oedema (p. 165)	Cardiac disease Abnormal ECG Bilateral interstitial or alveolar shadowing on chest X-ray
Pneumonia (p. 206)	Fever Productive cough Pleuritic chest pain Focal shadowing on chest X-ray
Exacerbation of chronic obstructive pulmonary disease (p.198)	Increase in sputum volume, tenacity or purulence Previous chronic bronchitis: sputum production daily for 3 months of the year, for 2 or more consecutive years Wheeze with reduced peak flow rate
Pulmonary embolism (p. 183)	Pleuritic or non-pleuritic chest pain Haemoptysis Risk factors for venous thromboembolism present (signs of DVT commonly absent)

Table 5.2 *Continued*

Diagnosis	Features
Pneumothorax (p. 217)	Sudden breathlessness in young otherwise fit adult
	Breathlessness following invasive procedure, e.g. subclavian vein puncture
	Pleuritic chest pain
	Visceral pleural line on chest X-ray, with absent lung markings between this line and the chest wall
Cardiac tamponade (p. 175)	Raised JVP
	Pulsus paradoxus > 20 mmHg
	Enlarged cardiac silhouette on chest X-ray
	Known carcinoma of bronchus or breast
Laryngeal obstruction	History of smoke inhalation or the ingestion of corrosives
	Palatal or tongue oedema
	Anaphylaxis
Tracheobronchial obstruction	Stridor (inspiratory noise) or monophonic wheeze (expiratory 'squeak')
	Known carcinoma of the bronchus
	History of inhaled foreign body
	$Pa\text{CO}_2$ >5 kPa in the absence of chronic obstructive pulmonary disease
	Wheeze unresponsive to bronchodilators
Large pleural effusion	Distinguished from pulmonary consolidation on the chest X-ray by:
	Shadowing higher laterally than medially
	Shadowing does not conform to that of a lobe or segment
	No air bronchogram
	Trachea and mediastinum pushed to opposite side

Acute breathlessness

Table 5.3 Arterial blood gases and pH in breathlessness with a normal chest X-ray

Disorder	Pa_{O_2}	Pa_{CO_2}	PHa *
Acute asthma	Normal/low	Low	High
Acute exacerbation of COPD	Usually low	May be high	Normal or low
Pulmonary embolism	Normal/low (without pre-existing cardiopulmonary disease)	Low	High
Pre-radiological pneumonia†	Low	Low	High
Sepsis sydrome	Normal/low	Low	Low
Metabolic acidosis	Normal	Low	Low
Hyperventilation without organic disease	High/normal	Low	High

* Respiratory alkalosis may be offset by a metabolic acidosis. Figure 43.1 (p. 357) allows identification of mixed acid–base disturbances.

† Most commonly due to viruses or *Pneumocystis carinii* (p. 383).

Problems

Breathlessness with a raised JVP

• This combination may be seen in pulmonary embolism, congestive heart failure with biventricular involvement, chronic hypoxic lung disease complicated by cor pulmonale, and cardiac tamponade.

• If there is pulsus paradoxus or a large cardiac silhouette on chest X-ray, echocardiography should be obtained urgently to confirm or exclude a pericardial effusion with tamponade. Never attempt pericardiocentesis (p. 447) without echocardiographic confirmation of a pericardial effusion except where there is imminent cardiac arrest.

Is it pneumonia or pulmonary oedema?

• Differentiation may sometimes be difficult, as wheeze may occur in both; pulmonary oedema may be localized and when severe (alveolar) may produce an air-bronchogram; and the radiological signs of pulmonary oedema are modified by the presence of lung disease, e.g. chronic obstructive pulmonary disease. The two may also coexist as patients with heart failure are at increased risk of pneumonia.

• Pulmonary oedema is unlikely if there are no clinical or ECG features to suggest significant cardiac disease.

• If in doubt, treat for both, with antibiotics and diuretic. If fever and a productive cough are absent and the white cell count is $< 15 \times 10^9/L$, give frusemide alone and assess the response. Repeat the chest X-ray the following day.

• Arrange echocardiography to clarify the diagnosis.

Breathlessness with a normal chest X-ray

• The history and arterial blood gases (Table 5.3) give the clue.

• Before you diagnose primary hyperventilation, you must exclude an underlying organic cause of tachypnoea including diabetic ketoacidosis and asthma. Arterial blood gases and pH should be checked, and the patient admitted for further investigation if these are abnormal.

Acute breathlessness

6 The unconscious patient

• When faced with an unconscious patient, remember *Airway—Breathing—Circulation—Diagnosis*.

• In young adults, the commonest cause of non-traumatic coma is poisoning and, in the elderly, stroke (Fig. 6.1)

Priorities

1 Airway, breathing and circulation

• Check the carotid or femoral pulse: if absent, follow the guidelines for resuscitation (Chapter 1).

• Clear the airway. Remove false teeth if loose and aspirate the pharynx, larynx and trachea with a suction catheter.

• If there is no reflex response (gagging or coughing) to the suction catheter, or the respiratory rate is <8/min, a cuffed endotracheal tube should be inserted, preferably by an anaesthetist. Before this is done, ventilate the patient using a bag-valve-mask system with 100% oxygen.

• If the patient responds to the suction catheter, and the respiratory rate is >8/min, give 60% oxygen by mask (unless carbon monoxide poisoning is suspected (Appendix 11.6, p. 123), in which case give oxygen 10 L/min by a tightly fitting facemask with a circuit which minimizes rebreathing). Unless you suspect neck trauma, place the patient in the recovery position (Fig. 6.2), to reduce the risks of airway obstruction and inhalation of vomit.

• Attach an ECG monitor, put in a peripheral IV cannula, measure arterial oxygen saturation, listen over both lungs, and check the blood pressure.

• If systolic BP is <90 mmHg and there are no signs of pulmonary oedema, give IV fluid (saline or colloid) 500 ml over 15–30 min.

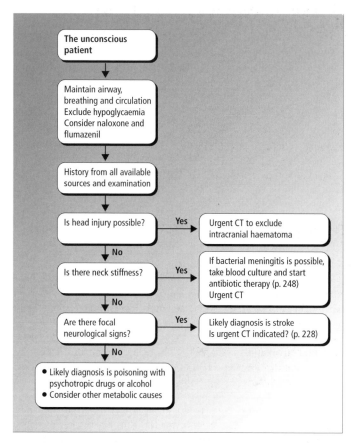

Fig. 6.1 Approach to the unconscious patient.

2 Exclude hypoglycaemia

Check blood glucose immediately by stick test. If blood glucose is <5 mmol/L, give dextrose 25 g IV (50 mL of dextrose 50% solution), via a large vein. In chronic alcoholics, there is a remote risk of precipitating Wernicke's encephalopathy by a glucose load; prevent this by giving thiamine 100 mg IV before or shortly after the dextrose.

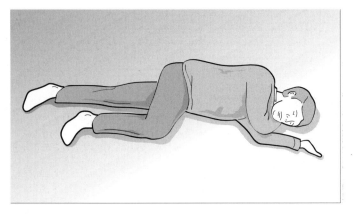

Fig. 6.2 The recovery position.

3 Treat prolonged or recurrent major fits

Treat with IV diazepam or lorazepam (see p. 263). For further management of status epilepticus, see Chapter 33.

4 Consider naloxone

• If the respiratory rate is <12/min or the pupils are pinpoint or there is other reason to suspect opioid poisoning, give naloxone.

• Give up to 4 doses of 800 μg IV every 2–3 min until the respiratory rate is around 15/min.

• If there is a response, start an IV infusion: add 2 mg to 500 mL dextrose 5% or saline (4 μg/mL) and titrate against the respiratory rate and conscious level. The plasma half-life of naloxone is 1 h, shorter than that of most opioids.

• If there is no response to naloxone, opioid poisoning is excluded.

5 Consider flumazenil

• If coma is a complication of the therapeutic use of benzodiazepine in hospital, give flumazenil.

• Give 200 μg IV over 15 s; if needed, further doses of 100 μg can be given at 1-min intervals up to a total dose of 2 mg.

Table 6.1 Urgent investigation of the comatose patient

Blood glucose
Creatinine, urea, sodium, potassium and calcium
Plasma osmolality *
Full blood count
Prothrombin time if liver failure suspected or coma remains unexplained
Arterial blood gases and pH (see Table 6.2)
Gastric lavage (see p. 113) if poisoning suspected† or coma remains unexplained
Chest X-ray
Blood culture if temperature < 36 or > 38°C
ECG if there is hypotension, coexistent heart disease or suspected ingestion of cardiotoxic drugs (anti-arrhythmics, tricyclic antidepressants)

* The normal range of plasma osmolality is 280–300 mosmol/kg. If the measured plasma osmolality (by freezing-point depression method) exceeds calculated osmolality (from the formula [2(Na + K) + urea + glucose]) by 10 mosmol/kg or more, consider poisoning with ethanol, ethylene glycol, isopropyl alcohol or methanol.

† If poisoning is suspected: save serum (10 mL), urine (50 mL) and vomit or gastric aspirate (50 mL) at 4°C for subsequent analysis.

- Flumazenil should not be given to other patients because of the risk of precipitating fits if there is mixed poisoning with benzodiazepines and tricyclics.

6 Arrange urgent investigation

The investigations needed are given in Table 6.1. A low $Paco_2$ is an important clue to several causes of coma (Table 6.2).

Further management

1 At this stage you should obtain a full history and perform a systematic examination. Your management depends on the neurological signs (Figs 6.1 and 6.3).

Table 6.2 Causes of coma with hyperventilation (low $Paco_2$)

Ketoacidosis: diabetic or alcoholic*
Liver failure*
Renal failure*
Bacterial meningitis
Poisoning with aspirin, carbon monoxide, ethanol, ethylene glycol, methanol, paracetamol or tricyclics*
Stroke complicated by pneumonia or pulmonary oedema
Brainstem stroke

* Associated with a metabolic acidosis.

- Document the level of consciousness in objective terms, using the Glasgow Coma Scale (see Appendix).
- Examine for signs of head injury (e.g. scalp laceration, bruising, bleeding from an external auditory meatus or from the nose).
- If there are signs of head injury, assume additional cervical spine injury until proved otherwise: the neck must be immobilized in a collar and X-rayed before you check for neck stiffness and the oculocephalic response.
- Check for neck stiffness.
- Record the size of pupils and their response to bright light.
- Check the oculocephalic response. This is a simple but important test of an intact brainstem. Rotate the head to left and right. In an unconscious patient with an intact brainstem, both eyes rotate in the opposite direction from movement of the head.
- Examine the limbs: tone, response to a painful stimulus (nailbed pressure), tendon reflexes and plantar responses.
- Examine the fundi.

2 The patient can now be placed in one of four groups.

Signs of head injury (with or without focal neurological signs)
- An intracranial haematoma must be excluded.
- Check for injury to other bones and organs.

The unconscious patient

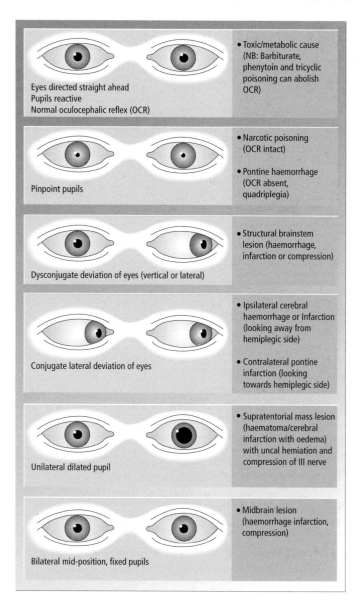

Fig. 6.3 Eye signs in the comatose patient.

Table 6.3 Causes of coma with neck stiffness

Bacterial meningitis
Encephalitis
Subarachnoid haemorrhage
Cerebral or cerebellar haemorrhage with extension into the subarachnoid space
Cerebral malaria

Note: In any of these conditions, neck stiffness may be lost with increasing coma.

- Correct hypotension (systolic BP <100 mmHg) with IV fluid or blood, guided by measurement of CVP.
- Arrange skull, cervical spine and chest X-rays and urgent CT.
- Discuss further management with a neurosurgeon.

Neck stiffness (with or without focal neurological signs) (Table 6.3)
- If the clinical features suggest bacterial meningitis, take blood for culture and start antibiotic therapy (p. 248).
- Malaria must be excluded in patients who have recently travelled to or through an endemic area (p. 392).
- Arrange urgent CT (which must be done before lumbar puncture to exclude a space-occupying lesion).

Focal neurological signs but no head injury or neck stiffness
(Table 6.4)
- Exclude hypoglycaemia.
- The likely diagnosis is a stroke (p. 227)
- Arrange urgent CT if the diagnosis is unclear or there is the possibility of an intracranial haematoma or obstructive hydrocephalus

No head injury, neck stiffness or focal neurological signs (Table 6.5)
- The commonest diagnosis is poisoning with psychotropic drugs or alcohol intoxication, but other metabolic causes must be considered.

The unconscious patient

Table 6.4 Causes of coma with focal neurological signs but no head injury or neck stiffness

With brainstem signs (deviation of the eyes/abnormal pupils)
Brainstem compression due to large intracerebral haemorrhage or infarction with oedema
Brainstem stroke
Cerebellar stroke

Without brainstem signs
Hypoglycaemia (in some cases)
Liver failure (in some cases)

Table 6.5 Causes of coma without head injury, neck stiffness or focal neurological signs

Poisoning with psychotropic drugs or alcohol
Hypoglycaemia
Anoxic brain injury
Liver failure
Respiratory failure
Renal failure
Diabetic ketoacidosis
Myxoedema coma
Acute adrenal insufficiency
Severe hyponatraemia
Severe hypercalcaemia
After major tonic–clonic seizure

The unconscious patient

• If alcohol intoxication is possible, check blood alcohol level. Coma is unlikely to be due to alcohol alone if the level is <44 mmol/L (<200 mg/dL), and other causes must be sought.

Appendix

The Glasgow Coma Scale

• This is a scale based on the assessment of three clinical signs: eye-opening, motor response and verbal response (Table 6.6). It provides

Table 6.6 Glasgow Coma Scale

1 Eye-opening	Score
None—the eyes remain closed	1
To pain—the eyes open in response to a painful stimulus applied to the trunk or limb (a painful stimulus to the head usually provokes closing of the eyes)	2
To voice	3
Spontaneous—the eyes are open with blinking	4

2 Motor response	Score
None	1
Extensor response	2
Abnormal flexor response	3
Withdrawal	4
Localizing—uses limb to locate or resist the painful stimulus	5
Voluntary—obeys commands	6

3 Verbal response	Score
None—no sound whatsoever is produced	1
Incomprehensible—mutters or groans only	2
Inappropriate—intelligible but isolated words	3
Confused speech	4
Orientated speech	5

| *Total score* | 3–15 |

Reference: Teasdale G, Jennett B. Assessment of impaired consciousness and coma: a practical scale. *Lancet* 1974; **2**: 81–4.

The unconscious patient

a simple, rapid, objective and reproducible measure of the level of consciousness.

• To assess the motor response, ask the patient to move the limb. If there is no response, apply firm pressure to the nailbed. Test and record for each of the limbs. Test for a localizing response by pressure on the supra-orbital notch or sternal rub. For the purpose of assessment of conscious level, the best motor response is taken. Differences between the limbs will be important in identifying any focal neurological lesion.

• The score for eye-opening, motor response and verbal response is summed, although you should record the elements of the score as well, e.g. E2, M4, V2 (eye-opening 2, motor response 4, verbal response 2).

• Coma is defined as a score of 8 or below, and a reduced conscious level if the score is 9–14.

The unconscious patient

7 Transient loss of consciousness

You need to decide:
- if the patient has had syncope or a fit;
- the likely cause of syncope, based on clinical assessment and the ECG (Appendix);
- if hospital admission is needed.

Priorities

1 Was it syncope or a fit?

Distinguishing between vasovagal syncope, cardiac syncope (Stokes–Adams attack) and a fit requires a detailed history taken from the patient and any eye-witnesses. Characteristic features are given in Table 7.1. Be aware that involuntary movements (including tonic–clonic seizures, after 30 s of cardiac arrest) are common in syncope, and should not be interpreted as necessarily indicating epilepsy.

Points to cover in the history

Background
- Any previous similar attacks.
- Previous significant head injury (i.e. with skull fracture or loss of consciousness).
- Birth injury, febrile convulsions in childhood, meningitis or encephalitis.
- Family history of epilepsy.
- Cardiac disease (? previous myocardial infarction, hypertrophic or dilated cardiomyopathy, long QT interval (at risk of ventricular tachycardia)).
- Drug therapy.
- Alcohol or substance abuse.
- Sleep deprivation.

Table 7.1 Features differentiating a generalized fit from vasovagal and cardiac syncope (Stokes–Adams attack)

	Generalized fit	Vasovagal syncope	Cardiac syncope (Stokes–Adams attack)
Occurrence when sitting or lying	Common	Rare	May occur
Occurrence during sleep	Common	Does not occur	May occur
Prodromal symptoms	May occur, with focal neurological symptoms, automatisms or hallucinations	Typical, with dizziness, sweating, nausea, blurring of vision, disturbance of hearing, yawning	Often none Palpitation may precede syncope in tachyarrhythmias
Focal neurological features at onset	May occur (and signify focal cerebral lesion)	Never occur	Never occur
Tonic–clonic movements	Characteristic, occur within 30 s of onset	May occur after 30 s of syncope (secondary anoxic seizure)	May occur after 30 s of syncope (secondary anoxic seizure)
Facial colour	Flush or cyanosis at onset	Pallor at onset and after syncope	Pallor at onset, flush on recovery
Tongue biting	Common	Rare	Rare
Urinary incontinence	Common	Uncommon	May occur
Injury	May occur	Uncommon	May occur
Post-ictal confusion	Common	Uncommon	Uncommon

Loss of consciousness

Before the attack

• Prodromal symptoms: were these cardiovascular (e.g. dizziness, palpitation, chest pain) or focal neurological symptoms (aura)?

• Circumstances, e.g. exercising, standing, sitting or lying, asleep.

• Precipitants, e.g. coughing, micturition, head-turning.

The attack

• Were there any focal neurological features at the onset: sustained deviation of the head or eyes or unilateral jerking of the limbs?

• Was there a cry (may occur in tonic phase of fit)?

• Duration of loss of consciousness.

• Associated tongue biting, urinary incontinence or injury.

• Facial colour changes (pallor common in syncope, uncommon with a fit).

• Abnormal pulse (must be assessed in relation to the reliability of the witness).

After the attack

• Immediately well or delayed recovery with confusion or headache?

2 What is the likely cause of syncope? (Fig. 7.1)

• Clinical assessment and an ECG will establish the likely cause of syncope in around 50% of patients.

• Check full blood count, creatinine and electrolytes (including magnesium in patients taking diuretic or anti-arrhythmic therapy) and blood glucose.

• Obtain a chest X-ray if cardiovascular examination or the ECG is abnormal.

Points to cover in the examination

• Conscious level (confirm the patient is fully orientated).

• Pulse, blood pressure, temperature, respiratory rate, oxygen saturation.

• Systolic BP sitting or lying and after 2 min standing (a fall > 20 mmHg is abnormal; note if symptomatic or not).

• Arterial pulses (check major pulses for asymmetry or bruits).

• JVP (if raised, consider pulmonary embolism, pulmonary hypertension or cardiac tamponade).

• Heart murmurs (aortic stenosis and hypertrophic cardiomyopathy may cause exertional syncope; atrial myxoma may simulate mitral stenosis).

Loss of consciousness

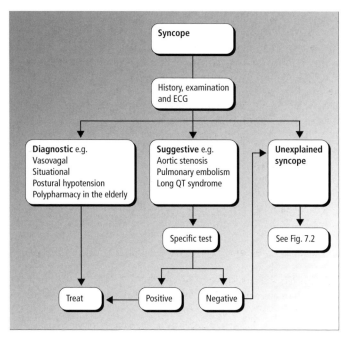

Fig. 7.1 Approach to the diagnosis of syncope. Reference: Linzer M *et al*. Diagnosing syncope. *Annals of Internal Medicine* 1997; **126**: 989–96 and **127**: 76–86.

Loss of consciousness

• Neck mobility (Does neck movement induce presyncope? Is there neck stiffness?).
• Presence of focal neurological signs: as a minimum, check visual fields, limb power, tendon reflexes and plantar responses.
• Fundi (for haemorrhages or papilloedema).
ECG abnormalities which may be relevant to the diagnosis are given in Table 7.2.

3 Admit or discharge?
Patients with vasovagal or situational syncope do not need admission. The majority of other patients with syncope will need to be admitted, at least for a period of 12–24 h observation.

Loss of consciousness

Table 7.2 Looking at the ECG after syncope. Note that abnormalities on the ECG will rarely prove the cause of syncope, but may provide evidence pointing to an underlying disorder

ECG feature	Possible significance
Sinus bradycardia (rate <50/min) or sinus pauses	May reflect sino-atrial disorder. Accept as the cause of syncope if definitely related to symptoms
First-degree AV block	Raises the possibility of intermittent second- or third-degree AV block
Second-degree AV block	Likely to be the cause of syncope: indication for pacing
Third-degree (complete) AV block	Likely to be the cause of syncope: indication for pacing
Atrial fibrillation	May reflect sino-atrial disorder or underlying structural heart disease
Paced rhythm	Pacemaker failure is rare but should be excluded (p. 34)
Short PR interval (<120 ms)	Look for other features of WPW syndrome (delta wave, widened QRS complex); if WPW present, discuss management with a cardiologist
Right axis deviation (QRS predominantly negative in lead I and positive in lead II)	Consider pulmonary hypertension or pulmonary embolism
Left axis deviation (QRS predominantly positive in lead I and negative in lead II)	As an isolated abnormality, usually of no significance

Right bundle branch block (RBBB)	Consider pulmonary embolism
Left bundle branch block	May reflect structural heart disease or conducting system disease
Bifascicular block (RBBB + left axis deviation) with or without first-degree AV block	Significantly increases the likelihood that syncope was due to intermittent AV block
Pathological Q waves	Consider previous myocardial infarction. Q waves resembling those seen in myocardial infarction may be found in hypertrophic cardiomyopathy and WPW syndrome
Left ventricular hypertrophy	Consider aortic stenosis or hypertrophic cardiomyopathy
Dominant R wave in V1	Causes include right ventricular hypertrophy, right bundle branch block, WPW syndrome and posterior myocardial infarction
Right ventricular hypertrophy	Consider pulmonary hypertension
Long QT interval	At risk of torsade de pointes

WPW, Wolff–Parkinson–White syndrome.

Loss of consciousness

Admission definitely indicated
- Previous myocardial infarction or known cardiomyopathy (? ventricular tachycardia).
- Associated chest pain (? acute myocardial infarction or aortic dissection).
- Associated abrupt headache (? subarachnoid haemorrhage).
- Raised JVP (? pulmonary embolism, pulmonary hypertension, cardiac tamponade).
- Signs of significant valvular disease (? aortic stenosis, atrial myxoma).
- Signs of congestive heart failure (? ventricular tachycardia).
- Abnormal ECG.

Admission often indicated
- Sudden loss of consciousness with injury, or with associated rapid palpitation; or with exertion.
- Taking drugs ssociated with torsade (quinidine, disopyramide, procainamide, amiodarone, sotalol).
- Significant postural hypotension (fall in systolic BP > 20 mmHg).
- Age over 70.

4 Who should be monitored on the CCU?
- Patients with ECG evidence of conducting system disease, but without absolute indications for temporary pacing: sinus bradycardia < 50/min, not due to beta-blockade; sinus pauses of 2–3 s; bifascicular or trifascicular block.
- Patients at risk of ventricular tachycardia: previous myocardial infarction; cardiomyopathy; long QT interval.

5 When is temporary pacing indicated?
- Second-degree or complete AV block.
- Sinus pauses > 3 s.
- Sinus bradycardia < 40/min unresponsive to atropine (p. 31).
- Failure of permanent pacemaker system (p. 35).

Further management

Clinical assessment diagnostic or suggestive
- Arrange the appropriate test to confirm or exclude your clinical sus-

picion (e.g. echocardiography; ventilation–perfusion lung scan).
• If initial tests are inconclusive or negative, further investigation is as for unexplained syncope (Fig. 7.2).

Unexplained syncope
• Management is detailed in Fig. 7.2.
• Patients aged 60 or over with unexplained syncope should be tested for carotid sinus hypersensitivity (Table 7.3).
• Patients with unexplained syncope must be advised that they should not drive until the cause has been identified and corrected.

Table 7.3 Testing for carotid sinus hypersensitivity

Is indicated in patients aged 60 and over with unexplained syncope

Contraindications to the test include the presence of a carotid bruit, recent myocardial infarction, recent stroke or a history of ventricular tachycardia

Begin with the patient lying

Attach an ECG monitor with a printer and check the blood pressure

The carotid sinus lies at the level of the upper border of the thyroid cartilage just below the angle of the jaw

Perform carotid sinus massage for up to 15 s whilst recording a rhythm strip. Press posteriorly and medially over the artery (first on the right, and if this is negative on the left) with your thumb or index and middle fingers

If the test is negative, repeat with the patient sitting

An abnormal response is defined by a sinus pause > 3 s or a drop in systolic blood pressure > 50 mmHg. If these occur, discuss with a cardiologist whether pacemaker implantation is indicated

Loss of consciousness

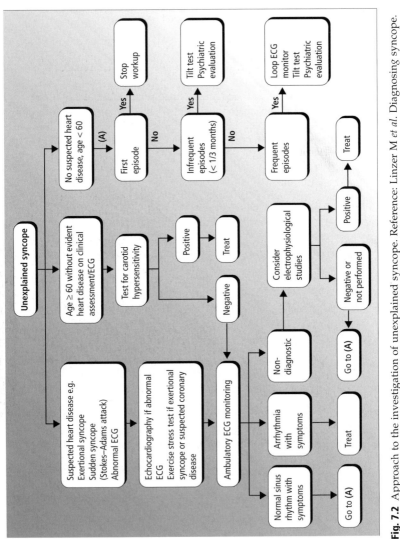

Fig. 7.2 Approach to the investigation of unexplained syncope. Reference: Linzer M *et al.* Diagnosing syncope. *Annals of Internal Medicine* 1997; **126**: 989–96 and **127**: 76–86.

Appendix

Table 7.4 Causes of syncope

Common	Less common
Cardiovascular	
Vasovagal syncope	Aortic stenosis
Situational syncope*	Pulmonary embolism
Postural hypotension due to drugs	Carotid sinus hypersensitivity
Arrhythmias	Pulmonary hypertension
	Aortic dissection
	Acute myocardial infarction
	Hypertrophic cardiomyopathy
	Atrial myxoma
	Postural hypotension due to other causes
	Cardiac tamponade
Neurological	
Epilepsy (misdiagnosed as syncope)	Subarachnoid haemorrhage
	Subclavian steal syndrome
	Vertebrobasilar TIA
	Migraine
Others	
Psychiatric causes	Rapid haemorrhage
	Hypoglycaemia

* Situational syncope: syncope occurring in relation to coughing, micturition, defecation or swallowing, without another cause apparent on examination or ECG.

Loss of consciousness

8 Acute confusional state

- Infection and drugs are the most common causes of an acute confusional state.
- Consider the diagnosis in any patient labelled as difficult, uncooperative or a 'poor historian'.
- An approach to the patient with suspected acute confusional state is given in Fig. 8.1.

Priorities

1 **Assess the mental state**: does the patient really have an acute confusional state (and not dementia, a functional psychosis or severe depression)?
- Check for **clouding of consciousness** (reduced alertness, impaired attention and concentration), **disorientation in time** (and often also for place and person) and **impaired short-term memory** (Table 8.1).
- The duration of the patient's abnormal mental state, as assessed by a reliable witness, often helps distinguish acute confusional state from dementia (which may of course coexist). Other features which differentiate between these diagnoses are given in Table 8.2.
- Vivid visual or auditory hallucinations suggest alcohol withdrawal.

2 Your **clinical assessment** is directed at identifying the cause of the acute confusional state (Appendix 8.1).
- If the patient was admitted with an acute confusional state, find out exactly what medications were being taken prior to admission (if necessary, contact the patient's primary care physician to check which drugs were prescribed, and ask relatives to collect all medications in the home). If the confusional state has developed in hospital, check the drug chart.

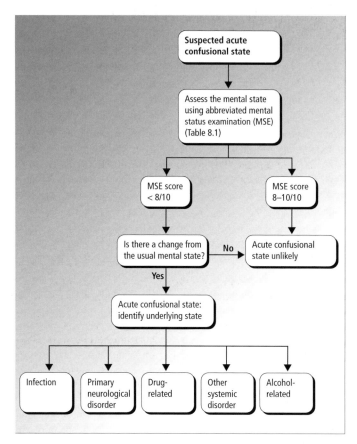

Fig. 8.1 Approach to the patient with suspected acute confusional state.

• Many drugs may cause an acute confusional state in the elderly, notably benzodiazepines, tricyclic antidepressants, analgesics (including NSAIDs, particularly indomethacin), lithium, steroids and drugs for Parkinsonism.

• Check the temperature (remember that infection may also cause a low temperature (<36°C)), pulse, blood pressure,

---

Table 8.1 Abbreviated mental status examination of the elderly

---

Age

Time (to nearest hour)

Address for recall at end of test—this should be repeated by the patient to ensure it has been heard correctly: 42 West Street

Year

Name of hospital

Recognition of 2 people (e.g. doctor, nurse)

Date of birth (day and month sufficient)

Year of 1st World War

Name of present monarch

Count backwards 20 to 1

Each correct answer scores one mark. The healthy elderly score 8–10

Reference: Qureshi KN, Hodkinson HM. Evaluation of a ten-question mental test in the institutionalized elderly. *Age and Ageing* 1974; **3**: 152–7.

respiratory rate (a sensitive sign of pneumonia) and oxygen saturation.

• Check for focal chest signs, abdominal tenderness or guarding, urinary retention, faecal impaction, pressure sores and signs of cellulitis.

• Are there abnormal neurological signs? As a minimum, check for neck stiffness (in flexion and extension), lateralized weakness, tendon reflexes and plantar responses.

• Consider non-convulsive status epilepticus if there are mild clonic movements of the eyelids, face or hands, or simple automatisms. Diazepam (10 mg IV) may terminate the status with improvement in conscious level. Seek advice from a neurologist.

• Are there signs suggesting acute liver failure (jaundice, asterixis ('liver flap'), hepatic fetor, stigmata of chronic liver disease)? See p. 295 for further management of acute liver failure.

• In patients with suspected alcohol abuse, check for other signs of Wernicke's encephalopathy: nystagmus, VI nerve palsy (unable to

Table 8.2 Clinical features of acute confusional state, dementia and acute functional psychosis

Characteristic	Acute confusional state	Dementia	Acute functional psychosis
Onset	Sudden	Insidious	Sudden
Course over 24 h	Fluctuating, nocturnal exacerbation	Stable	Stable
Consciousness	Reduced	Stable	Stable
Attention	Globally disordered	Normal, except in severe cases	May be disordered
Orientation	Usually impaired	Often impaired	May be impaired
Cognition	Globally impaired	Globally impaired	May be selectively impaired
Hallucinations	Usually visual or visual and auditory	Often absent	Predominantly auditory
Delusions	Fleeting, poorly systematized	Often absent	Sustained, systematized
Psychomotor activity	Increased, reduced or shifting unpredictably	Often normal	Varies from psychomotor retardation to severe hyperactivity
Speech	Often incoherent, slow or rapid	Difficulty finding words, perseveration	Normal, slow or rapid
Involuntary movements	Often asterixis or coarse tremor	Often absent	Usually absent
Physical illness or drug toxicity	One or both present	Often absent	Usually absent

Reference: Lipowski ZJ. Delirium in the elderly patient. *New England Journal of Medicine* 1989; **320**: 578–82.

Acute confusional state

Table 8.3 Investigation in acute confusional state

Blood glucose

Creatinine, urea, sodium, potassium and calcium

Liver function tests

Thyroid function tests

Full blood count

Prothrombin time if suspected liver disease

Blood culture if temperature <36 or >38°C

Urine stick test, microscopy and culture

ECG

Chest X-ray

Arterial blood gases if arterial oxygen saturation <90% or there are new chest signs

Cranial CT if confusional state followed fall or head injury, or there are new focal neurological signs or papilloedema

abduct the eye) and ataxia (wide-based gait; may be unable to stand or walk).

3 Check blood glucose, and test a urine specimen if available for glucose, blood and protein. If there is fever or low temperature, new focal chest signs or oxygen saturation is <90% breathing air, arrange a chest X-ray. Other investigations needed are given in Table 8.3.

Further management

1 **Specific treatment** is directed at the underlying cause.

• Stop any drugs which may be causing or contributing to confusion unless essential.

• Management of alcohol withdrawal is summarized in Appendix 8.2.

• Correct electrolyte abnormalities (sodium, potassium and calcium) (p. 336).

- If the cause of the confusional state remains unclear, but infection cannot be excluded, start antibiotic treatment (p. 103) after blood and urine cultures have been taken.
- Seek advice from a geriatrician or psychogeriatrician if the confusional state does not respond to treatment of the presumed cause.

2 Supportive measures
- The patient should ideally be nursed in a quiet area of the ward.
- Avoid physical restraints. If necessary, place the mattress on the floor rather than risk the patient falling out of bed.

3 Sedation should only be used if the patient is at risk of self-injury or if aggressive behaviour prevents treatment. Oral administration (syrup may be easier than tablets) is usually preferable to IM or IV. Recommended drugs are:
- haloperidol 0.5–3 mg PO or 2.5–5 mg IM, up to 6 hly, or
- droperidol 5–10 mg PO or 5 mg IM, up to 6 hly.

Discontinue sedative drugs as soon as possible.

Appendix 8.1 Causes of acute confusional state

1 Infection
- Urinary or respiratory tract infection are the commonest causes.
- Endocarditis and biliary tract sepsis should be considered in the febrile patient without localizing signs.
- Exclude malaria if there has been recent travel to an endemic region (p. 392).

2 Drug-related
- Many drugs may cause an acute confusional state in the elderly, notably benzodiazepines, tricyclic antidepressants, analgesics (including NSAIDs, particularly indomethacin), lithium, steroids and drugs for Parkinsonism.
- Benzodiazepine withdrawal may also cause a confusional state.

3 Alcohol-related
- Intoxication or withdrawal; see Appendix 8.2.

Acute confusional state

4 Primary neurological disorders
- Head injury.
- Post-ictal state.
- Non-dominant parietal lobe stroke.
- Subdural haematoma (p. 235).
- Subarachnoid haemorrhage (p. 243).
- Non-convulsive status epilepticus.
- Herpes encephalitis (p. 252).
- Meningitis (p. 247).
- Raised intracranial pressure.

5 Other systemic disorders
- Hypoglycaemia (p. 319).
- Hyperglycaemic states (ketoacidosis (p. 328) and non-ketotic hyperglycaemia (p. 335).
- Respiratory failure (p. 204).
- Heart failure.
- Acute liver failure (p. 295).
- Advanced acute renal failure (p. 302).
- Hypertensive encephalopathy (p. 161).
- Addisonian crisis (p. 364).
- Severe hypothyroidism (p. 373) or thyrotoxicosis (p. 369).
- Porphyria.
- Severe hyponatraemia (p. 338).
- Hypercalcaemia (p. 348).
- Hypothermia (p. 373).

Appendix 8.2 Alcohol withdrawal syndrome

Features
- **Signs of autonomic hyperactivity** (appear within hours of the last drink, usually peaking within 24–48 h): tremor, sweating, nausea, vomiting, anxiety, agitation.
- **Major seizures** ('rum fits') (usually occurring within 12–48 h).
- **Alcohol withdrawal delirium** ('delirium tremens'): auditory and visual hallucinations, acute confusional state, marked autonomic hyperactivity.

Delirium tremens can be life-threatening (due to complications such as hyperthermia, hypovolaemia, electrolyte derangement and respiratory infection) but only occurs in 5% of patients with alcohol withdrawal syndrome. In most cases, the symptoms of alcohol withdrawal are mild and do not require specific treatment. They pass within 2–7 days of the last drink.

Management

• General supportive measures: fluid replacement if needed; exclusion of hypoglycaemia; treatment of intercurrent illness; vitamin supplements (vitamin B compound, strong, 2 tablets daily, thiamine 100 mg 12-hly PO, and vitamin C 50 mg 12-hly PO).

• Patients with signs of Wernicke's encephalopathy (confusional state with nystagmus, VI nerve palsy (unable to abduct the eye) and ataxia (wide-based gait; may be unable to stand or walk)) should be treated with IV thiamine ('Pabrinex' IV high-potency injection, containing thiamine 250 mg per 10 mL (2 ampoules)): one pair of ampoules 12-hly for 5–7 days, given slowly over 10 min (may cause anaphylaxis).

• Alcohol withdrawal seizures are typically self-limiting and do not require specific treatment (see p. 269).

• If there is delirium tremens or severe agitation, start a benzodiazepine (safer than chlormethiazole).

• Arrange appropriate follow-up (e.g. referral to an alcohol problems clinic).

Acute confusional state

9 Headache

• Most patients with headache have tension-type headache or migraine. A minority have life-threatening disorders such as subarachnoid haemorrhage or bacterial meningitis.
• A careful and detailed clinical assessment is the key to diagnosis.

Clinical assessment of the patient with headache

History
• Is the headache acute, or chronic and recurrent?
• If acute, was the onset sudden?
• Is the headache still present? How long has it lasted?
• Was there syncope at the onset?
• How severe is the headache? Is it the worst headache ever?
• Distribution (unilateral, diffuse, localized)?
• Associated systemic, neurological or visual symptoms (ask about blurring, transient blindness, diplopia, scotomata, fortification spectra): did these precede or follow the headache?
• Medication history and possible exposure to toxins.
• Recent travel abroad?
• Is the patient immunocompromised or has a known malignancy?
• Family history of migraine or subarachnoid haemorrhage.

Examination
• Temperature.
• Pulse and blood pressure.
• Conscious level.
• Neck stiffness (in flexion and extension).
• Focal neurological signs.
• Horner syndrome (partial ptosis and constricted pupil: if present, consider carotid artery dissection (p. 230)).

- Visual acuity and fields.
- Fundi (? papilloedema or retinal haemorrhages).
- Sinus tenderness.
- Temporal artery thickening or tenderness (in patients over 50 with suspected temporal arteritis).

Headache with reduced conscious level or focal neurological signs

- Causes are given in Table 9.1.
- The mode of onset of symptoms will help distinguish between vascular (acute onset), infectious (subacute) and neoplastic (chronic) disease.
- If the patient is febrile, take blood cultures and start antibiotic therapy to cover bacterial meningitis (p. 247). CT should be performed before lumbar puncture.
- Discuss further management with a neurologist.

Table 9.1 Headache with reduced conscious level or focal neurological signs

Stroke
Subarachnoid haemorrhage
Chronic subdural haematoma
After major seizure
Acute hydrocephalus
Intracranial space-occupying lesion (e.g. neoplasm, abscess, subdural empyema)
Meningitis
Encephalitis
Cerebral malaria
Hypertensive encephalopathy

Headache

Headache with fever but no focal neurological signs

- Causes are given in Table 9.2.
- If neck stiffness is present, a lumbar puncture should be done to

exclude meningitis or subarachnoid haemorrhage. Cryptococcal meningitis may not give rise to neck stiffness and so, in immunocompromised patients, LP is indicated even in the absence of this sign.

• Consider malaria and typhoid in patients who have returned from abroad (Chapter 49).

Table 9.2 Headache with fever but no focal neurological signs

Meningitis (neck stiffness is not an invariable feature especially in cryptococcal meningitis)

Subarachnoid haemorrhage

Encephalitis

Systemic infectious disease (including malaria and typhoid in patients who have returned from abroad)

Local infection, e.g. sinusitis and otitis media

Headache with papilloedema but no focal neurological signs

• Causes are given in Table 9.3.

• If the diastolic BP is >120 mmHg and there are retinal haemorrhages or exudates, the working diagnosis is accelerated-phase hypertension: start antihypertensive therapy (p. 160).

• If the BP is normal, arrange CT and discuss further management with a neurologist.

Table 9.3 Headache with papilloedema but no meningeal or focal neurological signs

Accelerated-phase hypertension

Hypertensive encephalopathy

Intracranial space-occupying lesion (e.g. neoplasm in non-dominant frontal lobe)

Cerebral venous sinus thrombosis

Benign intracranial hypertension

Headache

Headache with local signs

• Causes are given in Table 9.4.

Table 9.4 Headache with local signs

Acute sinusitis
Acute angle-closure glaucoma
Temporal arthritis
Temporomandibular joint dysfunction
Cervicogenic headache (headache referred from disorder of the cervical spine)

Acute sinusitis
• Suspect from associated fever, facial pain especially on bending over, mucopurulent nasal discharge, and tenderness on pressure over the affected sinus.
• Obtain X-rays of the sinuses, looking for mucosal thickening, a fluid level or opacification.
• Treatment is with coamoxiclav (or erythromycin and metronidazole if allergic to penicillin) and steam inhalations.
• Discuss management with an ENT surgeon.

Acute angle-closure glaucoma
• Suspect from blurred vision with reduced visual acuity due to corneal clouding, red eye, pupil fixed in the mid-position.
• Refer urgently to an ophthalmologist.

Temporal arteritis
• See p. 98.

Table 9.5 Headache with no abnormal signs

Tension-type headache
Medication misuse (chronic consumption of large amounts of analgesics for
   tension-type headache)
Migraine
Drug related (e.g. nitrates, nicorandil, dihydropyridine calcium antagonists)
Toxin exposure (e.g. carbon monoxide poisoning)
Temporal arteritis
Subarachnoid haemorrhage
Benign thunderclap headache (assumes subarachnoid haemorrhage excluded)
Brief benign headache occurring during exertion or sexual intercourse

Headache with no abnormal signs

• Causes are given in Table 9.5. Always consider subarachnoid haemorrhage and temporal arteritis. Note that a first episode of severe headache cannot be reliably diagnosed as migraine or tension-type headache: diagnostic criteria require more than nine episodes for tension-type headache and more than four episodes for migraine without aura.

Subarachnoid haemorrhage (Table 9.6, p. 97)
• If there are no abnormal signs, but the headache was abrupt in onset and severe, subarachnoid haemorrhage must be excluded by CT, followed by examination of the CSF if the CT is normal or equivocal. CT is most sensitive for detection of subarachnoid haemorrhage if done within 12 h of onset of headache.
• Xanthochromia is the most reliable method of differentiating between subarachnoid haemorrhage and traumatic tap, and is always found 12 h to 2 weeks after the haemorrhage. Lumbar puncture should therefore be delayed >12 h after the onset of headache unless meningitis is a possibility.

Table 9.6 Clinical features of aneurysmal subarachnoid haemorrhage

History

Onset of headache: abrupt, maximal at onset, 'thunderclap' headache

Severity of headache: usually 'worst of life' or very severe

Qualitative characteristics: first headache ever of this intensity, unique or
  different in patients with prior headaches

Associated symptoms: transient loss of consciousness, diplopia, fit, focal
  neurological symptoms*

Background

Cigarette smoking

Hypertension

Alcohol consumption (especially after recent binge)

Personal or family history of subarachnoid haemorrhage*

Polycystic kidney disease*

Heritable connective tissue diseases: Ehlers–Danlos syndrome type IV,
  pseudoxanthoma elasticum, fibromuscular dysplasia*

Sickle cell disease, alpha$_1$-antitrypsin deficiency

Examination

Retinal or subhyaloid haemorrhages (retinal haemorrhages with curved lower
  and straight upper borders)*

Neck stiffness*

Focal neurological signs

Low-grade fever

* Patients with these features are at very high risk of having an intracranial
aneurysm. Ask advice on management from a neurologist, even if CT/LP are
negative.

Reference: Edlow JA, Caplan LR. Avoiding pitfalls in the diagnosis of subarachnoid
hemorrhage. *New England Journal of Medicine* 2000; **342**: 29–36.

Headache

Temporal arteritis
• Consider in any patient over 50 with headache, which will usually be of days or a few weeks in duration.
• Associated symptoms include malaise, weight loss, jaw claudication, scalp tenderness, and visual changes (amaurosis fugax, diplopia and partial or complete loss of vision).
• If the ESR is >50 mm/h and/or the temporal artery is thickened or tender (feel 2 cm above and 2 cm forward from the external auditory meatus), start prednisolone. For patients without visual symptoms, give 40 mg daily; with visual symptoms, give 60–80 mg daily.
• Arrange for a temporal artery biopsy to be done within 48 h of starting prednisolone.

Migraine
• Diagnostic criteria are given in Table 9.7. The first migraine headache usually occurs between the ages of 10 and 30.

Table 9.7 Diagnostic criteria for migraine

Migraine without aura
Attacks lasting 4–72 h
At least two of the following characteristics: unilateral; pulsating; moderate to
  severe; aggravated by movement
At least one associated symptom: nausea or vomiting; photophobia; phonophobia

Migraine with aura
One or more transient focal neurological aura symptoms
Gradual development of aura symptom over >4 min, or several symptoms in
  succession
Aura symptoms last 4–60 min
Headache follows or accompanies aura within 60 min

Reference: Ferrari MD. Migraine. *Lancet* 1998; **351**: 1043–51.

• Treatment of an acute attack is with dispersible aspirin or paracetamol and an antiemetic, e.g. metoclopramide 10 mg IM or domperidone (available in suppository form).

• If the headache does not respond to analgesic, use a triptan (5HT$_1$ agonist).

Headache

10 Sepsis syndrome

• Make a working diagnosis of sepsis syndrome (Table 10.1) if a patient has unexplained hypoxaemia, oliguria or confusional state associated with fever or reduced body temperature (<36°C). Sepsis syndrome is often complicated by hypotension (septic shock).
• *Escherichia coli, Staphylococcus aureus* and *epidermidis* and *Streptococcus pneumoniae* (pneumococcus) are the commonest pathogens.
• A good outcome depends on prompt diagnosis, vigorous fluid resuscitation, appropriate initial antibiotic therapy and drainage of any infected collection.

Priorities

1 If systolic BP is <90 mmHg, give colloid IV 500 ml over 15–30 min. See p. 36 for further management of hypotension. Give oxygen 35% and check oxygen saturation: increase inspired oxygen to 60% if oxygen saturation is <90%.
2 Examine for a focus of infection.
  • The clinical setting may make it obvious, e.g. signs of pneumonia (p. 206) or meningitis (p. 247) or recent instrumentation of urinary or biliary tract.
  • Check for neck stiffness, focal lung crackles or bronchial breathing, heart murmur, abdominal tenderness or guarding, arthritis, cellulitis, soft tissue abscess and signs of infection at the site of IV lines.
  • Obtain a surgical opinion if you suspect an abdominal or pelvic source of sepsis.
3 Investigations required urgently are given in Table 10.2.
4 Start antibiotic therapy as soon as blood has been taken for culture, based on the likely source of sepsis (Table 10.3). Take into account

Table 10.1 Definitions

Condition	Definition
Sepsis	Clinical evidence of infection Temperature >38 or <36˚C Heart rate >90/min Respiratory rate >20/min
Sepsis syndrome	Sepsis plus altered organ perfusion Hypoxaemia Oliguria Confusion
Septic shock	Sepsis syndrome plus hypotension (systolic BP <90 mmHg or a decrease from baseline systolic BP of >40 mmHg) despite volume replacement
Refractory septic shock	Septic shock that does not respond to therapy with IV fluid and inotropic/vasopressor therapy within 1 h

previous isolates from the patient, and the local pattern of antibiotic resistance in patients with hospital-acquired infection:
- Gentamicin levels need to be monitored and doses should be reduced in renal impairment (see BNF).
- Substitute aztreonam or ciprofloxacin for gentamicin if gentamicin resistance is prevalent.
- Substitute vancomycin for flucloxacillin if methicillin-resistant *Staphylococcus aureus* (MRSA) infection is possible. Serum levels of vancomycin should be measured.

5 Transfer the patient to the ITU if:
- systolic BP remains <90 mmHg after fluid replacement (see Chapter 3), or
- Pao_2 is <8 kPa (oxygen saturation <90%) despite an inspired oxygen concentration of 60%.

Sepsis syndrome

Table 10.2 Urgent investigation of the patient with sepsis syndrome and septic shock

---

Full blood count (the white cell count may be low in overwhelming bacterial sepsis; a low platelet count may reflect disseminated intravascular coagulation, p. 104)

Clotting screen if purpura or jaundice, prolonged oozing from puncture sites, bleeding from surgical wounds or low platelet count

Creatinine, sodium and potassium

Blood glucose (hypoglycaemia can complicate sepsis, especially in patients with liver disease)

Amylase (if abdominal pain or tenderness)

Chest X-ray

Arterial gases and pH

Blood culture (at least 2 sets)*

Urine microscopy and culture

Ascitic fluid microscopy and culture (p. 297)

Stool culture (if diarrhoea or recent foreign travel)

CSF examination if suspected meningitis (p. 247)

Joint aspiration if suspected septic arthritis (p. 387)

Blood film for malaria if recent travel to or through an endemic area (p. 392)

ECG if age > 60 or known cardiac disease

---

* If suspected IV line-related sepsis (central venous line, pulmonary artery catheter, indwelling IV catheter): take blood for culture via the line and a further sample from a peripheral vein; change the central venous line or pulmonary artery catheter and send the tip for culture. See p. 427.

Problems

Sepsis in the neutropenic patient

• Patients with neutrophil counts $< 0.5 \times 10^9/\mathrm{L}$ are at high risk of bacterial infection, particularly from Gram-negative rods and *Staphylococcus aureus* and *epidermidis*.

Table 10.3 Initial antibiotic therapy for sepsis syndrome

Suspected source of sepsis	Initial antibiotic therapy (IV, high dose)
Bacterial meningitis	Table 30.2, p. 248
Community-acquired pneumonia	Table 24.4, p. 211
Hospital-acquired pneumonia	Table 24.5, p. 212
Aspiration (inhalation) pneumonia	Amoxycillin clavulanate or fluoroquinolone + clindamycin or metronidazole
Endocarditis (not associated with IV drug use)	Benzylpenicillin (or vancomycin if penicillin allergic) + low-dose gentamicin
Endocarditis associated with IV drug use or within 2 months of cardiac valve surgery	Flucloxacillin (or vancomycin if penicillin allergic or suspected MRSA) + low-dose gentamicin
Peritonitis	Cefotaxime (or gentamicin) + metronidazole
Biliary tract sepsis	Cefotaxime or gentamicin
Urinary tract infection	Cefuroxime + gentamicin
IV line related	Flucloxacillin (or vancomycin if penicillin allergic or suspected MRSA) + gentamicin
Septic arthritis	Table 48.4, p. 390
Cellulitis	Benzylpenicillin + flucloxacillin (or coamoxiclav alone)
No localizing signs: neutropenic	Azlocillin + gentamicin (or ceftazidime alone)
No localizing signs: not neutropenic	Cefotaxime + gentamicin

Sepsis syndrome

- If the neutropenic patient has a single temperature >38°C, or two spikes of fever of >37.5°C during a 24-h period, the likely cause is bacterial infection and antibiotic therapy should be started.
- Search for a focus of infection. Examination should include the entire skin including the perineum and perianal region, indwelling IV line and other IV sites, and the mouth, teeth and sinuses.

Table 10.4 Possible causes of fever associated with IV drug use

Infection at injection sites

Thrombophlebitis

Endocarditis (especially right-sided) (which may be complicated by septic
    pulmonary embolism)

Pulmonary tuberculosis

Hepatitis B or C

Septic arthritis

Pyrogen reaction

AIDS-related infection, e.g. cryptococcal meningitis, *Pneumocystis carinii* pneumonia

- Investigations required urgently are given in Table 10.2.
- Several antibiotic regimens have been shown to be effective in neutropenic patients without localizing signs: an antipseudomonal penicillin plus an aminoglycoside (e.g. azlocillin + gentamicin); or monotherapy with a third-generation cephalosporin (e.g. ceftazidime) or aztreonam.
- Ask for advice from a haematologist.

Sepsis syndrome associated with IV drug use
- Several causes of fever must be considered (Table 10.4).
- Right-sided endocarditis may not give rise to abnormal cardiac signs.
- Antibiotic therapy must cover staphylococci (Table 10.3).

Disseminated intravascular coagulation
- Disseminated intravascular coagulation (DIC) is a complication of sepsis due to Gram-positive and Gram-negative organisms (as well as a number of non-infective disorders).
- Suspect in patients with sepsis syndrome (usually with septic shock) who develop purpura, prolonged oozing from puncture sites, bleeding from surgical wounds or bleeding from the gastrointestinal and respiratory tracts.

• Confirm by a low platelet count ($<100 \times 10^{12}/L$), prolonged prothrombin and activated partial thromboplastin times, and a high plasma concentration of fibrin degradation products. Monitor these indices.
• Ask advice on management from a haematologist.
• Give vitamin K 10 mg IV to reverse possible vitamin K deficiency which may contribute to the coagulopathy.
• If there is active bleeding or an invasive procedure is needed, give fresh frozen plasma and platelet concentrates.
• There is no conclusive evidence for the use of heparin in the treatment of DIC, but this should be considered if there is thromboembolism.

Sepsis syndrome

11 Poisoning

If you need advice about the management of poisoning, contact a Poisons Centre (Appendix 11.1) or access the TOXBASE web site (HTTP://www.spib.axl.co.uk) (user name and password needed for access).

Priorities

The unconscious patient

1 **Attend first to the airway, breathing and circulation.**

• Check the carotid or femoral pulse: if absent, follow the guidelines for resuscitation (Chapter 1).

• Clear the airway. Remove false teeth if loose, and aspirate the pharynx, larynx and trachea with a suction catheter.

• If there is no reflex response (gagging or coughing) to the suction catheter, or the respiratory rate is <8/min, a cuffed endotracheal tube should be placed, preferably by an anaesthetist. Before this is done, ventilate the patient using a bag-valve-mask system with 100% oxygen.

• If the patient responds to the suction catheter, and the respiratory rate is >8/min, give 60% oxygen by mask (unless carbon monoxide poisoning is suspected (Appendix 11.6), in which case give oxygen 10 L/min by a tightly fitting facemask with a circuit which minimizes rebreathing). Unless you suspect neck trauma, place the patient in the recovery position (Fig. 6.2, p. 66) to reduce the risks of airway obstruction and inhalation of vomit.

• Attach an ECG monitor, put in a peripheral IV cannula, measure arterial oxygen saturation, listen over both lungs and check the blood pressure.

• If systolic BP is <90 mmHg and there are no signs of pulmonary oedema, give IV fluid (saline or colloid) 500 mL over 15–30 min.

2 Exclude hypoglycaemia. Check blood glucose immediately by stick test. If blood glucose is <5 mmol/L, give dextrose 25 g IV (50 mL of dextrose 50% solution), via a large vein. In chronic alcoholics, there is a remote risk of precipitating Wernicke's encephalopathy by a glucose load; prevent this by giving thiamine 100 mg IV before or shortly after the dextrose.

3 Treat prolonged or recurrent major fits with diazepam 10–20 mg IV or lorazepam 2–4 mg IV.

4 Consider naloxone.

- If the respiratory rate is <12/min, or the pupils are pinpoint or there is other reason to suspect opioid poisoning, give **naloxone**.

- Give up to 4 doses of 800 μg IV every 2–3 min until the respiratory rate is around 15/min.

- If there is a response, start an IV infusion: add 2 mg to 500 mL dextrose 5% or saline (4 μg/mL) and titrate against the respiratory rate and conscious level. The plasma half-life of naloxone is 1 h, shorter than that of most opioids.

- If there is no response to naloxone, opioid poisoning is excluded.

5 Obtain the history from all available sources: ambulance personnel, friends and family, primary care physician and hospital records.

6 Make a systematic examination.

- Points to cover in the neurological examination of the unconscious patient are given on pp. 68–9. Check also for possible complications of coma (hypothermia, pressure necrosis of skin or muscle, corneal abrasions, inhalation pneumonia).

- The clinical features may give clues to the poison (Table 11.1). Is there evidence of substance abuse? Check for needle marks in the antecubital fossae, neck, supraclavicular areas, groins, dorsum of feet and under the tongue.

7 Investigations needed are given in Table 11.2. The results may provide further clues to the toxin.

8 Criteria for admission to ITU include:

- Endotracheal tube placed.
- Glasgow Coma Scale score of 8 or below.
- Hypoventilation ($Paco_2$ > 6 kPa).
- Pao_2 < 7 kPa breathing air.
- Major arrhythmias or significant overdose with a drug known to have a high risk of causing arrhythmias (e.g. tricyclic antidepressant).

Poisoning

Table 11.1 Clues to the poison

Feature	Poisons to consider
Coma	Barbiturates, benzodiazepines, ethanol, opioids, trichloroethanol, tricyclics
Fits	Amphetamines, cocaine, dextropropoxyphene, insulin, oral hypoglycaemics, phenothiazines, theophylline, tricyclics, lead
Constricted pupils	Opiates, organophosphates, trichloroethanol
Dilated pupils	Amphetamines, cocaine, phenothiazines, quinine, sympathomimetics, tricyclics
Arrhythmias	Anti-arrhythmics, anticholinergics, phenothiazines, quinine, sympathomimetics, tricyclics
Hypertension	Amphetamines, cocaine
Pulmonary oedema	Carbon monoxide, ethylene glycol, irritant gases, opioids, organophosphates, paraquat, salicylates, tricyclics
Ketones on breath	Ethanol, isopropyl alcohol, alcoholic or starvation ketoacidosis (p. 359)
Hypothermia	Barbiturates, ethanol, opioids, tricyclics
Hyperthermia	Amphetamines and MDMA, anticholinergics, cocaine, monoamine oxidase inhibitors
Hypoglycaemia	Insulin, oral hypoglycaemics, ethanol, salicylates
Hyperglycaemia	Theophylline, organophosphates, salbutamol
Renal failure	*Amanita phalloides*, ethylene glycol, paracetamol, salicylates, prolonged hypotension, rhabdomyolysis
Hypokalaemia	Salbutamol, salicylates, theophylline
Metabolic acidosis	Carbon monoxide, ethanol, ethylene glycol, methanol, paracetamol, salicylates, tricyclics
Raised plasma osmolality	Ethanol, ethylene glycol, isopropyl alcohol, methanol
Rhabdomyolysis	Carbon monoxide, ethanol, opioids, solvents

Table 11.2 Urgent investigation of the unconscious patient with suspected poisoning

---

Blood glucose, sodium, potassium and creatinine

Plasma osmolality*

Paracetamol and salicylate levels (as mixed poisoning is common)

Full blood count

Urinalysis (myoglobinuria due to rhabdomyolysis gives positive stick test for blood)

Arterial blood gases and pH

Chest X-ray

ECG if there is hypotension, coexistent heart disease or suspected ingestion of
    cardiotoxic drugs (anti-arrhythmics, tricyclics) or age > 60

If the substance ingested is not known, save serum (10 mL), urine (50 mL) and
    vomitus or first gastric aspirate (50 mL) at 4°C in case later analysis is needed

---

* The normal range of plasma osmolality is 280–300 mosmol/kg. If the measured plasma osmolality (by freezing-point depression method) exceeds calculated osmolality (from the formula [2(Na + K) + urea + glucose]) by 10 mosmol/kg or more, consider poisoning with ethanol, ethylene glycol, isopropyl alcohol or methanol.

- Recurrent seizures.
- Hypotension not responsive to IV fluid.

The conscious patient

1 Check baseline observations: conscious level (fully orientated or confused), pulse, blood pressure, respiratory rate, arterial oxygen saturation, temperature and blood glucose.

2 Establish:
- which poisons were taken, in what amount and over what period;
- if the patient has vomited since ingestion;
- current symptoms;
- associated physical or psychiatric illness.

3 Investigations needed will depend on the poisons and the presence of other physical illness. After poisoning with some drugs (Table 11.3), plasma levels should be checked.

Table 11.3 Poisoning in which plasma levels should be measured
(NB: Always check the units of measurement used by your laboratory)

Poison	Plasma level at which specific treatment is indicated	Treatment
Aspirin and other salicylates	Appendix 11.3	Fluids, HD, PD
Barbiturates	Discuss with Poisons Centre	RAC, HP
Digoxin	>4 ng/mL (>5 mmol/L)	Digoxin-specific antibody fragments
Ethylene glycol	>500 mg/L	Ethanol*, HD, PD
Iron	>3.5 mg/L†	Desferrioxamine
Lithium (plain tube)	>5 mmol/L	HD, PD
Methanol	>500 mg/L	Ethanol*, HD, PD
Paracetamol	Appendix 11.4	Acetylcysteine
Theophylline	>50 mg/L	RAC, HP, HD

HD, haemodialysis; HP, haemoperfusion; PD, peritoneal dialysis; RAC, repeated oral activated charcoal.

* Ethanol or 4-methyl pyrazole are the first-line antidotes to prevent the formation of toxic metabolites.

† Also measure plasma iron level if clinical evidence of severe iron toxicity (hypotension, nausea, vomiting, diarrhoea) or after massive ingestion (>20 mg elemental iron/kg body weight; one 20 mg tablet of ferrous sulphate contains 6 mg elemental iron).

4 **If the patient refuses treatment and is at risk of harm**, you need to ask the help of senior medical staff and a psychiatrist. Figure 11.1 gives an algorithm showing what to do.

Further management

Reducing absorption
1 **Activated charcoal** (50 g mixed with 200 mL of water) should be given if a significant amount of any poison has been ingested within

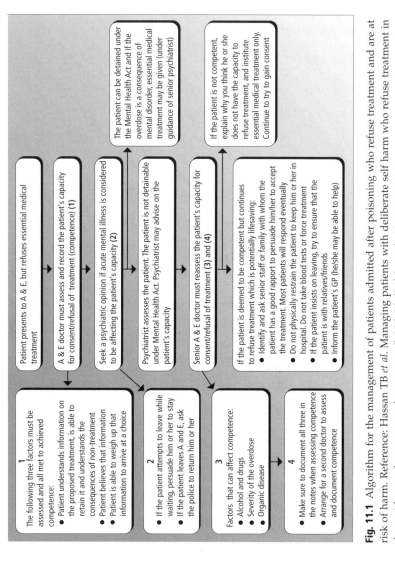

Fig. 11.1 Algorithm for the management of patients admitted after poisoning who refuse treatment and are at risk of harm. Reference: Hassan TB *et al.* Managing patients with deliberate self harm who refuse treatment in the accident and emergency department. *British Medical Journal* 1999; **319**: 107–9.

The following text appears within the algorithm:

Patient presents to A & E, but refuses essential medical treatment

A & E doctor must assess and record the patient's capacity for consent/refusal of treatment (competence) **(1)**

Seek a psychiatric opinion if acute mental illness is considered to be affecting the patient's capacity **(2)**

Psychiatrist assesses the patient. The patient is not detainable under Mental Health Act. Psychiatrist may advise on the patient's capacity

Senior A & E doctor must reassess the patient's capacity for consent/refusal of treatment **(3)** and **(4)**

If the patient is deemed to be competent but continues to refuse treatment which is potentially lifesaving:
- Identify and ask senior staff or family with whom the patient has a good rapport to persuade him/her to accept the treatment. Most patients will respond eventually
- Do not physically restrain the patient to keep him or her in hospital. Do not take blood tests or force treatment
- If the patient insists on leaving, try to ensure that the patient is with relatives/friends
- Inform the patient's GP (he/she may be able to help)

The patient can be detained under the Mental Health Act and if the overdose is a consequence of mental disorder, essential medical treatment may be given (under guidance of senior psychiatrist)

If the patient is not competent, explain why you think he or she does not have the capacity to refuse treatment, and institute essential medical treatment only. Continue to try to gain consent

1
The following three factors must be assessed and all met to achieved competence:
- Patient understands information on the proposed treatment, is able to retain it and understands the consequences of non-treatment
- Patient believes that information
- Patient is able to weigh that information to arrive at a choice

2
- If the patient attempts to leave while waiting, persuade him or her to stay
- If the patient leaves A and E, ask the police to return him or her

3
Factors that can affect competence:
- Alcohol and drugs
- Severity of the overdose
- Organic disease

4
- Make sure to document all three in the notes when assessing competence
- Arrange for a second doctor to assess and document competence

Table 11.4 Charcoal adsorption in poisoning with different agents

Repeated dosing indicated	Single dose only indicated	Charcoal not indicated
Barbiturates	Antihistamines	Acids
Carbamazepine	Paracetamol	Alkalis
Dapsone	Salicylates	Carbamate
Digoxin	Tricyclics	Cyanide
Phenytoin	Other poisons unless	Ethanol
Quinine	charcoal contraindicated	Ethylene glycol
Sustained-release		Hydrocarbons
preparations		Iron
Theophylline		Lithium
		Methanol
		Organophosphates

1 h (or longer if modified-release preparations or drugs with anti-cholinergic effects have been taken), and gastric lavage or oral antidotes (Appendix 11.2) are not indicated. Exceptions to this are poisoning with substances which are poorly adsorbed by charcoal (Table 11.4).

• Because of the risk of inhalation, activated charcoal should not be given to a patient with a reduced conscious level unless the airway is protected by a cuffed endotracheal tube.

2 Gastric lavage
Gastric lavage should be performed:

• if a potentially dangerous dose of a poison has been ingested within 1 h (or within 4 h in the case of aspirin and other salicylates), or

• if the patient is unconscious and the time of ingestion is not known, provided the airway is protected by a cuffed endotracheal tube to prevent inhalation pneumonitis.

Table 11.5 Technique of gastric lavage

If the patient is unconscious, a cuffed endotracheal tube should be placed first
to protect the airway

Suction apparatus should be to hand

Tip the trolley head down, with the patient lying on his or her left side

Use a wide-bore tube (Jacques gauge 30 in adults) which has been lubricated (e.g.
with KY jelly)

Insert the tube. The gastro-oesophageal junction is about 40 cm from the incisor
teeth in an adult. Confirm that the tube is in the stomach by aspirating and
confirming the aspirate is acidic with litmus paper

Run in 300–600 mL of water warmed to body temperature and then drain out.
Repeat 3–4 times or more if the washings still contain tablets

Leave activated charcoal (50 g in 200 mL water) in the stomach, unless
contraindicated (see Table 11.4)

Gastric lavage should not be performed:
  • after ingestion of corrosives (acids, alkalis, kettle descaler, bleach)
  or petroleum derivatives (petrol, paraffin, 'turps substitute', white
  spirit and kerosene), or
  • in patients with oesophageal varices or stricture, or previous
  gastric surgery.
The procedure is described in Table 11.5: if the patient is conscious,
verbal consent must be obtained.
3 Induced emesis with ipecacuanha is not of benefit in adults and
should not be used.

Increasing elimination
1 Drugs whose elimination can be increased by repeated dosing with
activated charcoal are given in Table 11.4. Give 50 g initially then 25 g
4-hly by mouth or nasogastric tube until recovery or until plasma drug
levels have fallen to within the safe range.
2 Other methods (haemodialysis, haemoperfusion, whole bowel irri-
gation) may be indicated in selected cases. Discuss management with
a Poisons Centre.

Poisoning

Is a specific antidote or treatment indicated?
• See Appendix 11.2. Discuss the case with a Poisons Centre first, unless you are familiar with the poison and its antidote, as some antidotes may be harmful if given inappropriately.
• The management of aspirin, paracetamol, digoxin and carbon monoxide poisoning is given in Appendices 11.3–11.6.

Supportive treatment
1 Unconscious patients not requiring endotracheal intubation or transfer to ITU (see above) should be nursed in the recovery position in a high-dependency area.
2 In all patients with severe poisoning, monitor
   • Conscious level (initially hourly).
   • Respiratory rate (initially every 15 min).
   • Oxygen saturation by pulse oximeter (continuous display).
   • ECG monitor (continuous display).
   • Blood pressure (initially every 15 min).
   • Temperature (initially hourly).
   • Urine output (put in a bladder catheter if the poison is potentially nephrotoxic or if the patient is unconscious).
   • Arterial blood gases and pH (initially 2-hly) if the poison can cause metabolic acidosis (Table 11.1) or there is suspected acute respiratory distress syndrome (p. 168) or after inhalation injury.
   • Blood glucose if the poison may cause hypo- or hyperglycaemia (initially hourly) or in paracetamol poisoning presenting after 16 h (initially 4-hly).
3 Management of problems commonly seen after poisoning is outlined in Table 11.6.

Psychiatric assessment
1 This should be performed when the patient has recovered from the physical effects of the poisoning. Points to be covered are:
   • The circumstances of the overdose: carefully planned, indecisive or impulsive; taken alone or in the presence of another person; action taken to avoid intervention or discovery; suicidal intent admitted?
   • Past history of self-poisoning or self-injury; psychiatric history or contact with psychiatric services; alcohol or substance abuse.

Table 11.6 Problems encountered in the patient with poisoning

Problem	Comment and management
Coma	If associated with focal neurological signs or evidence of head injury, CT must be done to exclude intracranial haematoma
Cerebral oedema	May occur after cardiac arrest, in severe carbon monoxide poisoning, in fulminant hepatic failure from paracetamol (p. 298), and in MDMA poisoning, due to hyponatraemia. Results in hypertension and dilated pupils. Give mannitol 20% 100–200 mL (0.5 g/kg) IV over 10 min, provided urine output is >30 mL/h. Check plasma osmolality: further mannitol may be given until plasma osmolality is 320 mosmol/kg Hyperventilate to a $Pa\text{CO}_2$ of 4 kPa (30 mmHg)
Fits	Due to toxin or metabolic complications. Check blood glucose, arterial gases and pH, plasma sodium, potassium and calcium. Treat prolonged or recurrent major fits with diazepam IV up to 20 mg. See p. 263 for further management
Respiratory depression	Half-life of most opiates is longer than that of naloxone and repeated doses or an infusion may be required. Elective ventilation may be preferable
Inhalation pneumonia	Treatment includes tracheobronchial suction, consideration of bronchoscopy to remove particulate matter from the airways, physiotherapy and antibiotic therapy (Table 24.7, p. 215).
Hypotension	Usually reflects vasodilatation, but always consider other causes (e.g. gastrointestinal bleeding). Get an ECG if the patient has taken a cardiotoxic poison, has known cardiac disease or is aged >60
Arrhythmias	Due to toxin or metabolic complications. Check arterial gases and pH, and plasma potassium, calcium and magnesium. See p. 10 for further management
Renal failure	May be due to prolonged hypotension, nephrotoxic poison, haemolysis or rhabdomyolysis. See p. 302 for further management
Gastric stasis	Place a nasogastric tube in comatose patients to reduce the risk of regurgitation and inhalation
Hypothermia	Manage by passive rewarming (p. 375)

Table 11.7 Patients with self-poisoning at high risk of suicide

Middle-aged or elderly male
Widowed/divorced/separated
Unemployed
Living alone
Chronic physical illness
Psychiatric illness, especially depression
Alcohol or substance abuse
Circumstances of poisoning: massive; planned; taken alone; timed so that
    intervention or discovery unlikely
Suicide note written or suicidal intent admitted

- Family history of depression or suicide.
- Social circumstances.
- Mental state: evidence of depression or psychosis?

2 Patients at increased risk of suicide (Table 11.7) and those with overt psychiatric illness should be discussed with a psychiatrist. Follow-up by the primary care physician or psychiatric services should be arranged before discharge.

Appendix 11.1 Poisons Information Centres

Telephone numbers of Poisons Information Centres (which may be consulted day or night) are:

- **Belfast**   44   (028) 9024 0503
- **Birmingham**   44   (0121) 507 5588 or (0121) 507 5589
- **Cardiff**   44   (029) 2070 9901
- **Dublin**   353   (01) 837 9964
- **Edinburgh**   44   (0131) 536 2300
- **London**   44   (020) 7635 9191
- **Newcastle**   44   (0191) 282 0300

Appendix 11.2 Specific antidotes

- Discuss the case with a Poisons Centre first, unless you are familiar with the poison and its antidote, as some antidotes may be harmful if given inappropriately.
- Specific antidotes are given in Table 11.8.

Table 11.8 Specific antidotes

Poison	Antidote
Anticholinergic agents	Physostigmine.
Arsenic	Dimercaprol
Benzodiazepines	Flumazenil
Beta-blockers	Glucagon
Calcium antagonists	Calcium gluconate
Cyanide	Dicobalt edetate alone or Sodium nitrite + sodium thiosulphate
Digoxin	Digoxin-specific antibody fragments
Ethylene glycol	Ethanol or 4-methylpyrazole
Fluoride	Calcium gluconate
Iron	Desferrioxamine
Lead	Dimercaprol or penicillamine
Mercury	Dimercaprol or penicillamine
Methanol	Ethanol or 4-methylpyrazole
Opiates	Naloxone
Organophosphates	Atropine
Paracetamol	Acetylcysteine or methionine (Appendix 11.4)
Paraquat	Fuller's earth
Thallium	Berlin Blue
Warfarin	Vitamin K or fresh frozen plasma (see Table 50.6, p. 408)

NB: Discuss the case with a Poisons Centre first, unless you are familiar with the poison and its antidote, as some antidotes may be harmful if given inappropriately.

Table 11.9 Investigation after poisoning with aspirin and other salicylates

Full blood count

Prothrombin time (may be prolonged)

Creatinine, sodium and potassium (hypokalaemia is common)

Blood glucose (hypoglycaemia may occur)

Arterial blood gases and pH (respiratory alkalosis in early stage, progressing to metabolic acidosis)

Plasma salicylate level (sample taken > 6 h after ingestion) (Table 11.10)

Chest X-ray (pulmonary oedema may occur)

Appendix 11.3 Poisoning with aspirin and other salicylates

- Ingestion of >10 g of aspirin may cause moderate or severe poisoning in an adult.
- Clinical features of severe poisoning include tremor, tinnitus, hyperventilation, nausea, vomiting and sweating.

Management

1 Gastric lavage should be performed if the patient is seen within 4 h of ingestion of >10 g. If gastric lavage is contraindicated or declined by the patient, give activated charcoal.

2 Investigation is given in Table 11.9. Further management depends on the plasma salicylate level (Table 11.10).

Mild poisoning
- Fluid replacement (oral or IV).

Moderate or severe poisoning
- Fluid replacement, preferably guided by measurement of the CVP (if the patient is aged over 60 or has cardiac disease).
- Put in a bladder catheter to monitor urine output.

Table 11.10 Plasma salicylate level (sample taken > 6 h after ingestion): interpretation and management

Plasma level (mg/L)	(mmol/L)	Interpretation	Action
150–250	1.1–2.8	Therapeutic	None required
250–350	1.8–3.6	Mild poisoning	Fluid replacement
500–750	3.6–5.4	Moderate poisoning	Urinary alkalinization
750–1000	5.4–7.2	Severe poisoning	Haemodialysis or peritoneal dialysis
>1000	>7.2	Massive poisoning	Haemodialysis or peritoneal dialysis

- Patients with moderate poisoning should be managed with urinary alkalinization (aim for urine pH over 7.0): give sodium bicarbonate 1.26% 500 mL + dextrose 5% 500 mL initially over 1 h. Check the urinary and arterial pH and CVP and adjust the infusion rate accordingly. Stop the infusion of bicarbonate if arterial pH rises above 7.55.
- Patients with severe or massive poisoning (plasma level >750 mg/L (>5.4 mmol/L) after rehydration or >1000 mg/L (>7.2 mmol/L) before rehydration) or renal failure or pulmonary oedema should be referred for haemodialysis. Peritoneal dialysis can be used but is less effective.
- Correct hypokalaemia with IV potassium (p. 346).
- Give vitamin K 10 mg IV to reverse hypoprothrombinaemia.

Appendix 11.4 Paracetamol poisoning

- Moderate or severe poisoning in an adult may follow ingestion of >7.5 g of paracetamol, or of >5 g if there is hepatic enzyme induction due to chronic alcohol abuse or drug therapy (carbamazepine, phenobarbitone, phenytoin, rifampicin), or if there is depletion of hepatic glutathione as in anorexia, chronic alcohol abuse and AIDS.

• Acute liver failure and acute renal failure (due to acute tubular necrosis) are potential complications of paracetamol poisoning, occurring at 36–72 h after ingestion.

• Severe poisoning may give no symptoms in the first 24 h. Nausea and vomiting, right upper quadrant pain, jaundice and encephalopathy may develop after 24 h in patients with hepatotoxicity.

• Acetylcysteine (AC) replenishes mitochondrial and cytosolic glutathione and is the preferred antidote. Oral methionine may be used if AC is not available, or if there is a risk that the patient will otherwise leave without any treatment.

Management

1 If the patient is unconscious (because of mixed poisoning with psychotropic drugs or alcohol), gastric lavage should be performed. Give activated charcoal to conscious patients who present within 1 h after taking >7.5 g (or >5 g if at increased risk of liver damage).

2 Table 11.11 summarizes further management. The acetylcysteine infusion regimen is given in Table 11.12.

3 The plasma paracetamol level is a poor guide to the risk of hepatotoxicity in patients who have taken staggered overdoses, and if the total dose taken is >12 g, or the patient is at increased risk of liver damage, acetylcysteine should be given.

4 Minor reactions to acetylcysteine (nausea, flushing, urticaria and pruritus) are relatively common, and usually settle when the peak rate of infusion is passed. If there is a severe reaction (angio-oedema, wheezing, respiratory distress, hypotension and hypertension), stop the infusion temporarily and give an antihistamine (chlorpheniramine 10 mg IV over 10 min).

5 Make early contact with a liver unit if the patient has evidence of severe hepatotoxicity (Table 11.13). In such patients (before transfer):

• Start a course of acetylcysteine if not previously administered.

• Give dextrose 10% 1 L 12-hly IV to prevent hypoglycaemia, and monitor blood glucose 4-hly.

• Monitor conscious level 4-hly.

• Monitor CVP and urine output: correct hypovolaemia with colloid.

• Check prothrombin time 12-hly and plasma creatinine daily.

• Start prophylaxis against gastric stress ulceration with omeprazole 40 mg daily IV or by mouth or by nasogastric tube.

Poisoning

Table 11.11 Management of paracetamol poisoning

Patient seen within 8 h after overdose
Give activated charcoal 50 g if <1 h since overdose of >15 mg/kg
Take blood for plasma paracetamol level at or after 4 h since ingestion
Start acetylcysteine (AC) (Table 11.12) if the plasma paracetamol level is above the
    treatment line (Fig. 11.2)
If the plasma paracetamol level is not available by 8 h, begin AC if
    >15 mg/kg of paracetamol has been taken
Discontinue AC if the plasma paracetamol level is below the treatment line
On completion of AC treatment, check the prothrombin time, alanine
    transaminase/aspartate transaminase activities and plasma creatinine
If the patient is asymptomatic and the investigation results are normal, there is no
    risk of serious complications and the patient may be discharged

Patient seen 8–15 h after overdose
Take blood for plasma paracetamol level, prothrombin time, alanine
    transaminase/aspartate transaminase activities, plasma creatinine and bilirubin,
    acid–base status (venous sample) and full blood count
Start AC immediately (Table 11.12) if >150 mg/kg paracetamol has been taken
Discontinue AC if the plasma paracetamol level is below the treatment line (Fig.
    11.2)
On completion of AC treatment repeat investigations (except paracetamol level)
If the patient is asymptomatic and the investigation results are normal, there is little
    risk of serious complications and the patient may be discharged

Patient seen 15–24 h after overdose
Give standard AC course (Table 11.12) if >150 mg/kg paracetamol has been taken
Take blood on admission for plasma paracetamol level, prothrombin time, alanine
    transaminase/aspartate transaminase activities, plasma creatinine, bilirubin and
    phosphate, acid–base status (venous sample) and full blood count
Repeat the above investigations at the end of the AC course
If the investigations are abnormal or if the patient is symptomatic, consider
    continuing AC treatment (100 mg/kg in 1 L 5% dextrose over 16 h, repeated until
    recovery). Repeat investigations as appropriate

Table 11.11 *Continued*

Patient seen >24 h after overdose

Take blood on admission for plasma paracetamol level, prothrombin time, alanine transaminase/aspartate transaminase activities, plasma creatinine, bilirubin and phosphate, acid–base status (venous sample) and full blood count

If the patient has taken >150 mg/kg paracetamol, is symptomatic or has abnormal investigation results, give a standard course of AC (Table 11.12)

Repeat the above investigations at the end of the AC course

If the patient has, or is at risk of developing fulminant hepatic failure, consider continuing AC treatment (100 mg/kg in 1 L 5% dextrose over 16 h, repeated until recovery

Reference: Vale JA, Proudfoot AT. Paracetamol (acetaminophen) poisoning. *Lancet* 1995; **346**: 547–552.

Table 11.12 Acetylcysteine (AC) regimen in paracetamol poisoning

150 mg/kg in 200 mL dextrose 5% IV over 15 min, then
50 mg/kg in 500 mL dextrose 5% IV over 4 h, then
100 mg/kg in 1 L dextrose 5% IV over 16 h

Table 11.13 Paracetamol poisoning: indications of severe hepatotoxicity

Rapid development of grade 2 encephalopathy (confused but able to answer questions)
Prothrombin time >20 s at 24 h, >45 s at 48 h or >50 s at 72 h
Increasing plasma bilirubin
Increasing plasma creatinine
Falling plasma phosphate
Arterial pH <7.3 more than 24 h after ingestion

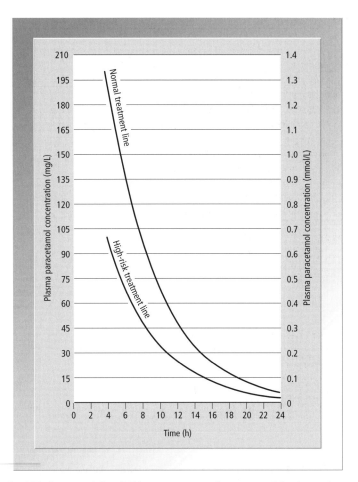

Fig. 11.2 Treatment thresholds in paracetamol poisoning. Use the high-risk (lower) treatment line in patients with:
• chronic alcohol abuse;
• hepatic enzyme induction from therapy with carbamazepine, phenobarbitone, phenytoin, or rifampicin;
• chronic malnutrition or recent starvation (within 24 h);
• HIV positive or AIDS.
Graph reproduced with permission of the University of Wales College of Medicine Therapeutics and Toxicology Centre.

Table 11.14 Severe digoxin poisoning: calculation of the dose of digoxin-specific antibody fragments (Digibind, GlaxoWellcome)

Setting	Dose
Acute ingestion of unknown amount	Give 20 vials (800 mg)
Acute ingestion of known amount	Digoxin load (mg) = dose ingested (mg) x 0.8 (to take account of incomplete absorption). Number of vials of Digibind needed = digoxin load (mg)/0.6
Toxicity during chronic therapy, steady-state digoxin level not known	Give 6 vials
Toxicity during chronic therapy, steady-state digoxin level known	Number of vials of Digibind needed = plasma digoxin level (ng/mL) x body weight (kg)/100

Table 11.15 Acute carbon monoxide poisoning: clinical features

Blood carboxyhaemoglobin (%)	Clinical features which may be seen
< 10	No symptoms – acute poisoning excluded if exposure was within 4 h
10–50	Headache, nausea, vomiting, tachycardia, tachypnoea
> 50	Coma, fits, cardiorespiratory arrest

• See Chapter 37 for other aspects of the management of acute liver failure.

Appendix 11.5 Digoxin poisoning

• Digoxin toxicity causes nausea, vomiting, diarrhoea, confusional state and a wide range of tachy- and bradyarrhythmias.

Management

1 Give repeated doses of activated charcoal (p. 110) to reduce absorption of digoxin (preceded by gastric lavage if seen within 1 h of ingestion).

2 Check electrolytes and creatinine and send a sample for later digoxin assay; recheck plasma potassium hourly (hyperkalaemia indicates severe toxicity and should be treated with dextrose and insulin (p. 345) if >6 mmol/L).

3 Admit to the CCU for ECG monitoring.

4 Give digoxin-specific antibody fragments (Table 11.14) if:
   • there is sustained ventricular tachycardia or third-degree (complete) AV block;
   • plasma potassium is >5 mmol/L or rising.

5 Manage arrhythmias along standard lines (Chapter 2), bearing in mind these points:
   • If DC cardioversion is needed for supraventricular arrhythmias, start with a 25-J shock (as there is an increased risk of provoking ventricular arrhythmias).
   • For second- or third-degree AV block, use temporary pacing: avoid isoprenaline because of the risk of ventricular arrhythmias.

Appendix 11.6 Carbon monoxide poisoning

• May occur from inhalation of car exhaust fumes, fumes from inadequately maintained or ventilated heating systems (including those using natural gas), smoke from all types of fires and methylene chloride in paint strippers (by hepatic metabolism).

• The severity of poisoning depends on the concentration of carbon

monoxide in the inspired air, the length of exposure and the presence of anaemia or cardiorespiratory disease.
• Clinical features of acute poisoning are given in Table 11.15.

Management

1 If carbon monoxide poisoning is suspected, give 100% oxygen (10 L/min) using a tightly fitting facemask with a circuit which minimizes rebreathing.
  • Unconscious patients should be intubated and ventilated mechanically with 100% oxygen. Cerebral oedema may occur and is treated with mannitol and mild hyperventilation (Table 11.6).
2 Attach an ECG monitor and record a 12-lead ECG.
  • Severe poisoning may result in myocardial ischaemia, with anginal chest pain, ST segment depression and arrhythmias.
3 Check the carboxyhaemoglobin (COHb) level in venous blood (heparinized sample).
  • If acute carbon monoxide poisoning is confirmed (COHb > 10%), recheck 2-hly and continue 100% oxygen until two consecutive samples contain <5%.
4 Check arterial blood gases and pH (metabolic acidosis is usually present) and arrange a chest X-ray.
5 Although its effectiveness is disputed, generally accepted indications for hyperbaric oxygen therapy are:
  • Carboxyhaemoglobin level >40% at any time.
  • Coma.
  • Neurological symptoms or signs other than mild headache.
  • Evidence of myocardial ischaemia or arrhythmias.
  • Pregnancy.
Contact a Poisons Centre to discuss the management of severe poisoning and for the location of the nearest centre which can provide hyperbaric oxygen therapy.

12 The critically ill patient

You may be called to see a patient who is clearly very ill, but in whom the diagnosis is not immediately apparent, or who is deteriorating rapidly despite treatment.

• You are likely to need assistance, so don't delay calling for this. You want help before cardiorespiratory arrest has occurred. Contact your senior cover to discuss management and assessment on the ward by the critical care team.

• Key features of the critically ill patient are severe respiratory, cardio-vascular or neurological derangement, usually reflecting multiorgan disease.

Priorities

Remember Airway—Breathing—Circulation

1 Attach an ECG monitor, put in a peripheral IV cannula, check arterial oxygen saturation, give oxygen 40–60%, listen over both lungs and measure the blood pressure. Check the temperature.

2 Make a rapid but systematic assessment of the airway, breathing, circulation, neurological status and abdomen.

3 Arrange urgent investigation (Table 12.1).

Airway and breathing

• Make sure the airway is clear. If the patient is unconscious, remove false teeth if loose and aspirate the pharynx, larynx and trachea with a suction catheter. If there is no reflex response (gagging or coughing) to the suction catheter or the respiratory rate is <8/min, a cuffed endo-tracheal tube should be inserted, preferably by an anaesthetist. Before

Table 12.1 Urgent investigation of the critically ill patient

ECG
Chest X-ray
Arterial blood gases and pH
Creatinine, sodium and potassium
Blood glucose
Full blood count
Clotting screen if low platelet count, suspected coagulation disorder, jaundice or
    purpura
Group and save (cross-match 6 units if haemorrhage suspected)
Blood culture ($\times 2$)
Serum amylase (raised in pancreatitis, perforated ulcer, mesenteric ischaemia and
    severe sepsis) if abdominal pain or tenderness
Urine stick test, microscopy and culture
Cranial CT if reduced conscious level or focal signs
Lumbar puncture (after CT) if suspected meningitis

this is done, ventilate the patient using a bag-valve-mask system with 100% oxygen.
- What is the respiratory rate? Rates <10 or >40/min signify critical illness.
- Is arterial oxygen saturation <90% despite breathing 40% oxygen? This indicates severe impairment of gas exchange.

Circulation

- Remember that a 'normal' blood pressure may be maintained by vasoconstriction and does not mean that organ perfusion is adequate. Signs of low cardiac output include confusion and agitation, cold extremities, sweating, oliguria and metabolic acidosis.
- Heart rates <40 or >150/min with signs of low cardiac output require urgent correction: see Fig. 2.1 (p. 11).

The critically ill patient

Table 12.2 The JVP in hypotension

Hypotension with a high JVP
  Biventricular failure
  Pulmonary embolism
  Right ventricular infarction
  Cardiac tamponade
  Tension pneumothorax

Hypotension with a normal or low JVP
  Hypovolaemia
  Sepsis
  Drugs or poisons
  Left ventricular failure

• If systolic BP is <80 mmHg, or has fallen by more than 40 mmHg and there are signs of low cardiac output, urgent correction is needed. Look carefully at the JVP, which may provide an important clue to the diagnosis (Table 12.2). If there are no signs of pulmonary oedema, give IV fluid (saline or colloid) 500 mL over 15 min. If hypovolaemia or vasodilatation is likely (suspect vasodilatation if the pulses are bounding), lay the patient flat and elevate the foot of the bed. For further management of hypotension, see Chapter 3.

Neurological status

• What is the **conscious level** (assessed using the Glasgow Coma Scale (Table 6.6, p. 72))? If the Glasgow Coma Scale score is <9, discuss endotracheal intubation with an anaesthetist.
• If the conscious level is reduced, you must **exclude hypoglycaemia** by immediate stick test. If blood glucose is <5 mmol/L, give dextrose 25 g IV (50 mL of dextrose 50% solution), via a large vein.
• If the respiratory rate is <12/min or the pupils are pinpoint, or there is other reason to suspect opioid poisoning, give naloxone. Give up to

Table 12.3 Common causes of critical illness

Neurological
   Severe stroke (p. 227)
   Bacterial meningitis (p. 247)

Cardiovascular
   Acute myocardial infarction with cardiogenic shock (p. 137)
   Major pulmonary embolism, especially with coexisting cardiopulmonary
      disease (p. 183)
   Aortic dissection (p. 156)
   Cardiac tamponade (p. 175)

Respiratory
   Exacerbation of chronic obstructive pulmonary disease with severe respiratory
      failure (p. 198)
   Severe pneumonia (p. 206)
   Tension pneumothorax (p. 217)

Abdominal
   Generalized peritonitis (Table 36.4, p. 292)
   Mesenteric infarction (Table 36.5, p. 292)
   Severe pancreatitis (Table 36.6, p. 292)

Others
   Septic shock (p. 100)
   Severe poisoning (e.g. with salicylates, paracetamol or tricyclics) (p. 106)
   Severe diabetic ketoacidosis (p. 328) or hyperosmolar non-ketotic
      hyperglycaemia (p. 335)
   Severe anaphylaxis (p. 414)

4 doses of 800 µg IV every 2–3 min until the respiratory rate is around 15/min. Further doses may be needed (see p. 107).

• If you suspect benzodiazepine overdose may be the cause, give **flumazenil**, 200 µg IV over 15 s; if needed, further doses of 100 µg can be given at 1-min intervals up to a total dose of 2 mg.

• If there are **recurrent or prolonged major seizures**, treat with diazepam 10–20 mg IV or lorazepam 2–4 mg IV: see Chapter 33.

• Check for neck stiffness.
• Make a rapid assessment of limb tone and power: is there **lateralized weakness**?

Abdomen

• Check for abdominal tenderness and guarding.
• If the patient has severe abdominal pain or generalized abdominal tenderness, and is shocked (systolic BP < 90 mmHg with cold skin), the likely diagnosis is **generalized peritonitis, mesenteric infarction or severe pancreatitis** (Tables 36.4–36.6, p. 292).

Further management

This is directed by the dominant clinical problem or likely diagnosis. Common causes of critical illness are given in Table 12.3.

Section 2
Specific Problems

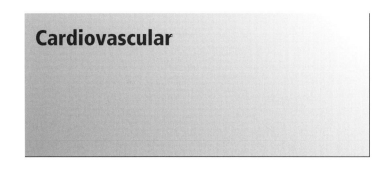

Cardiovascular

13 Acute myocardial infarction

The working diagnosis is based on the history and ECG. The history is usually of acute central chest pain lasting 20 min or more, but other presentations include acute epigastric pain with vomiting, acute confusional state, pulmonary oedema, ventricular tachycardia and postoperative hypotension. Management is summarized in Figs 13.1 and 13.2.

Priorities

1 Attach an ECG monitor, give oxygen and record a 12-lead ECG. Make sure a defibrillator is near because VF is a common early complication. Check the pulse and blood pressure. Major arrhythmias should be treated along standard lines (Chapter 2).

2 Put in a peripheral IV cannula, take blood (Table 13.1) and relieve pain with diamorphine. Give 5 mg (2.5 mg if the patient is small or elderly) IV over 3–5 min, with further doses of 2.5 mg every 10–15 min until pain free. An antiemetic should also be given (e.g. prochlorperazine 12.5 mg or metoclopramide 10 mg IV).

3 Take a brief history focusing on the time of onset of the pain, and any past history of ischaemic heart disease. Complete your examination. Check the JVP and lung bases, listen for a murmur and check the major pulses.

4 Give aspirin 300 mg (chewed), unless the patient is already taking this or it is contraindicated, and glyceryl trinitrate sublingually (1 tablet or 2 puffs of spray).

5 Give an intravenous beta-blocker unless there is pulmonary oedema, systolic blood pressure is <100 mmHg or heart rate is <60/bpm (e.g. metoprolol 5–15 mg IV or atenolol 5–10 mg IV).

6 Is the patient suitable for thrombolysis? The questions you need to ask yourself are:

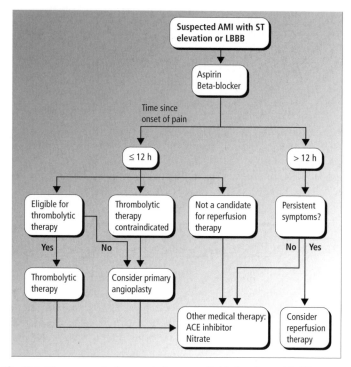

Fig. 13.1 Management of suspected myocardial infarction with ST elevation or left bundle branch block not known to be old.

• Does the ECG show regional ST elevation (>1 mm in 2 or more adjacent leads) or left bundle branch block, not known to be old?
• Is it within 12 h of the onset of pain (within 24 h if chest pain and/or ST elevation are still present especially after anterior infarction).
• Could the ST elevation be due to a diagnosis other than acute myocardial infarction, e.g. acute pericarditis (p. 172), or physiological early repolarization (p. 50)?
• Are there any major contraindications to thrombolysis (Table 13.2)?

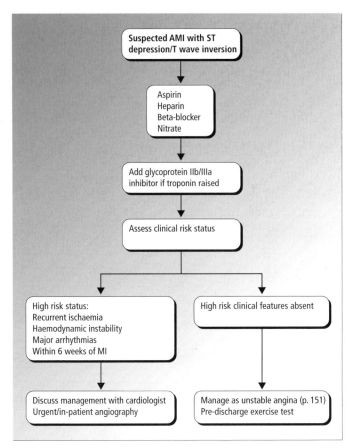

Fig. 13.2 Management of suspected myocardial infarction with ST depression/T wave inversion.

Table 13.1 Investigation in suspected myocardial infarction

Needed urgently
ECG (repeat daily for 3 days or if pain recurs)
Chest X-ray
Creatinine, sodium and potassium (recheck potassium if significant arrhythmia
  occurs or after large diuresis)
Blood glucose (diabetes should be managed by insulin infusion (p. 323)
Plasma markers of myocardial necrosis (p. 53)

For later analysis
Full blood count
Cholesterol (value is representative if checked within 24 h of infarction and enables
  patients with hypercholesterolaemia to be identified before discharge)

7 Which thrombolytic? (Table 13.3) There is no universal consensus and you should be guided by your local protocol. There is no compelling advantage to alteplase except in patients who have had streptokinase in the last 4 days to 12 months.

Problems encountered during thrombolysis are discussed in Table 13.4.

8 Consider primary angioplasty if rapid access to an interventional centre is available. The indications are evolving but include:

- ST elevation but thrombolysis contraindicated;
- cardiogenic shock;
- early presentation within 6 h of the onset of pain;
- expected time to angioplasty <90 min.

9 If the patient is a known diabetic or the blood glucose is >11 mmol/L, see p. 323 for further management of diabetes after myocardial infarction.

10 Patients with suspected M1 who do not have ST elevation or new left bundle branch block should receive aspirin and heparin (unfractionated or LMW heparin (p. 403)), plus a glycoprotein IIb/IIIa inhibitor (tirofiban or eptifibatide) if plasma troponin is raised.

Table 13.2 Thrombolytic therapy: contraindications

Absolute

Active internal bleeding

Suspected aortic dissection

Prolonged or traumatic cardiopulmonary resuscitation

Recent head trauma or known intracranial neoplasm

Trauma or surgery within the previous 2 weeks which could be a source of rebleeding

Diabetic haemorrhagic retinopathy or other haemorrhagic ophthalmic condition

Pregnancy

Recorded blood pressure >200/120 mmHg

History of cerebrovascular accident known to be haemorrhagic

Relative

Recent trauma or surgery (>2 weeks)

History of chronic severe hypertension with or without drug therapy

Active peptic ulcer

History of cerebrovascular accident

Known bleeding diathesis or current use of anticoagulants

Significant liver dysfunction

If there are one or more relative contraindications to thrombolytic therapy, you must weigh the risks and benefits of therapy for the individual before deciding whether or not it should be given

Acute myocardial infarction

11 At this point you need to review the haemodynamic effects of the infarction.

Recognize cardiogenic shock from the following:

- Systolic blood pressure <90 mmHg.
- Heart rate either >100/min or <40/min.
- Breathlessness or Sao_2 < 90%.
- Skin cool and sweating.
- Agitation or confusion.
- Oliguria.

Acute myocardial infarction

Table 13.3 Thrombolytic therapy

Streptokinase

Suitable for the majority of patients

Adjunctive heparin not needed if aspirin is given

Give streptokinase 1.5 MU as an IV infusion over 1 h

Give aspirin 300 mg PO (chewed), followed by 150 mg daily for 3 months, 75 mg daily thereafter

Alteplase (tissue plasminogen activator (tPA)): standard regimen

Use if the patient has received streptokinase within the previous 4 days to 12 months

Adjunctive heparin and aspirin should be given

Give alteplase 1.5 mg/kg as an IV infusion over 3 h

Give heparin 5000 U IV bolus, followed by a continuous IV infusion to maintain APTT 1.5–2.5 times control (p. 404) for at least 2 days

Give aspirin 300 mg PO (chewed), followed by 150 mg daily for 3 months, 75 mg daily thereafter

Alteplase: accelerated regimen

May be of additional benefit in patients < 50 with large anterior infarcts presenting within 4 h who are normotensive (systolic BP < 140 mmHg), i.e. low risk of haemorrhagic stroke

Adjunctive heparin and aspirin should be given as above

Give alteplase 15 mg IV bolus, followed by 0.75 mg/kg (maximum 50 mg) over 30 min, followed by 0.5 mg/kg (maximum 35 mg) over the next 60 min

---

These patients have a poor prognosis and early revascularization should be discussed with a cardiologist unless there is a prompt response to medical management.

Hypotension without pulmonary oedema

The two possibilities are **hypovolaemia** and **right ventricular infarction**. Hypovolaemia may be due to sweating, vomiting or previous diuretic therapy.

Table 13.4 Thrombolytic therapy: problems

Hypotension during streptokinase infusion
Usually reversed by elevating the foot of the bed or slowing the infusion

Allergic reaction to streptokinase
Give chlorpheniramine 10 mg IV and hydrocortisone 100 mg IV (prophylactic
   treatment not needed)

Oozing from puncture sites
If venepuncture is necessary, use a 22 G (blue) needle and compress the puncture
   site for 10 min
Central venous lines should be inserted via an antecubital fossa vein
   (percutaneously or by cut-down)
For arterial puncture, use a 23 G (orange) needle in the radial or brachial artery and
   compress the puncture site for at least 10 min

Uncontrollable bleeding
Stop the infusion of thrombolytic
Transfuse whole fresh blood if available or fresh frozen plasma
As a last resort, give tranexamic acid 1 g (10 mg/kg) IV over 10 min

Symptomatic bradycardia unresponsive to atropine
If temporary pacing is required within 24 h of thrombolytic therapy, the wire should
   ideally be placed via an antecubital fossa vein
If there is no suitable superficial vein, the options are a cut-down (seek help from a
   cardiologist if you are not familiar with this) or placement via the femoral vein
   (p. 425)

Acute myocardial infarction

• Check the JVP—it will be low in hypovolaemia and high in right
ventricular infarction. If in doubt, either put in a central line to measure
the CVP or obtain an urgent echocardiogram to assess right and left
ventricular function.
• For both, initial treatment is with IV fluid. Give colloid 500 mg IV
over 15–30 min, followed by a further 500 mg over 30–60 min if systolic
BP remains <100 mmHg and there are no clinical signs of pulmonary
oedema.

• Sinus bradycardia or AV block commonly complicates right ventricular infarction. If unresponsive to atropine 0.6–1.2 mg IV, put in a pacing wire (p. 438).

Right ventricular infarction

• If blood pressure remains low despite giving 1 L of fluid, start an infusion of dobutamine (p. 484).

• If hypotension persists, put in a pulmonary artery catheter catheter (p. 429). In right ventricular infarction, the right atrial pressure will be high (12–20 mmHg) and equal to or greater than the wedge pressure or pulmonary artery diastolic pressure.

• Give more fluid if necessary to raise the wedge pressure/pulmonary artery diastolic pressure to around 15 mmHg. You run the risk of causing pulmonary oedema if you give large volumes of fluid (>1 L) without monitoring of the wedge pressure if there is a large associated inferior left ventricular infarct.

Hypotension with pulmonary oedema

• Increase inspired oxygen aiming for an oxygen saturatation >90% ($Pao_2 > 8$ kPa). Consider using a continuous positive airways pressure (CPAP) system if these targets are not met despite an inspired oxygen of 60%.

• Start inotropic/vasopressor therapy (Table 13.5).

• Put in a urinary catheter. Target urine output is >30 mL/h.

• Arrange urgent echocardiography to assess left ventricular function and to exclude papillary muscle or ventricular septal rupture.

Table 13.5 Choice of inotropic/vasopressor therapy in cardiogenic shock due to myocardial infarction

Systolic BP (mmHg)	Choice of therapy
>90	Dobutamine (p. 484)
80–90	Dopamine (p. 484)
<80	Noradrenaline (p. 481)

• Diuretics are relatively ineffective in patients with cardiogenic shock, but can be used once the cardiac output has increased (as shown by improvement in the patient's mental state and skin perfusion).

• Providing the systolic BP has increased to at least 100 mmHg, start a nitrate infusion, initially at low dose (e.g. isosorbide dinitrate 2 mg/h).

• If the patient is not improving, discuss management with a cardiologist. Consider placing a pulmonary artery catheter (p. 429) to allow more accurate titration of therapy. Adjust the doses of inotrope and nitrate, aiming for a PA diastolic/wedge pressure of 15–20 mmHg with a systolic BP of >100 mmHg.

Mild pulmonary oedema without hypotension

• Give frusemide 40–80 mg IV.

• Give nitrate by IV infusion (e.g. isosorbide dinitrate 2 mg/h, increasing by 2 mg/h every 15–30 min until breathlessness is relieved or systolic blood pressure falls below 100 mmHg or to a maximum of 10 mg/h) or buccal administration (glyceryl trinitrate buccal tablet, 5 mg).

• Start an angiotensin-converting enzyme inhibitor, e.g. ramipril 1.25 mg b.d.

Bradyarrhythmias and atrioventricular block

• For details of diagnosis and management, see Chapter 2.

• Atropine 0.6–1.2 mg IV is the first-line treatment of symptomatic bradycardia.

• Generally accepted indications for temporary pacing are given in Table 13.6. Discuss the case with a cardiologist if you are uncertain about the need for pacing.

Tachyarrhythmias

• For details of diagnosis and management, see Chapter 2. Tachyarrhythmias complicating acute myocardial infarction are managed along standard lines, bearing in mind the following points:

• In patients with significant arrhythmias, plasma potassium should be kept at 4–5 mmol/L.

• Regular broad-complex tachycardia (>120/min) after infarction is almost always ventricular tachycardia rather than SVT with aberrant

Table 13.6 Indications for temporary pacing in acute myocardial infarction

Asystole (after restoration of spontaneous rhythm)

Complete heart block

Right bundle branch block with new left anterior hemiblock or left posterior hemiblock*

New left bundle branch block

Mobitz type II second-degree AV block

Mobitz type I (Wenckebach) second-degree AV block with hypotension not responsive to atropine

Sinus bradycardia with hypotension or recurrent sinus pauses not responsive to atropine

Atrial or ventricular overdrive pacing for recurrent ventricular tachycardia (seek advice from a cardiologist)

* Left anterior hemiblock gives left axis deviation (S wave > R in lead II); left posterior hemiblock gives right axis deviation (S wave > R in lead I).

conduction. If in doubt, assume it is VT (and treat with lignocaine or synchronized DC shock).

Further management

1 General

• Bed/chair rest with ECG monitoring for 24 h is followed by a programme of mobilization.

• Oxygen can be discontinued if the chest X-ray shows clear lung fields and there are no complications of infarction.

• Fever (up to 38°C) and a neutrophil leucocytosis (up to 12–15 × 10^9/L) are common systemic responses to infarction, usually peaking at 3–4 days. Other causes of fever after infarction include pericarditis and thrombophlebitis at the cannula site.

• Patients with an uncomplicated course and suitable home circumstances can be discharged after 5 days.

2 Drug therapy (Table 13.7)

• Heparin should be used routinely for 48 h after alteplase or if there is atrial fibrillation.

• Aspirin 150 mg daily (for 3 months, 75 mg daily thereafter) should be continued in all patients.

• An oral beta-blocker should be continued indefinitely unless contraindicated.

• An ACE inhibitor should be started if there is clinical heart failure or for the indications in Table 13.7.

• A statin should be started if the total cholesterol level on admission was >5 mmol/L.

3 Recurrent pain

• A bruised sensation is common for 1–2 days and should not be over-interpreted especially after resuscitation.

• Pericarditis occurs in 20% of patients and causes pain which is similar to the initial infarct, but usually less severe and affected by posture and respiration. A pericardial rub may not be heard. Give aspirin up to 600 mg 6-hly. If this fails to relieve pain, give a non-steroidal anti-inflammatory agent, e.g. indomethacin 25–50 mg 8-hly.

• **Reinfarction** (prolonged chest pain with fresh ST elevation) should be treated with further thrombolytic therapy. Use alteplase if streptokinase has been given more than 4 days previously. Continuing or recurrent pain even without new ST segment changes and which is not clearly pericarditic may be an indication for angiography and should be discussed with a cardiologist.

4 New murmur

• A pericardial rub may be mistaken for a murmur.

• A soft midsystolic murmur is benign and does not require echocardiography unless there is heart failure or hypotension. Louder murmurs suggest aortic stenosis and require echocardiography.

• Pansystolic murmurs require echocardiography. They may result from ischaemic mitral regurgitation or less commonly (about 2% of acute infarcts) papillary muscle or ventricular septal rupture.

• Ventricular septal rupture usually causes sudden haemodynamic deterioration, with pulmonary oedema and often cardiogenic shock, but may occasionally cause little compromise or may present late with deteriorating renal function.

Acute myocardial infarction

Table 13.7 Summary of drug therapy after myocardial infarction

Drug	Comment
Aspirin	Aspirin 300 mg PO stat at presentation, followed by 150 mg daily for 3 months, and 75 mg daily thereafter
	If there is definite hypersensitivity to aspirin, give clopidogrel 75 mg once daily
Heparin	Heparin by infusion should be given:
	• Routinely after alteplase for 48 h
	• For atrial fibrillation (followed by warfarin if atrial fibrillation persists)
	• For left ventricular thrombus shown on echocardiography (followed by warfarin for 3 months)
	Patients who are not receiving heparin by infusion and who are immobile should receive subcutaneous heparin 7500 units 12-hly.
Beta-blocker	An oral beta-blocker should be given unless there is:
	• Clinical evidence of heart failure
	• Definite asthma
	• Second- or third-degree AV block or bradycardia < 50/min
	If beta-blockade is contraindicated and there is no evidence of heart failure, consider diltiazem or verapamil as alternatives
Angiotensin-converting enzyme inhibitor	Selection of patients to receive an ACE inhibitor remains controversial, but the following groups are generally agreed:
	• Clinical heart failure
	• Large anterior infarct
	• Second infarction
	• Left ventricular ejection fraction < 40% on echocardiography
	The ideal time to start treatment has not been defined but 24 h after infarction is reasonable
Statin	Start a statin if total cholesterol measured before or within 24 h of the infarct was > 5 mmol/L. Target total cholesterol < 5 mmol/L, LDL-cholesterol < 3 mmol/L

- Discuss with a cardiologist if there is a ventricular septal rupture or the patient is unwell with a murmur.

5 Fever

See Table 13.8.

6 Exercise stress testing

- The majority of late deaths occur in the first 3 months after discharge. Your aim is to identify those patients whose prognosis will be improved by early revascularization.
- A treadmill exercise test should be performed before or soon after discharge in all patients unless unsuitable for revascularization, e.g.

Table 13.8 Fever after myocardial infarction

Due to the infarct itself
Pericarditis
Thrombophlebitis at cannula site
Infection related to a Swan–Ganz catheter or pacing wire
Deep vein thrombosis
Urinary tract infection
Pneumonia (consider inhalation pneumonia after resuscitation (p. 214)

Table 13.9 Discharge check-list after myocardial infarction

Aspirin 150 mg daily for 3 months, 75 mg daily thereafter
Beta-blocker unless contraindicated
ACE inhibitor if there has been clinical heart failure or LVEF is < 40%
A statin if total cholesterol > 5 mmol/L
Advice on smoking cessation, diet, lifestyle and work
Exercise rehabilitation arranged
Exercise stress test performed or arranged

advanced age, comorbidity. High-risk features are ST depression >2mm or chest pain before 6min of the Bruce protocol.

• Indications for myocardial perfusion scan or stress echocardiogram include:

• patients unable to exercise;
• left bundle branch block;
• equivocal exercise test results.

7 Rehabilitation and secondary prevention

• If total cholesterol measured before or within 24h of the infarct was >5mmol/L, start statin (choice of agent and starting dose according to local guidelines). Patients should be given advice on a lipid-lowering diet. Target LDL-cholesterol is <3mmol/e (total cholesterol <5mmol/e), measured 2 months after the infarct.

• Treat hypertension, aiming for a BP of 140/85mmHg or less (130/80 or less if diabetic).

• Patients who were cigarette smokers should be given advice on how to quit.

• Liaise between hospital rehabilitation team and practice nurse over follow-up.

• Psychiatric abnormalities are common after myocardial infarction and may need specialist referral

• Invite to a rehabilitation programme for advice about coronary risk management, exercise and psychosocial support.

14 Unstable angina

- Describes the clinical syndromes which range in severity from a change in the pattern of exertional angina to preinfarction angina with prolonged rest pain.
- The cause is usually rupture of a coronary arterial plaque, and the formation of a non-occlusive platelet-rich 'white' thrombus.
- The risk of myocardial infarction or death (which is around 12% within 6 months of presentation) is determined by clinical features, ECG findings and the presence of plasma markers of myocardial necrosis: risk stratification based on these characteristics guides management (Fig. 14.1).

Priorities

1 Detailed history

Take a detailed history of the chest pain, examine the patient and record an ECG. Give sublingual glyceryl trinitrate if there is pain at rest. Investigation is shown in Table 14.1.

Features supporting a diagnosis of unstable angina are given below. If none of these is present, unstable angina is much less likely and other causes of chest pain must be considered (Chapter 4):

- Preceding similar exertional chest pain.
- Known coronary artery disease (previous myocardial infarction or angiographically proved coronary disease).
- Risk factors for coronary artery disease (multiple factors or single major factor such as non-insulin-dependent diabetes or familial hypercholesterolaemia).
- Abnormal ECG with ST depression and/or T wave inversion. Dynamic ST/T changes associated with episodes of chest pain are a particularly important diagnostic feature. Even minor changes must be regarded as suspicious in patients who are are at medium or high risk of having coronary disease.

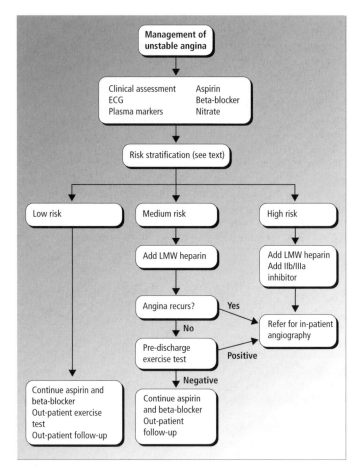

Fig. 14.1 Management of unstable angina.

2 Patients can now be assigned to one of three groups

Low risk

• New-onset or worsening exertional angina, but no episodes of severe or prolonged (>20 min) chest pain in the preceding 2 weeks; **and**

Table 14.1 Investigation in unstable angina

ECG on admission, daily for 2 days and if pain recurs
Chest X-ray
Plasma markers of myocardial necrosis (p. 53)
Creatinine, sodium and potassium
Glucose
Plasma cholesterol
Full blood count (to exclude anaemia)

- normal ECG or minor T wave changes only; **and**
- plasma markers of myocardial necrosis not present.

Medium risk
- One or more episodes of severe or prolonged chest pain in the preceding 2 weeks; **or**
- abnormal ECG (ST depression, deep anterior T wave inversion, left bundle branch block); **or**
- plasma markers of myocardial necrosis present.

High risk
- Ongoing chest pain with ST/T abnormalities; **or**
- recent myocardial infarction (within 6 weeks); **or**
- haemodynamic instability (pulmonary oedema, hypotension); **or**
- abnormal ECG (ST depression, deep anterior T wave inversion, left bundle branch block) **and** plasma markers of myocardial necrosis present.

3 Initial management
Low-risk patients
- Send home on treatment with aspirin, a beta-blocker or calcium antagonist, and sublingual nitrate as required (Table 14.2).
- Tell the patient to return to hospital if symptoms worsen.
- Arrange follow-up by the primary care physician within 3 days.
- Arrange an exercise test and out-patient follow-up within 2 weeks.

Table 14.2 Drug therapy in unstable angina

Drug	Comments
Aspirin	300 mg PO (chewed) stat, followed by 150 mg daily for 3 months, 75 mg daily thereafter. Give clopidogrel 75 mg daily if definite aspirin allergy
Heparin (unfractionated or low molecular weight)	Low-molecular-weight heparins have the advantages of subcutaneous administration and no requirement for monitoring of the activated partial thromboplastin time • Enoxaparin 100 units/kg 12-hly SC or • Dalteparin 120 units/kg 12-hly SC (maximum 10 000 units 12-hly) or • Unfractionated heparin by IV infusion: see p. 404
Platelet glycoprotein IIb/IIIa receptor inhibitor	Indicated in high-risk patients • Abciximab • Tirofiban • Eptifibatide
Beta-blocker	First-line treatment unless there is a major contraindication • Atenolol 50–100 mg daily PO or equivalent dose of other beta-blocker
Calcium antagonist	Diltiazem or verapamil should be used if beta-blocker contraindicated • Diltiazem 90–180 mg 12-hly PO or • Verapamil 40–120 mg 8-hly PO Avoid agents associated with reflex tachycardia (e.g. nifedipine); these should not be started without prior beta-blockade
Nitrate	Indicated for symptomatic relief. Use IV if haemodynamically unstable • IV nitrate • Isosorbide mononitrate 10–40 mg 12-hly daily PO • Buccal nitrate 2–5 mg 8-hly

Medium-risk patients
• Admit to the general ward.
• Start aspirin, heparin and a beta-blocker or calcium antagonist (Table 14.2). Aim for a resting heart rate around 50/min.
• If chest pain recurs, manage as high risk.

High-risk patients
• Admit to the CCU.
• If there is chest pain at rest, give nitrate by IV infusion or buccal administration (Table 14.2).
• Start aspirin, heparin and a platelet IIb/IIIa receptor inhibitor. Start a beta-blocker or calcium antagonist (Table 14.2).
• The management of pulmonary oedema and hypotension is given on p. 144. Hold off beta-blockade until resolution of the acute episode and consider checking LV function by echocardiography first.

Further management

Medium-risk patients
• Bed or chair rest for 12–24h followed by a programme of mobilization.
• If there is no recurrence of chest pain, arrange an exercise stress test before discharge.
• Institute secondary prevention as after myocardial infarction (p. 150).
• Discuss further management with a cardiologist before discharging the patient if angina occurs on mobilization or if the exercise test shows evidence of myocardial ischaemia at a low workload (under 6min of the Bruce protocol, or equivalent).

High-risk patients
• Discuss further management with a cardiologist.
• Angiography with a view to coronary revascularization will be indicated in the majority.
• Institute secondary prevention as after myocardial infarction (p. 150).

Unstable angina

15 Aortic dissection

- Consider the diagnosis in any patient with chest or upper abdominal pain of instantaneous onset.
- Dissections are either distal (only involving the descending thoracic aorta) or proximal (entry-point in or retrograde extension to the ascending thoracic aorta) (Fig. 15.1).

Priorities

1 **Put in an IV cannula and relieve pain** with diamorphine 5 mg IV (2.5 mg in the small or elderly) with further doses every 15 min as required. Obtain an ECG to exclude acute myocardial infarction as an alternative cause for the pain. Very rarely, aortic dissection can involve the right coronary artery causing inferior infarction.

2 **Complete your clinical assessment**, with careful attention to the following points:

History

- Was the pain instantaneous in onset (like a hammer-blow or a light turning on)?
- Did the pain radiate along the course of the aorta or its major branches?
- Were there associated neurological symptoms (e.g. syncope)?
- Is the patient at increased risk of dissection because of hypertension, Marfan syndrome, aortic root dilatation, bicuspid aortic valve or pregnancy?

Examination

- Blood pressure in both arms (the normal difference in systolic pressure is < 15 mmHg).
- Elevation of the JVP and arterial paradox as signs of tamponade.
- Presence and symmetry of the peripheral pulses.

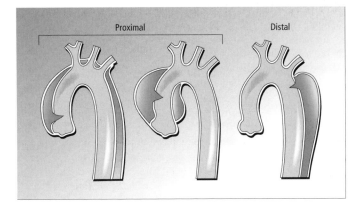

Fig. 15.1 Classification of aortic dissection.

- Early diastolic murmur of aortic regurgitation (due to distortion or dilatation of the aortic root).
- Limb power and tendon reflexes.

3 **Obtain a chest X-ray.**
- Abnormalities which may be seen are shown in Table 4.2.
- A PA film alone is normal in around 50% of cases.
- AP (anteroposterior) films commonly show apparent widening of the mediastinum in normal subjects and this feature in isolation should not be given undue weight.

4 **If readily available, transthoracic echocardiography should be done**, looking for:
- An intimal flap (seen in 50% of proximal dissections).
- Dilatation of the ascending aorta to 5 cm or more.
- Aortic regurgitation.
- Pericardial fluid (which is an ominous sign signifying retrograde extension into the pericardial space).

5 **The diagnosis of aortic dissection** is likely if the pain was of instantaneous onset and:
- there is an intimal flap; or
- there is pericardial fluid; or
- one or more major pulses are absent or asymmetric; or

- the chest X-ray shows a characteristic abnormality (Table 4.2, p. 51); or:
- there is aortic regurgitation; or:
- the ascending aorta is >5 cm in diameter.

6 **If the working diagnosis is aortic dissection**, start hypotensive treatment (Table 15.1).

- Make sure adequate analgesia has been given.
- BP should be monitored continuously with an intra-arterial line if you use nitroprusside.
- Put in a bladder catheter to monitor urine output.
- Aim to reduce systolic blood pressure to 100–120 mmHg, providing the urine output remains >30 mL/h.

7 **Discuss further management** with a cardiothoracic surgeon.

- Patients with clinically definite dissection should usually be transferred immediately to a regional cardiothoracic centre for further investigation, unless they would not be candidates for surgery because of advanced age or severe comorbidity.
- Proximal dissections require urgent repair. Distal dissections will usually be managed medically unless there are complications and provided that retrograde extension is excluded.

Aortic dissection

Table 15.1 Hypotensive therapy for acute aortic dissection

Labetolol infusion
- Make up a solution of 1 mg/mL by diluting the contents of 2 ampoules (200 mg) to 200 mL with normal saline or dextrose 5%
- Start the infusion at 15 mL/h and increase it every 15 min as necessary

or

- Nitroprusside plus propranolol

Nitroprusside infusion
- Make up a solution of 100 µg/mL by adding 50 mg to 500 mL dextrose 5%
- Start the infusion at 6 mL/h (10 µg/min) and increase it by steps of 10 µg/min every 5 min as necessary

Propranolol
- Give 0.1 mg/kg IV every 4–6 h

- The early death rate is very high and time should not be lost arranging investigation locally.

8 **If no other cause for the chest pain is found**, and aortic dissection remains a possibility, further investigation is needed: either computed tomography with contrast or transoesophageal echocardiography as available. Pitfalls to be aware of are:

- CT can miss an intimal flap if the contrast is too dense.

- The clinical picture of aortic dissection may be due to **aortic mural haematoma** (without an intimal flap) in 15% of cases, which may be missed on computed tomography. Transoesophageal echocardiography in trained hands shows:
  - Aortic wall >4 mm thick.
  - Echolucencies caused by blood in the aortic wall.
  - Fascial planes in the aortic wall which 'shear' during systole.

Management of mural haematoma is the same as for dissection. Continue hypotensive therapy and discuss further management with a cardiothoracic surgeon.

Further management of distal aortic dissection

If, after discussion, the decision is to manage locally, this means that the patient has a dissection unequivocally involving only the descending thoracic aorta.

1 Transfer the patient to an ITU or CCU, and continue IV hypotensive therapy. Start oral therapy (Chapter 16), which should include a beta-blocker unless there are major contraindications.

2 Maintain adequate pain relief (initially with a combination of opiate and non-steroidal anti-inflammatory drug).

3 Discuss with a cardiothoracic surgeon if:

- Severe pain continues or recurs.
- A large pleural effusion develops.
- The urine output falls. If not due to excessive hypotensive therapy or hypovolaemia, this suggests involvement of the renal arteries and is an ominous sign.
- There is evidence of other branch artery involvement (e.g. abdominal pain with bloody diarrhoea due to ischaemic colitis).

Aortic dissection

16 Severe hypertension

- Defined by a diastolic blood pressure >120 mmHg.
- Emergency intravenous therapy is rarely required and is potentially dangerous. Abrupt reduction of blood pressure may cause stroke, myocardial infarction or renal failure.

Priorities

1 Make a clinical assessment
History

- Is the patient known to have hypertension? What treatment has been given? What is the compliance with treatment? What investigations have been done to exclude an underlying cause for hypertension? Is there associated cardiac or renal disease?
- Has the patient had a recent stroke or subarachnoid haemorrhage? In this setting, lowering the blood pressure may worsen the neurological deficit: discuss management with a neurologist before starting hypotensive therapy.
- Are there features to suggest **hypertensive encephalopathy** (which is rare) (Table 16.1)? It may be difficult to distinguish between hypertensive encephalopathy, subarachnoid haemorrhage (p. 242) and stroke. Hypertensive encephalopathy is favoured by the gradual onset of symptoms and the absence (or late appearance) of focal neurological signs. If there is diagnostic doubt, a CT scan should be obtained to exclude cerebral or subarachnoid haemorrhage before starting IV therapy.
- Does the patient have acute chest pain (consider **aortic dissection** (p. 156)) or breathlessness (consider **pulmonary oedema** due to left ventricular failure)?

Examination

- Measure the blood pressure in both arms.

Table 16.1 Clinical features of hypertensive encephalopathy

Early features
　Headache
　Nausea and vomiting
　Confusional state
　Retinal haemorrhages, exudates or papilloedema

Late features
　Focal neurological signs
　Fits
　Coma

Table 16.2 Urgent investigation in the patient with severe hypertension

Creatinine, sodium and potassium
Urinalysis (plus urine microscopy if abnormal)
Chest X-ray
ECG

- Check for signs of heart failure and aortic regurgitation.
- Check the presence and symmetry of the major pulses (and check for radio-femoral delay).
- Listen for carotid, abdominal and femoral bruits.
- Examine the abdomen (?palpable kidneys, ?abdominal aortic aneurysm).
- Examine the fundi. Retinal haemorrhages, exudates or papilloedema (not due to other causes) define accelerated phase or 'malignant' hypertension.

2 **Urgent investigation is given in Table 16.2.**
3 **Are there indications for emergency treatment of hypertension?**
- Hypertensive encephalopathy.

Table 16.3 Intravenous therapy for hypertensive emergencies

Use labetalol unless there is left ventricular failure
Make up a solution of 1 mg/mL by diluting the contents of 2 ampoules (200 mg) to 200 mL with normal saline or dextrose 5%
Start the infusion at 15 mL/h and increase it every 15 min

The alternative is nitroprusside (intra-arterial pressure monitoring needed)
Make up a solution of 100 μg/mL by adding 50 mg to 500 mL dextrose 5%
Start the infusion at 6 mL/hour (10 μg/min) and increase it by steps of 10 μg/min every 5 min

Severe hypertension

- Acute aortic dissection (see p. 156 for the specific management of this).
- Left ventricular failure with alveolar pulmonary oedema.
4 **If so, transfer the patient to the CCU or ITU.**
- Put in an arterial line to allow continuous monitoring of the blood pressure and a urinary catheter to monitor urine output. Give oxygen if the patient is breathless or oxygen saturation is <90%.
- Give frusemide 40–80 mg IV if there is left ventricular failure or encephalopathy.
- Start IV therapy aiming to reduce diastolic BP to no less than 100–110 mmHg within 1 h (Table 16.3).
- Start appropriate oral therapy (Table 16.4).

Further management

1 Admit the patient with:
- retinal haemorrhages, exudates or papilloedema;
- renal failure;
- interstitial pulmonary oedema;
- diastolic pressure >130 mmHg.
2 Start oral therapy (Table 16.4)
- Aim to reduce diastolic BP to around 110 mmHg over the first 24 h.

Table 16.4 Initial oral therapy for severe hypertension.

Clinical features	Drug therapy
Interstitial pulmonary oedema	Frusemide 20 mg PO (higher doses will be needed in patients with impaired renal function); plus
	Nifedipine 10–20 mg 8-hly PO
Phaeochromocytoma suspected	Labetalol 100–200 mg 12-hly PO
Beta-blockers contraindicated	Nifedipine 10–20 mg 8-hly PO; or
	Hydralazine 25–50 mg 8-hly PO
Other patients	Atenolol 50 mg daily PO

Table 16.5 Clinical features and pointers to diagnosis of renal artery stenosis

Age < 50 with no family history of hypertension (fibromuscular dysplasia)
Peripheral arterial disease
Refractory hypertension
Deteriorating blood pressure control in compliant, long-standing hypertensive patients
Renal impairment with ACE inhibition
Renal impairment with minimal proteinuria
'Flash' pulmonary oedema
> 1.5 cm difference in kidney size on ultrasound
Low plasma sodium and potassium (due to secondary hyperaldosteronism)

Reference: McLaughlin K et al. Renal artery stenosis. British Medical Journal 2000; **320**, 1124–7.

- Recheck the blood pressure every 30 min. If the diastolic BP is unchanged after 4 h, repeat the dose or add another drug.
3 Look for causes of secondary hypertension. Consider:
  - Drugs, e.g. corticosteroids, oral contraceptives.

- Coarctation of the aorta (radio-femoral delay).
- Renal artery stenosis (Table 16.5).
- Intrinsic renal disease (raised creatinine, abnormal urinalysis or microscopy).
- Phaeochromocytoma (paroxysmal headache, sweating or palpitation; family history of endocrinopathy; hypertensive crisis following anaesthesia or administration of contrast).
- Primary hyperaldosteronism (hypokalaemia).
- Cushing syndrome (truncal obesity, thin skin with purple abdominal striae, proximal myopathy).

4 Seek expert advice from a nephrologist if there is:
- renal failure or other evidence of intrinsic renal disease (>2+ proteinuria and/or red cell casts in the urine);
- suspected renal artery stenosis (Table 16.5).

17 Pulmonary oedema

Pulmonary oedema may be due to:

• high pulmonary capillary pressure from cardiac or renal disease, iatrogenic fluid overload or acute central nervous system disease, notably subarachnoid haemorrhage (Tables 17.1 and 17.2);

• increased pulmonary capillary permeability—the acute respiratory distress syndrome (ARDS) or 'shock lung' (see Appendix).

Priorities

1 Give oxygen 35–60%. Pulse oximetry may be unreliable due to peripheral vasoconstriction, and you should check arterial blood gases if there is no improvement within 30 min.

2 Check the blood pressure, pulse and JVP, and listen to the heart and lungs.
   • If there is any diagnostic doubt, obtain a chest X-ray before starting drug treatment. Inspiratory crackles are not always present; wheeze is common and may lead to the misdiagnosis of asthma.

3 Attach an ECG monitor and treat major arrhythmias (p. 10).

4 Put in a peripheral IV cannula and give the following drugs:
   • diamorphine 2.5–5.0 mg (or morphine 5.0–10.0 mg) by slow IV injection;
   • frusemide 40–80 mg IV;
   • sublingual or buccal nitrate, if systolic BP is >90 mmHg.

5 If pulmonary oedema is due to overtransfusion, venesect using a large-bore cannula or a blood donation set.

6 Record a 12-lead ECG (looking for evidence of acute myocardial infarction or other cardiac disease, e.g. left ventricular hypertrophy, left bundle branch block) and obtain chest X-ray to confirm the clinical

Table 17.1 Causes of pulmonary oedema due to high pulmonary capillary pressure

Cardiac
   Acute myocardial infarction or severe myocardial ischaemia
   Acute myocarditis
   Acute aortic regurgitation (aortic dissection, infective endocarditis, chest trauma)
   Acute mitral regurgitation (infective endocarditis, ruptured chordae or papillary
      muscle, chest trauma)
   Ventricular septal rupture after myocardial infarction (p. 147)
   Severe mitral stenosis
   Left atrial myxoma
   Severe aortic stenosis

Renal
   Acute or chronic renal failure
   Renal artery stenosis (p. 163)

Iatrogenic fluid overload

Acute central nervous system disease
   Subarachnoid haemorrhage

diagnosis and exclude other causes of breathlessness. Other investigations needed are given in Table 17.3.

7 Has the patient got ARDS rather than cardiogenic pulmonary oedema?
Suspect ARDS if:
- the patient has risk factors for ARDS (Table 17.4);
- the ECG is normal;
- the chest X-ray shows diffuse bilateral shadowing (often sparing the costophrenic angles), but without cardiomegaly or distension of upper lobe pulmonary veins.

Diagnostic criteria for ARDS are given in Table 17.5.
Management of ARDS is outlined in the Appendix.

8 Has the patient got renal failure (p. 302)? In patients with a blood urea >20 mmol/L or creatinine >200 μmol/L, standard doses of frusemide are often ineffective.
- Try a frusemide infusion (100 mg over 60 min by syringe pump).

Table 17.2 Precipitants of pulmonary oedema in patients with previously stable valve or left ventricular disease

Acute myocardial infarction or myocardial ischaemia
Arrhythmia (the onset of atrial fibrillation is a common precipitant of pulmonary
   oedema in patients with severe mitral or aortic stenosis)
Drugs with a negative inotropic effect (e.g. beta-blockers)
Poor compliance with diuretic therapy
Drugs causing fluid retention (e.g. NSAIDs, steroids)
Iatrogenic fluid overload

Table 17.3 Urgent investigation in pulmonary oedema

ECG (arrhythmia? evidence of acute myocardial infarction or ischaemia? evidence of
   other cardiac disease, e.g. left ventricular hypertrophy, left bundle branch block?)
Chest X-ray (to confirm the clinical diagnosis and exclude other causes of
   breathlessness)
Arterial blood gases and pH (if not improving after 30 min)
Creatinine, sodium, potassium and glucose
Echocardiography if acute valve lesion or ventricular septal rupture suspected (in
   other patients, echocardiography should be done within 48 h)

- If this fails, dialysis or haemofiltration may be needed. Discuss management with a nephrologist. In extreme circumstances, venesect 500 mL while renal replacement therapy is being arranged.

Further management of cardiogenic pulmonary oedema

1 Further drug therapy depends on the blood pressure
- Systolic BP must be rapidly increased to >90 mmHg to maintain coronary, cerebral and renal perfusion.

Table 17.4 Causes of acute respiratory distress syndrome

Direct lung injury	Indirect lung injury
Common causes	*Common causes*
Pneumonia	Sepsis
Aspiration of gastric contents	Severe trauma with shock and multiple transfusions
Less common causes	*Less common causes*
Pulmonary contusion	Cardiopulmonary bypass
Fat emboli	Drug overdose
Near-drowning	Acute pancreatitis
Inhalational injury	Transfusions of blood products
Reperfusion pulmonary oedema after lung transplantation or pulmonary embolectomy	

Reference: Ware LB, Matthay MA. The acute respiratory distress syndrome. *New England Journal of Medicine* 2000; **342**: 1334–49.

Table 17.5 Diagnostic criteria for acute respiratory distress syndrome

Antecedent history of precipitating condition
Refractory hypoxaemia (e.g. $Pao_2 < 8\,kPa$ despite Fio_2 40%)
Bilateral pulmonary infiltrates on chest X-ray
Pulmonary artery wedge pressure $<18\,mmHg$ (with normal colloid oncotic pressure) or no evidence of cardiac cause of pulmonary oedema

• Stop drugs with a negative inotropic effect (see p. 32 for reversal of beta-blockade).
• Consider placement of a pulmonary artery catheter (p. 429) if inotropic/vasopressor therapy is needed: discuss this with a cardiolo-

gist or ITU physician. Intra-aortic balloon counterpulsation may be indicated for patients with pulmonary oedema due to myocardial ischaemia, acute mitral regurgitation or ventricular septal rupture.

• Diuretics are relatively ineffective in patients with hypotension and pulmonary oedema (cardiogenic shock), but can be used once the cardiac output has increased (as shown by improvement in the patient's mental state and skin perfusion).

Systolic BP > 110 mmHg
• Give another dose of frusemide 40–80 mg IV.
• Start a nitrate infusion. If the patient remains breathless, increase the infusion rate every 15–30 min providing systolic BP is >110 mmHg.

Systolic BP 90–110 mmHg
• Start a dobutamine infusion at 5 μg/kg/min (p. 484). Dobutamine can be given via a peripheral line. Increase the dose by 2.5 μg/kg/min every 10 min until systolic BP is >110 mmHg or a maximum dose of 20 μg/kg/min has been reached.
• A nitrate infusion can be added if systolic BP is maintained at >110 mmHg.

Systolic BP 80–90 mmHg
• Start a dopamine infusion at 10 μg/kg/min (p. 484). Dopamine must be give via a central line. Increase the dose by 5 μg/kg/min every 10 min until systolic BP is >110 mmHg. If systolic BP remains <90 mmHg despite dopamine 20 mcg/kg/min, use noradrenaline instead.
• A nitrate infusion can be added if systolic BP is maintained at >110 mmHg.

Systolic BP < 80 mmHg
• Start a noradrenaline infusion at 2.5 μg/kg/min (p. 481). Noradrenaline must be given via a central line. Increase the dose by 2.5 μg/kg/min every 10 min until systolic BP is >110 mmHg.
• A nitrate infusion can be added if systolic BP is maintained at >110 mmHg.

2 Maintain oxygenation

• Check arterial gases and pH. If arterial pH is less than 7.1 due to metabolic acidosis, give sodium bicarbonate 50 mL of 8.4% solution over 15–30 min (severe metabolic acidosis has a negative inotropic effect and facilitates ventricular arrhythmias).

• Increase the inspired oxygen concentration if necessary to maintain Pao_2 around 10 kPa.

• Continuous positive airways pressure delivered through a tight-fitting facemask can improve oxygenation and reduce the need for mechanical ventilation, and may be helpful in patients with severe pulmonary oedema.

• Mechanical ventilation is indicated if Pao_2 is <8 kPa despite 60% oxygen or $Paco_2$ is rising, if recovery from the underlying cause is possible. Discuss this with an ITU physician.

3 Monitor urine output

• The urine output is a good guide to the cardiac output and should ideally be >30 mL/h (>0.5 mL/kg/h).

• Put in a urinary catheter if systolic BP is <90 mmHg or if no urine is passed after 1 h.

4 Decide what has caused or precipitated the attack (Tables 17.1 and 17.2)

• As a general rule, all patients with pulmonary oedema should have echocardiography to determine left ventricular function and exclude significant valve disease or an intracardiac shunt.

• Discuss further management with a cardiologist if pulmonary oedema was due to acute myocardial ischaemia or structural heart disease.

• Ask advice from a nephrologist if pulmonary oedema was due to renal failure or suspected renal artery stenosis (Table 16.5).

Appendix

Management of the acute respiratory distress syndrome

ARDS (Table 17.5) is the result of pulmonary endothelial damage, usually occurring as part of multiple organ failure. Patients with suspected ARDS should be referred early to the ITU. The key elements in management are the following:

Maintenance of oxygenation
• Keep Pao_2 9–11 kPa by adjusting the inspired oxygen concentration (Fio_2).
• Ventilation will be needed if Pao_2 is <7 kPa despite Fio_2 60%. Ventilation in the prone position improves oxygenation.
• Haemoglobin should be kept around 10 g/dL (to give the optimum balance between oxygen-carrying capacity and blood viscosity).

Fluid balance
• Pulmonary artery wedge pressure should be kept at 10–15 mmHg (measured with the ventilator temporarily disconnected as ventilation (especially with PEEP) causes a variable increase in PAWP).
• Renal failure is commonly associated with ARDS and may be managed by haemofiltration.

Prevention and treatment of sepsis
• Sepsis is a common cause and complication of ARDS.
• Culture blood, tracheobronchial aspirate and urine daily. Treat presumed infection with broad-spectrum antibiotic therapy.

Pulmonary oedema

18 Pericarditis

Consider the diagnosis in any patient with:
- central chest pain which is worse on inspiration and relieved by sitting forward;
- pericardial friction rub (pericarditis may be painless);
- unexplained enlargement of the cardiac shadow on the chest X-ray (reflecting a pericardial effusion).

Causes are given in Table 18.1.

Priorities

1 Relieve pain: an NSAID is usually sufficient (e.g. indomethacin 25–50 mg 8-hly PO). Severe pain may require an opiate.

2 Obtain an ECG. The diagnosis is based on the clinical features supported by the ECG (Table 4.1). Note that:
- The ECG is rarely helpful in pericarditis after myocardial infarction (the commonest cause of pericarditis seen in hospital).
- The changes on the initial ECG may be impossible to distinguish from those of acute myocardial infarction. If there is diagnostic doubt, thrombolytic therapy must not be given.
- Other investigation is given in Table 18.2.

3 Is there evidence of **cardiac tamponade** (raised JVP, pulsus paradoxus >20 mmHg)? See p. 175 for further management of tamponade.

Further management

1 If the patient is ill, always consider **bacterial pericarditis**:
- Bacterial pericarditis is usually due to spread of intrathoracic infection, e.g. following thoracic surgery or trauma, or complicating bacterial pneumonia.

Pericarditis

Table 18.1 Causes of pericarditis

Idiopathic

Infectious diseases (viral, bacterial, fungal and tuberculous)

Acute myocardial infarction

Rheumatic diseases, e.g. systemic lupus erythematosus

Advanced renal failure

Pericardial surgery, trauma or irradiation

Dressler/post-cardiotomy syndrome

Drugs — procainamide, hydralazine

Neoplastic diseases (most commonly carcinoma of the bronchus or breast)

Table 18.2 Investigation in suspected pericarditis

Chest X-ray — ?enlarged cardiac shadow, ?interstitial pulmonary oedema, ?consolidation

ECG (see Table 4.1, p. 50)

Plasma markers of myocardial necrosis (see Table 4.3, p. 53)

Creatinine, sodium and potassium

Full blood count

ESR and C-reactive protein

Echocardiogram (if cardiac tamponade suspected or cardiac silhouette enlarged — ?effusion or myocarditis)

Blood for viral serology (for later analysis)

Blood culture (if suspected bacterial infection)

Autoantibody screen (for later analysis)

Pericarditis

• Start antibiotic therapy with flucloxacillin and gentamicin IV after taking blood cultures.

• Obtain an echocardiogram to look for an effusion or evidence of endocarditis.

• Perform pericardiocentesis (p. 447) if there is an effusion large enough to be drained safely (echo-free space >2 cm). Send fluid for

Gram stain and culture. Consider tuberculous or fungal infection if the effusion is purulent but no organisms are seen on Gram stain.

• Discuss further management with a cardiologist or cardiothoracic surgeon.

2 Has the patient had recent cardiac surgery, raising the possibility of **Dressler (post-cardiotomy) syndrome**?

• Dressler syndrome occurs in 15% of patients, usually 2–4 weeks after surgery (range 1 week to 3 months) (and is also a recognized but nowadays rare (<1%) late complication of myocardial infarction).

• It is an acute self-limiting illness with fever, pleuritis and pericarditis. The ECG may show typical changes of pericarditis or only non-specific ST/T abnormalities. The chest X-ray may show an enlarged cardiac silhouette (due to pericardial effusion), bilateral pleural effusions and transient pulmonary infiltrates. The ESR is raised (often >70 mm/h).

• Obtain an echocardiogram because pericardial effusion is common.

• If pain has not settled after 48 h of treatment with aspirin or an NSAID, consider prednisolone (initially 40 mg daily PO, tapered over 1 month).

3 Presumed viral (or 'idiopathic') pericarditis is the likely diagnosis in young and otherwise healthy adults. It may be preceded by a flu-like illness and is usually a self-limiting disorder lasting 1–3 weeks.

• Echocardiography is not indicated unless the JVP is raised or the chest X-ray shows an enlarged cardiac silhouette.

• Give aspirin or an NSAID until the pain has resolved.

• Recurrent pericarditis may occur in 15–40% of patients, and can be prevented by treatment with prednisolone or colchicine.

19 Cardiac tamponade

Consider cardiac tamponade if there is:
- hypotension or breathlessness and
- a raised jugular venous pressure.

Have a high level of suspicion after the insertion of a central line or in the presence of predisposing conditions (Table 19.1).

Echocardiography is needed urgently in suspected tamponade.

Priorities

1 Give oxygen, attach an ECG monitor and put in a peripheral venous cannula. Your examination should include an assessment of arterial paradox.
- Inflate the blood-pressure cuff above systolic BP.
- Slowly deflate the cuff, watching the chest, and note the pressure at which sounds are first heard in expiration alone.
- Continue deflating the cuff and note the pressure at which sounds are heard thoughout expiration and inspiration.
- A difference in these systolic pressures of >10 mmHg is abnormal.

2 Obtain an ECG and chest X-ray to exclude other diagnoses (Table 19.2), and an urgent echocardiogram, looking for:
- The presence, size and distribution (circumferential or loculated) of a pericardial effusion: safe aspiration requires an effusion of >2 cm thickness along the chosen needle path.
- Echo-correlates of tamponade (diastolic collapse of the free wall of the right ventricle, a fall in mitral inflow velocity on inspiration and engorgement of the inferior vena cava).

Be aware that a pleural effusion or dilated right ventricle may be misdiagnosed on echocardiography as a pericardial effusion.

Table 19.1 Causes of cardiac tamponade

Malignant disease (most commonly carcinoma of the bronchus or breast)
Acute myocardial infarction (with free wall rupture or haemopericardium as a
    complication of anticoagulation)
Diagnostic procedures with cardiac perforation
Dressler/post-cardiotomy syndrome
Idiopathic pericarditis
Uraemic pericarditis
Pyogenic or tuberculous pericarditis
Aortic dissection
Rheumatic diseases, e.g. systemic lupus erythematosus

Table 19.2 Causes of hypotension with a raised JVP

Cardiac tamponade
Severe biventricular failure
Pulmonary embolism
Right ventricular infarction
Other causes of right ventricular failure
Acute severe asthma
Tension pneumothorax

3 Discuss with a cardiologist before attempting aspiration in the following circumstances:
• Signs of tamponade but only small pericardial effusion (echo separation <1.5 cm). This can occur with effusive–constrictive pericarditis in malignancy, autoimmune conditions and after viral infection. Percutaneous drainage is potentially hazardous and may not relieve the symptoms.
• Early after cardiac surgery. It may be more appropriate to drain the effusion surgically.

- If there is severely impaired left ventricular function: pericardio-centesis may lead to further ventricular dilatation.

4 Perform pericardiocentesis if a large effusion is present (echo separation 2 cm or more) and there are clinical signs of tamponade. The technique of pericardial aspiration is described in detail on p. 447.

- If systolic pressure is <90 mmHg and the effusion cannot be drained immediately, treat with IV colloid or blood together with an infusion of noradrenaline (p. 481) via a central line.

Further management

This is directed at the underlying cause (Table 19.1).

- Patients with malignant effusions will usually require further inter-vention to prevent recurrent tamponade, e.g. chemotherapy or creation of a pericardial window.
- If the patient has Dressler syndrome (2–4 weeks after cardiac surgery, high ESR) start prednisolone 40 mg PO daily.
- For recurrent idiopathic effusion consider prednisolone or colchicine.

Cardiac tamponade

20 Deep vein thrombosis

Deep vein thrombosis (DVT) is common (with an incidence of approximately 1 per 1000 each year), but leg swelling is usually due to other causes (see Appendix).

Management

History and clinical signs
The history and clinical signs are a guide to the probability of DVT (Table 20.1). Pay particular attention to:
- Risk factors for DVT (Table 20.2).
- Is the swelling unilateral or bilateral?
  - Bilateral swelling suggests a systemic aetiology, e.g. heart failure or hypoalbuminaemia or IVC obstruction.
- What is the degree and extent of swelling?
  - Unilateral swelling extending above the knee suggests DVT.
- Skin redness?
  - If along the course of the vein, this suggests DVT, but if over an area of skin, with tenderness, cellulitis is more likely.
- Is there evidence of heart failure or liver failure?
- Could trauma be the cause?
  - History of trauma.
  - Localized swelling with bruising.
- Are there symptoms of pulmonary embolism?

Further investigation
This is necessary to prove the diagnosis if DVT is clinically likely.
- Ultrasonography and venography are the most widely available tests.

Table 20.1 Estimating the probability of DVT

Clinical features	Score
History	
Active cancer (treatment ongoing, or within previous 6 months, or palliative)	1
Paralysis, paresis or recent plaster immobilization of the legs	1
Recently bedridden for more than 3 days, or major surgery within 4 weeks	1
Examination	
Localized tenderness along the distribution of the deep venous system	1
Entire leg swollen	1
Calf swelling by >3 cm when compared with asymptomatic leg (measured 10 cm below tibial tuberosity)	1
Pitting oedema (greater in the symptomatic leg)	1
Collateral superficial veins (non-varicose)	1
Alternative diagnosis?	
An alternative diagnosis is as likely or more likely than DVT	−2
Score	
Score 3 or more: high probability of DVT	
Score 1 or 2: moderate probability of DVT	
Score 0 or less: low probability of DVT	

Reference: Wells PS *et al*. Value of assessment of pretest probability of deep-vein thrombosis in clinical management. *Lancet* 1997; **350**: 1795–8.

Deep vein thrombosis

Treatment

If DVT is proved, initial treatment consists of:

• Bed rest with elevation of the leg for 24–48 h or until swelling is resolving.

• Compression stocking to reduce the risk of post-phlebitic syndrome.

• Analgesia with NSAID if needed.

• Give heparin by IV infusion (p. 404) or low-molecular-weight heparin.

Table 20.2 Risk factors for DVT

Age > 50	
Previous DVT or pulmonary embolism	
Surgery	Major abdominal or pelvic
	Hip or knee
Malignant disease	Especially metastatic or abdominal or pelvic
Immobility	Prolonged travel
	Severe illness or disability
Pregnancy and puerperium	
Local trauma	Fracture
Haematological	Deficiency of antithrombin III, protein C or S or resistance to activated protein C
	Presence of factor V Leiden or prothrombin G20210A mutation
	High level of factor VIII
	Polycythaemia, thrombocytosis
Others	Oral contraceptive
	Antiphospholipid syndrome, Behcet syndrome, nephrotic syndrome, hyperhomocysteinaemia

• Warfarin should be started (p. 407) during heparin therapy, overlapping for 3–4 days: during this period, check both the APTT and International Normalized Ratio (INR) daily. Heparin can be stopped after 5 days provided the INR is >2.0. Warfarin is usually given for 3 months after a first DVT (target INR 2.0–3.0). Indefinite treatment may be indicated after recurrent thromboembolism (target INR 3.0–4.5).

Why has this patient had a DVT?
• Consider the risk factors (Table 20.1).
• Women with unexplained DVT/PE should have examination of the breasts and a pelvic examination plus pelvic ultrasound if a clinical abnormality is found.
• Men should have digital examination of the prostate and measurement of prostate-specific antigen.

Table 20.3 Investigation in DVT

Chest X-ray
ECG if symptoms of pulmonary embolism
Full blood count and ESR
Biochemical profile including liver function tests
In patients < 50 with unexplained or recurrent DVT, or family history of
    thromboembolism, check antithrombin III, protein C and S levels, factor VIII level,
    presence of factor V Leiden and prothrombin G20210A mutation, autoantibody
    screen and anticardiolipin antibody

• Patients under 50 or with a strong family history of DVT/PE should be screened for a thrombophilic disorder (Table 20.3): seek expert advice from a haematologist.

You suspected DVT, but the venogram was negative

• Consider other causes of leg swelling (Appendix).

• Unexplained asymmetric leg swelling with a negative venogram is a recognized syndrome and carries a benign prognosis. No treatment is necessary.

Appendix

Causes of leg swelling

Venous/lymphatic

• Deep vein thrombosis.
• Superficial thrombophlebitis.
• IVC obstruction (e.g. by tumour).
• Varicose veins with chronic venous hypertension.
• Post-phlebitic syndrome.
• Congenital lymphoedema.
• After vein harvesting for coronary bypass grafting.
• Dependent oedema (e.g. in paralysed limb).
• Severe obesity with compression of iliofemoral veins by abdominal fat.

Deep vein thrombosis

Musculoskeletal
- Calf haematoma.
- Ruptured Baker's cyst.
- Muscle tear.

Skin
- Cellulitis (recognized by tenderness, erythema and induration of the skin).

Systemic (oedema is bilateral, but may be asymmetric)
- Congestive heart failure.
- Liver failure.
- Renal failure.
- Nephrotic syndrome.
- Hypoalbuminaemia.
- Chronic respiratory failure.
- Pregnancy.
- Idiopathic oedema of women.
- Calcium antagonists.
- Other drugs causing salt/water retention.

21 Pulmonary embolism

Consider the diagnosis in any patient (Table 21.1) with:
• acute breathlessness, or worsening of chronic breathlessness (e.g. in COPD or heart failure);
• circulatory collapse;
• pleuritic chest pain or haemoptysis.

One or more predisposing factors for venous thromboembolism (Table 20.2) are present in 80–90% of patients with pulmonary embolism. Pulmonary embolism is rare in patients aged under 40 with no risk factors.

Management is summarized in Fig. 21.1

Priorities

1 Make a rapid clinical assessment:
• Pulse, blood pressure, JVP.
• Respiratory rate, pleural rub.
• Arterial oxygen saturation (if <90%, check arterial blood gases). Hypoxia is invariable with a large embolism, but normal arterial gases do not exclude a small embolism.
• Risk factors for thromboembolism, signs of DVT (see Table 20.2).

2 Obtain an ECG and chest X-ray. These are principally of value in excluding alternative diagnoses (e.g. myocardial infarction, pneumonia, pneumothorax).

In pulmonary embolism:
• The ECG will usually show only sinus tachycardia or minor ST/T wave changes. Evidence of right ventricular strain (right axis deviation, right bundle branch block) may be seen with major embolism.
• The chest X-ray is often normal or may show non-specific abnormalities such as an elevated hemi-diaphragm, a small pleural effusion or focal shadowing.

Pulmonary embolism

Table 21.1 Main clinical presentations of pulmonary embolism

	Circulatory collapse, previously well	Circulatory collapse, with underlying cardio-pulmonary disease	Pulmonary infarction	Isolated dyspnoea
Frequency	5%	10%	60%	25%
Pulmonary arterial occlusion	Extensive	Small/moderate	Small/moderate	Moderate/large
Examination	Hypotension, raised JVP	Hypotension; may have raised JVP; signs of underlying cardiopulmonary disease	Focal lung signs	Tachypnoea (>20/min)
Chest X-ray	Usually normal	May be abnormal	Often focal shadowing	Usually normal
ECG	Often acute RV strain (RAD, RBBB)	Unhelpful*	Normal	Non-specific abnormalities
Arterial blood gases	Markedly abnormal	Unhelpful*	May be normal	Usually abnormal

JVP, jugular venous pressure; RV, right ventricular; RAD, right axis deviation; RBBB, right bundle branch block.

* Because abnormalities are mainly due to underlying cardiopulmonary disease.

Reference: British Thoracic Society, Standards of Care Committee. Suspected pulmonary embolism: a practical approach. Thorax 1997; **52** (Suppl 4).

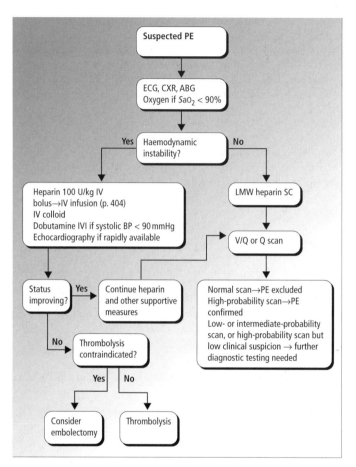

Fig. 21.1 Management of suspected pulmonary embolism.

• A normal ECG and chest X-ray do not exclude pulmonary embolism.

3 If pulmonary embolism is likely, or cannot be excluded, give 5000–10 000 units of unfractionated heparin by IV bolus (100 U/kg) if the patient is haemodynamically unstable, or low-molecular-weight heparin SC.

4 If you suspect acute major embolism (circulatory collapse with systolic BP < 90 mmHg and signs of low cardiac output):

• Connect an ECG monitor: atrial fibrillation or flutter may occur with major pulmonary emboli and should be treated with IV digoxin (p. 27).

• Start an infusion of colloid: run in fluid rapidly until systolic blood pressure is >90 mmHg. This will increase right ventricular filling and hence cardiac output.

• If the patient remains hypotensive after 500 mL of colloid, start dobutamine, at 10 µg/kg/min (p. 484). Increase it as needed up to 40 µg/kg/min until systolic BP is >90 mmHg. If systolic BP remains <90 mmHg, dopamine or noradrenaline should be used (p. 481).

• If the BP is <90 mmHg after 30–60 min and there is clinically definite pulmonary embolism, give thrombolysis (Table 21.2) provided there are no contraindications.

• Most deaths from acute major pulmonary embolism occur within 1 h, so pulmonary angiography is rarely practicable. Echocardiography is helpful, if it can be done immediately, in showing a dilated right ventricle, high pulmonary artery pressures and no left-sided disease capable of explaining the clinical features.

Further management

1 Continue heparin.

2 Confirm or exclude the diagnosis. Further investigation to confirm or exclude pulmonary embolism is essential. A scheme for this is shown in Fig. 21.1 and Table 21.3.

• A normal perfusion (Q) scan or ventilation/perfusion (V/Q) scan excludes the diagnosis of pulmonary embolism.

• A 'high-probability' scan confirms the diagnosis in patients in whom the clinical suspicion of pulmonary embolism is moderate or high.

• Further diagnostic testing is needed for patients in whom the scan shows a low or intermediate probability or in whom the clinical suspicion of pulmonary embolism is low but the scan is reported as 'high probability'.

Table 21.2 Thrombolytic therapy for acute major pulmonary embolism

Criteria to be met
Systolic BP < 90 mmHg after standard treatment for 30–60 min
Clinically definite embolism (compatible clinical picture, risk factor(s) for
    thromboembolism present (Table 20.2, p. 180), no other diagnosis likely)
No contraindication to thrombolytic therapy (Table 13.2, p. 141)

Regimens
Thrombolytic therapy can be given via a peripheral or central vein. If pulmonary
    angiography has been performed, leave the angiography catheter in place
    because of the risk of bleeding from the puncture site

Streptokinase
250 000 U IV over 30 min, followed by
100 000 U/h IV for 12–72 h

Alteplase
10 mg IV over 1–2 min IV, followed by
90 mg IV over 2 h (maximum total dose 1.5 mg/kg in patients < 65 kg)

Check the thrombin time (TT) or activated partial thromboplastin time (APTT) 3–4 h
    after stopping streptokinase or alteplase. When TT/APTT are less than twice
    control, restart heparin

3 Further diagnostic testing to confirm or exclude venous thromboembolism

Options are:

- Imaging of the leg veins by duplex ultrasound or contrast venography.
- Imaging of the pulmonary arteries by angiography, spiral computed tomography or magnetic resonance angiography.
- Measurement of plasma D-dimer (a breakdown product of cross-linked fibrin): a normal value excludes thrombosis, although a raised value is not specific for this.

You will have to make a judgement in individual cases as to how far to pursue the diagnosis and which test is most appropriate. For

Table 21.3 Combining the clinical probability with the perfusion or ventilation/perfusion scan result

Clinical probability of pulmonary embolism

Low	Moderate	High
Atypical clinical picture and major risk factors for VTE absent	Typical clinical picture but major risk factors for VTE absent or Atypical clinical picture but major risk factors for VTE present	Typical clinical picture and major risk factors for VTE present

Clinical probability of pulmonary embolism

Q or V/Q scan result	Low	Moderate	High
Normal	Pulmonary embolism excluded		
Low or Intermediate probability	Further diagnostic testing needed		
High probability	Further diagnostic testing needed	Pulmonary embolism confirmed	

VTE, venous thromboembolism.

patients with pre-existing cardiopulmonary disease who have inconclusive test results, anticoagulation should be given unless there are major contraindications, as their mortality if untreated is high.

4 If pulmonary embolism is confirmed, or the balance of risk : benefit favours anticoagulation:

• Warfarin should be started (Table 50.5, p. 407) during heparin therapy, overlapping for 3–4 days: during this period, check both the APTT and International Normalized Ratio (INR) daily.

- Heparin can be stopped after 5 days provided the INR is >2.0.
- Warfarin is usually given for 3–6 months after a first pulmonary embolism (target INR 2.0–3.0). Indefinite treatment may be indicated after recurrent thromboembolism

5 Look for a cause for the pulmonary embolism (see Table 20.2, p. 180).

Pulmonary embolism

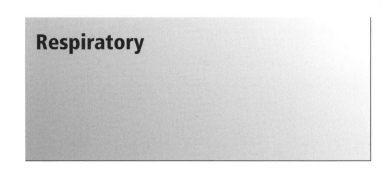

Respiratory

22 Acute asthma

- Asthma is the commonest cause of acute breathlessness with wheeze but other diagnoses should be considered, especially in older patients or if the response to treatment is poor (p. 60).
- The severity of an attack is easily underestimated.
- Management is summarized in Fig. 22.1.

Priorities

1 **Give oxygen 40–60% and salbutamol 5 mg or terbutaline 10 mg via an oxygen-driven nebulizer. Make a rapid assessment of the severity of the attack.** Is the patient fully conscious? Can he or she talk in complete sentences or just gasped words? Check peak flow, respiratory rate, arterial oxygen saturation, pulse rate and blood pressure. Listen over the lungs.

2 **Is the attack life-threatening?** Any of the following signs indicates a life-threatening asthmatic attack:

- Silent chest, cyanosis, feeble respiratory effort.
- Bradycardia or hypotension.
- Exhaustion, confusion or coma.
- Peak flow < 30% of predicted (p. 487) or previous best.

If one or more of these signs is present, put in an IV cannula, attach an ECG monitor and:

- Call an anaesthetist in case urgent ventilation is needed.
- Add ipratropium 0.5 mg to the nebulizer solution.
- Give hydrocortisone 200 mg IV.
- Give aminophylline 250 mg IV over 20 min (but not if the patient is already taking an oral theophylline) or salbutamol 250 µg IV over 10 min followed by an infusion (Table 22.1).

3 **Check blood gases if there are any features of a life-threatening attack or if arterial oxygen saturation is less than 92%.** In other

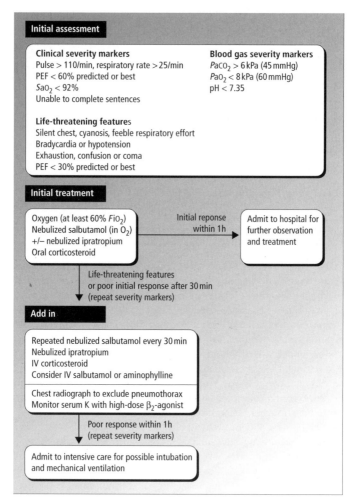

Initial assessment

Clinical severity markers
Pulse > 110/min, respiratory rate > 25/min
PEF < 60% predicted or best
Sao_2 < 92%
Unable to complete sentences

Blood gas severity markers
$Paco_2$ > 6 kPa (45 mmHg)
Pao_2 < 8 kPa (60 mmHg)
pH < 7.35

Life-threatening features
Silent chest, cyanosis, feeble respiratory effort
Bradycardia or hypotension
Exhaustion, confusion or coma
PEF < 30% predicted or best

Initial treatment

Oxygen (at least 60% Fio_2)
Nebulized salbutamol (in O_2)
+/– nebulized ipratropium
Oral corticosteroid

Initial reponse
within 1 h

Admit to hospital for
further observation
and treatment

Life-threatening features
or poor initial response after 30 min
(repeat severity markers)

Add in

Repeated nebulized salbutamol every 30 min
Nebulized ipratropium
IV corticosteroid
Consider IV salbutamol or aminophylline

Chest radiograph to exclude pneumothorax
Monitor serum K with high-dose β_2-agonist

Poor response within 1 h
(repeat severity markers)

Admit to intensive care for possible intubation
and mechanical ventilation

Fig. 22.1 Management of acute asthma. Adapted from international and UK guidelines. Reference: Lipworth BJ. Treatment of acute asthma. *Lancet* 1997; **350** (suppl II): 18–23.

Table 22.1 Bronchodilator infusions in acute severe asthma

Aminophylline
Loading dose: 250 mg IV over 20 min. Omit if the patient has been taking oral
    theophylline
Maintenance dose: 0.5 mg/kg/h by IV infusion. For an average-sized adult, add
    250 mg to 1 L of normal saline and infuse over 8 h. If you cannot check levels,
    halve the dose in patients with congestive heart failure or liver disease
Therapeutic range: 10–20 mg/L; nausea and vomiting are common toxic effects

Salbutamol
Add 5 mg (5 mL of 1 mg/mL solution) to 500 mL normal saline or 5% dextrose, giving
    a salbutamol concentration of 10 μg/mL
Loading dose: 250 μg (25 mL) IV over 10 min
Maintenance dose: start at 10 μg (1 mL)/min, increasing up to 30 μg (3mL)/min if
    needed
Check plasma potassium: hypokalaemia may occur

patients, arterial blood gases need not be checked (and to do so unnecessarily may deter asthmatics from seeking attention promptly for acute attacks). Arrange a chest X-ray to exclude pneumonia or pneumothorax.

4 **If the patient is not improving within 15–30 min:**
   • Give nebulized salbutamol more frequently up to every 15–30 min.
   • Add ipratropium 0.5 mg to the nebulizer solution and repeat 6-hly.
   • Give hydrocortisone 200 mg IV.
   • Consider upper airways obstruction (stridor, laryngeal oedema, raised $Paco_2$) and other causes of breathlessness (p. 60).
5 **If the patient is still not improving:**
   • Start an aminophylline infusion (unless the patient is taking an oral theophylline).

(for a small patient, give aminophylline 750 mg over 24 h; for a large patient, aminophylline 1500 mg in 24 h), or a salbutamol infusion (Table 22.1 p. 195).

• Transfer to the ITU if there is: deteriorating peak flow, worsening or persistent hypoxia or hypercapnia, or the patient is clearly exhausted.

Further management

1 Admit or discharge?
• The patient can be discharged after observation for 1 h if, after treatment with one nebulizer, the peak flow is > 75% of predicted or best known, and the exacerbation is isolated (e.g. caused by a failure to take medication). If in doubt, admit.

2 Otherwise admit to a ward where the patient can be adequately observed
• Start oral prednisolone 30–50 mg daily.
• Continue 35–60% humidified oxygen via a controlled delivery mask. Increase if necessary to keep arterial Po_2 around 10 kPa (75 mmHg).
• Continue nebulized salbutamol 2.5–5 mg (nebule or 0.5–1 mL of nebulizer solution diluted to 3 mL in normal saline) 4-hly.
• Ensure a fluid intake of 2–3 L/day given IV if necessary.

3 Monitoring
• Peak flow should be measured initially every 30 min to 1 h and after improvement every 6 h.
• Arterial gases should be rechecked if the peak flow is not improving; if $Paco_2$ was above 5 kPa on admission (recheck 20–30 min after institution of treatment); or if the patient's clinical condition worsens.
• Theophylline levels should be checked if an aminophylline infusion continues for > 24 h. The therapeutic range for theophylline is 10–20 mg/L.
• Check electrolytes the day after admission. Salbutamol and steroids may result in significant hypokalaemia. Give potassium supplements if the plasma level is < 3.5 mmol/L.

4 Antibiotics

• Only a minority of asthma attacks are provoked by bacterial infection and antibiotics are not routinely required.

• Give antibiotics as for pneumonia (p. 211) if there is focal shadowing on the chest X-ray or fever or purulent sputum.

5 If the patient is not improving or deteriorates

• Add ipratropium, aminophylline or IV salbutamol as above.

• Check that prednisolone has been started and IV hydrocortisone given.

• Exclude severe hypokalaemia.

• Get a chest X-ray to exclude pneumonia or pneumothorax.

• Seek advice from a chest physician.

6 Planning the discharge

• Switch from nebulized to inhaled bronchodilator therapy when peak flow is > 75% of predicted or best. Discharge if peak flow remains stable at or above this level, with < 25% diurnal variation in the 24 h before discharge, with the patient on the same medication that will be taken at home.

• Start inhaled steroid at least 24 h before discharge and check inhaler technique.

• Oral prednisolone should be given until the acute attack has completely resolved (no sleep disturbance, normal effort tolerance, and peak flow >80% of predicted normal or previous best). As a rule of thumb, steroids should be continued for double the length of time it takes for peak flow to return to this level, to a maximum of 21 days.

• Make sure the patient has a peak flow meter and written plan of management. Arrange follow-up with the primary care physician 1 week after discharge, and in the Chest Clinic within 4 weeks.

Patients with chronic obstructive pulmonary disease (COPD) are prone to acute tracheobronchitis, with worsening of respiratory symptoms. The working diagnosis of an acute exacerbation is based on the presence of:

• Increased breathlessness, wheeze and chest tightness.

• Increased cough, sputum volume and purulence.

Respiratory failure, with hypoxaemia and/or acute respiratory acidosis, is the major complication.

Priorities

1 Give **oxygen 28%** and **salbutamol 5 mg plus ipratropium 500 µg (via an air-driven nebulizer)** while you make a rapid clinical assessment of the patient (Table 23.1). Check **arterial blood gases** (within 1 h of starting oxygen) and arrange a **chest X-ray**. Other investigations are given in Table 23.2.

2 **If the patient is severely ill and does not respond to nebulized salbutamol and ipratropium:**

• Review the chest X-ray. Is there focal shadowing indicative of **pneumonia** (in which case start appropriate antibiotic therapy (p. 211)) or a **pneumothorax**? If a pneumothorax is present, an intercostal tube drain should be placed (p. 455).

• Give **aminophylline** 250 mg IV over 20 min (but not if the patient is already taking a theophylline). Follow this with an infusion of aminophylline 750–1500 mg over 24 h, according to body size.

• Give **hydrocortisone** 200 mg IV.

• Give an **antibiotic** IV (coamoxiclav, cefuroxime or cefotaxime (p. 211)).

Table 23.1 Clinical assessment of the patient with an acute exacerbation of chronic obstructive pulmonary disease (COPD)

History
Breathlessness: usual and recent change
Wheeze: usual and recent change
Sputum: usual volume/purulence and recent change
Effort tolerance: usual (e.g. ability to cope with activities of daily living unaided; distance walked on the flat; number of stairs climbed without stopping) and recent change
Previous acute exacerbations requiring hospital admission/ventilation
Previous lung function tests and arterial blood gases (from the notes): an FEV_1 60–80% of predicted signifies mild COPD; 40–60%, moderate COPD; less than 40%, severe COPD
Requirement for home nebulized bronchodilator and/or oxygen therapy
Concurrent illness, especially cardiac

Examination
Conscious level
Respiratory rate
Use of accessory muscles of respiration
Paradoxical abdominal breathing
Arterial oxygen saturation
Pulse rate, blood pressure, JVP, peripheral oedema
Peak expiratory flow rate
Lung signs
Peripheral oedema

Acute exacerbation of COPD

3 If there are clinical signs of **impending respiratory arrest** (feeble respiratory efforts, deteriorating conscious level), consider **endotracheal intubation and mechanical ventilation** (Table 23.3).
  • Get help urgently from an ITU physician or anaesthetist.
  • The decision for mechanical ventilation must take into account the functional capacity prior to the exacerbation, the likelihood of

Table 23.2 Investigation in acute exacerbation of COPD

Chest X-ray (check for focal shadowing indicative of pneumonia or pneumothorax)
Arterial blood gases and pH
ECG
Sputum culture
Blood culture if febrile or focal shadowing on chest X-ray
Creatinine, sodium, potassium and glucose
Full blood count

improvement with treatment (better if there is a clearly defined cause for the acute exacerbation), and the wishes of patient if these are known.

4 If there is **respiratory failure** (Pao_2 <7.5–8 kPa, Sao_2 <88–90% despite oxygen, or pHa <7.35), but mechanical ventilation is not indicated or appropriate, consider **non-invasive positive pressure ventilation (NIPPV)**. If mechanical ventilation is not appropriate and NIPPV not available, a doxapram infusion can be used as a last resort (Table 23.3). Discuss this with a chest or ITU physician.

Doxapram should be given as follows:
- Start the infusion at 1 mL/min (a 500-mL bottle contains 2 mg/mL in 5% dextrose).
- Check arterial blood gases and pH after 1 h.
- If Pao_2 remains <6.5 kPa or pHa < 7.25, increase the infusion rate to the maximum of 2 mL/min.

Further management

This consists of bronchodilator therapy, controlled oxygen, antibiotics and corticosteroids. Physiotherapy is of little value unless sputum is copious (>25 mL/day) or there is mucus plugging with lobar atelectasis.

Acute exacerbation of COPD

Table 23.3 Ventilatory support in acute exacerbations of COPD complicated by severe respiratory failure

Method	Indications	Contraindications	Comments
Non-invasive positive pressure ventilation (NIPPV)	PaO_2 <7.5–8 kPa despite supplemental oxygen Arterial pH <7.35	Decreased conscious level Respiratory rate <12/min Arterial pH <7.25 Copious secretions Orofacial abnormalities which prevent fitting of the mask	Around 20% of patients cannot tolerate NIPPV If arterial pH is <7.3, admit to ITU. Consider mechanical ventilation if no improvement in arterial pH and other variables within 1–2 h of starting NIPPV
Endotracheal intubation and mechanical ventilation	Impending respiratory arrest Deteriorating conscious level PaO_2 <7.5–8 kPa despite supplemental oxygen Arterial pH <7.25 Inability to protect airway or to clear copious secretions	Known severe COPD with severely impaired functional capacity and/or severe comorbidity Patient has expressed wish not to be ventilated	Potential complications of barotrauma, infection and inability to wean some patients from the ventilator
Doxapram	PaO_2 <7.5–8 kPa despite supplemental oxygen Arterial pH <7.35 NIPPV not available and mechanical ventilation not appropriate	Respiratory rate >20/min	Has not been proved to improve survival or reduce the need for mechanical ventilation

1 Bronchodilator therapy
- Salbutamol 2.5–5.0 mg by nebulizer up to 4-hly; and/or
- ipratropium 500 μg by nebulizer up to 4-hly;
- switch from nebulized to inhaled bronchodilator therapy when the patient is no longer needing supplemental oxygen.

2 Controlled oxygen
- Give oxygen if Sao_2 on air is $< 90\%/Pao_2 < 8$ kPa ($Sao_2 < 88\%$, $Pao_2 < 7.5$ kPa if known chronic respiratory failure).
- Start with an inspired oxygen of 28% (or 2 L/min by nasal prongs).
- Check arterial gases and pH 1 h after starting oxygen.
- Increase the inspired oxygen to 35% if Pao_2 is <7.5 kPa (<6.5 kPa if known chronic respiratory failure).
- If this oxygen level cannot be attained, or arterial pH falls below 7.35, consider assisted ventilation (Table 23.3): ask advice from a chest physician.

3 Antibiotics
- Are indicated if there is evidence of infection, as shown by fever, or increased sputum volume and purulence.
- Initial therapy is with amoxycillin 500 mg 8-hly PO. If the patient is allergic to penicillin or has received a penicillin in the previous month, use trimethoprim 200 mg 12-hly PO or ciprofloxacin 500 mg 12-hly PO. Modify therapy in the light of sputum and blood culture results. Give a 7-day course.
- If there is no response to amoxycillin, consider using coamoxiclav or ciprofloxacin. In ill patients, use cefuroxime or cefotaxime IV.

5 Corticosteroids
- Give prednisolone 30 mg daily for 7–10 days.

6 Planning the discharge
The following criteria should be met before discharge:
- Clinically stable off IV therapy for > 24 h.
- Bronchodilator therapy needed no more than 6-hly, with the patient on the same medication (nebulized or inhaled) that will be taken at home.
- Able to walk at least short distances unaided.

• Social support at home organized.
• Follow-up arranged in 4–6 weeks, preferably with a chest physician.

Problems

The patient is not improving despite treatment
Possibilities include:
• **Wrong diagnosis**: consider pneumonia, pulmonary embolism and pulmonary oedema. Other causes of respiratory failure with raised $Pa\text{CO}_2$ are given in Table 23.4.
• **Missed pneumothorax.**
• **Inadequately treated infection**. Consider changing to cefuroxime or cefotaxime IV and adding a macrolide.
• **Inadequate bronchodilator therapy.** Check that nebulizers are being run at the correct flow rate. Nebulized salbutamol and ipratropium can be given 2-hly if necessary, or salbutamol can be given by IV infusion 5–30 µg/min (see p. 195).

Cor pulmonale
• Fluid retention with peripheral oedema may occur in patients with COPD complicated by acute or chronic respiratory failure even without right ventricular dysfunction.
• The diagnosis of cor pulmonale is made from a raised JVP, enlarged cardiac silhouette on the chest X-ray, and ECG evidence of right ventricular hypertrophy (not an invariable feature).
• Obtain an echocardiogram to confirm right ventricular dysfunction, estimate pulmonary artery pressures and exclude left ventricular or aortic/mitral valve disease.
• Treat fluid retention with a diuretic. There is no definite evidence for the use of digoxin (unless indicated for rate control in atrial fibrillation) or ACE inhibitors in cor pulmonale.
• Resistant cor pulmonale raises the suspicion of obstructive sleep apnoea.

Arrhythmias
• Supraventricular arrhythmias are common in acute exacerbations of COPD.

Table 23.4 Causes of type II (ventilatory) respiratory failure (with high Pa_{CO_2} and low Pa_{O_2})

Site of lesion	Causes
Brain	Stroke
	Mass lesion with brainstem compression
	Encephalitis
	Sedative drugs
	Status epilepticus
Spinal cord	Cord compression
	Transverse myelitis
	Poliomyelitis, rabies
Peripheral nerve	Guillain–Barré syndrome
	Critical illness polyneuropathy
	Toxins
	Acute intermittent porphyria
	Vasculitis, e.g. SLE
	Diphtheria
Neuromuscular junction	Myasthenia gravis
	Eaton–Lambert syndrome
	Botulism
	Toxins
Muscle	Hypokalaemia
	Hypophosphataemia
	Rhabdomyolysis
Thoracic cage and pleura	Crushed chest
	Morbid obesity
	Kyphoscoliosis
	Ankylosing spondylitis
Lungs and airways	Upper airways obstruction
	Severe acute asthma
	Chronic obstructive pulmonary disease
	Severe pneumonia
	Severe pulmonary oedema

• Check plasma potassium: salbutamol and steroids may result in significant hypokalaemia. Give potassium replacement if plasma potassium is <3.5 mmol/L (p. 346).

• Treat atrial fibrillation/flutter with digoxin, combined if needed with verapamil or diltiazem (p. 27).

• Treat multifocal atrial tachycardia with verapamil if the ventricular rate is >110/min. DC cardioversion is ineffective (p. 31).

Acute exacerbation of COPD

24 Pneumonia

• Pneumonia usually presents with acute respiratory symptoms, but should always be considered in patients with unexplained sepsis or confusional state.

• Examination of the chest may be normal and, if you suspect pneumonia, a chest X-ray is needed.

Priorities

Make a clinical assessment of the patient and arrange urgent investigation (Table 24.1).

You need to answer four questions:

• Is this pneumonia?
• How severe is the pneumonia?
• What is the background?
• What should be your initial antibiotic therapy?

1 Is this pneumonia?

• Suspect pneumonia if there are acute respiratory symptoms (cough, purulent sputum, pleuritic chest pain or breathlessness) and fever. Associated non-respiratory symptoms (e.g. confusion, upper abdominal pain, diarrhoea) are common and may dominate the picture.

• Examination shows abnormal chest signs in 80% of patients with pneumonia (most often an increased respiratory rate (> 20/min) and focal crackles).

• Other diagnoses to consider, especially in patients with atypical features or who fail to respond to antibiotic therapy, are given in Table 24.2.

Table 24.1 Investigation of the patient with suspected pneumonia

Urgent (in all patients)
Chest X-ray*
Arterial blood gases and pH
Blood culture (x2)
Sputum (if available) for Gram stain and culture
Full blood count
Creatinine and electrolytes

Later (in selected patients)
Ziehl–Neelsen stain of sputum (*M. tuberculosis*)
Urine antigen test (*Legionella*)
HIV serology (with informed consent)
Serological testing (acute/convalescent) (*Mycoplasma*, *Legionella*)
Bronchoscopy (Table 24.6) and bronchoalveolar lavage

* The presence of focal shadowing on the chest X-ray is required to make the diagnosis of pneumonia, although this may initially be absent in patients who are severely neutropenic or hypovolaemic, and in early *Pneumocystis carinii* pneumonia. Other features to look for are: pleural effusion — if present, aspirate a sample and send for Gram stain and culture; cavitation, which is especially associated with tuberculosis and *Staphylococcus aureus* infection, but may also occur with Gram-negative and anaerobic infections; pneumothorax, which may occur in cavitating pneumonias and is particularly associated with *Pneumocystis carinii* pneumonia.

2 How severe is the pneumonia?

Features which indicate severe pneumonia are given in Table 24.3.
Admit the patient to ITU if any of the following are present:

- Respiratory rate > 30/min or exhaustion.
- Pa_{O_2} < 8 kPa (60 mmHg) despite breathing 60% oxygen.
- Pa_{CO_2} > 6 kPa (45 mmHg).
- Acidosis (arterial pH < 7.3).
- Hypotension (systolic BP < 90 mmHg) not responsive to IV fluid.

Table 24.2 Differential diagnosis of pneumonia

Pulmonary embolism
Pulmonary oedema (cardiogenic and non-cardiogenic (ARDS))
Bronchial carcinoma
Pulmonary vasculitis
Pulmonary haemorrhage
Acute extrinsic allergic alveolitis
Organizing pneumonitis
Sub-diaphragmatic abscess

Table 24.3 Features of severe community-acquired pneumonia

Clinical
Age >60
Underlying chronic lung disease or other chronic illness
Confusion
Systolic BP <90 mmHg or diastolic BP <60 mmHg
Respiratory rate >30/min
Extrapulmonary site of infection

Investigation
White cell count <4 or >20 x 10^9/L
Renal impairment (creatinine >120 μmol/L or urea >7 mmol/L)
Pao_2 <6.6 kPa breathing air
Acidosis
Atrial fibrillation
Multilobe involvement or significant pleural effusion on chest X-ray
Bacteraemia
Albumin <35 g/L

• Other organ failure or disseminated intravascular coagulation (suspect DIC if the platelet count is $< 100 \times 10^{12}/L$ (p. 104)).

3 What is the background?

A wide range of microbes may cause pneumonia, *Streptococcus pneumoniae* being the commonest. The setting of the pneumonia has a strong influence on the possible causes in an individual patient, and this will influence your choice of initial antibiotic therapy. Gram-negative rods, *S. aureus*, anaerobic bacteria and *Chlamydia pneumoniae* are more often the cause of pneumonia in hospital or nursing-home residents than in community-acquired pneumonia. Other points to consider are:

• Does the patient have **chronic obstructive pulmonary disease** (*S. pneumoniae, H. influenzae, Moxarella catarrhalis, Legionella* species) or **bronchiectasis** or **cystic fibrosis** (*Pseudomonas* species, *S. aureus)?*

• Has pneumonia followed **influenza** (*S. pneumoniae, S. aureus, S. pyogenes, H. influenzae*)?

• Is the patient **at risk of aspiration** because of a reduced conscious level or disordered swallowing (see Appendix) (anaerobic bacteria)

• Does the patient have **HIV** infection (see p. 381) (*Pneumocystis carinii, S. pneumoniae, H. influenzae, M. tuberculosis*)?

• Has there been recent **travel abroad** or hotel stay (*Legionella pneumophila*)?

• Has the patient had contact with **birds** (*Chlamydia psittaci*) or with **farm animals or cats** (*Coxiella burnetii*)?

• Is there a background of **chronic alcohol abuse** (*S. pneumoniae*, Gram-negative rods, *M. tuberculosis*) or **IV drug use** (*S. aureus*, anaerobic bacteria, *M. tuberculosis*)?

4 What should be your initial antibiotic therapy?

• Your initial therapy depends on the clinical setting and severity of the illness, and Gram stain of the sputum, if a specimen is available. Start antibiotic therapy as soon as blood has been taken for culture.

• To be a reliable guide to the selection of antibiotic, the sputum smear should have >25 polymorphonuclear leucocytes and <10 epithelial cells per low-power field, and >8–10 organisms compatible with a likely pulmonary pathogen per high-power field. Gram-positive diplococci suggest pneumococcal infection, Gram-positive cocci in clusters *S. aureus*, and Gram-negative pleomorphic coccobacilli *H. influenzae*.

• Antibiotics can be given orally unless the pneumonia is severe or there is vomiting.

• Choices for initial therapy of typical community- and hospital/nursing-home-acquired pneumonia are given in Tables 24.4 and 24.5.

Further management

1 Oxygen: humidified oxygen should be continued until Pao_2 is > 8 kPa (60 mmHg) with the patient breathing air, or O_2 saturation > 90%.

2 Fluid balance: insensible losses are greater than normal due to fever (allow 500 mL/day/°C) and tachypnoea. Patients with severe pneumonia should receive IV fluids (2–3 L/day) with a daily check of creatinine and electrolytes if abnormal on admission. Monitor the CVP if the patient is oliguric or if plasma creatinine is >200 µmol/L.

3 Analgesia for pleuritic pain: give paracetamol or an NSAID such as ibuprofen.

4 Physiotherapy: physiotherapy is indicated if patients are producing sputum but having trouble expectorating it, and in patients with bronchiectasis. Nebulized normal saline may also be helpful when sputum is thick and difficult to expectorate.

5 Bronchodilator therapy with nebulized salbutamol or ipratropium should be given to patients with chronic obstructive pulmonary disease or asthma (p. 198).

6 Antibiotic therapy. If IV therapy was started on admission, oral therapy can be substituted at 48–72 h, provided that the patient is improving and there is no vomiting or diarrhoea. Modify your initial therapy in the light of culture/serology results; if in doubt, ask advice from a microbiologist.

• Pneumococcal pneumonia: treat until afebrile for 3 days.

• Mycoplasmal, *Legionella* or *Chlamydia pneumoniae* pneumonias: treat for at least 2 weeks.

Table 24.4 Initial antibiotic therapy of community-acquired pneumonia

| Severity/Regimen | Comorbidity (chronic lung, cardiovascular, neurological, renal or liver disease, or diabetes mellitus) | |
	Absent	Present
Non-severe – Preferred	Amoxycillin 0.5–1.0 g 8-hly PO or Ampicillin 0.5 g 6-hly IV or Benzylpenicillin 1.2 g 6-hly IV	Amoxycillin/clavulanate 625 mg 8-hly PO or 1.2 g 8-hly IV
– Alternative	Erythromycin 250–500 mg 6-hly PO or IV	Clarithromycin 250–500 mg 12-hly PO or Sparfloxacin 200–400 mg daily PO or Cefuroxime 750 mg 8-hly IV
Severe – Preferred	Amoxycillin/clavulanate 1.2 g 8-hly IV and Erythromycin 0.5–1.0 g 6-hly IV or clarithromycin 0.5 g 12-hly IV and Rifampicin 600 mg 12-hly PO or IV	Cefotaxime 1 g 8-hly IV or ceftriaxone 2 g daily IV and Erythromycin 0.5–1.0 g 6-hly IV or clarithromycin 0.5 g 12-hly IV and Rifampicin 600 mg 12-hly PO or IV
– Alternative	Cefuroxime 1.5 g 8-hly IV and Erythromycin 0.5–1.0 g 6-hly IV or clarithromycin 0.5 g 12-hly IV and Rifampicin 600 mg 12-hly PO or IV	Meropenem 0.5 g 8-hly IV and Erythromycin 0.5–1.0 g 6-hly IV or clarithromycin 0.5 g 12-hly IV and Rifampicin 600 mg 12-hly PO or IV

Pneumonia

Reference: Finch R. Community acquired pneumonia. *Journal of Royal College of Physicians* 1998; **32**: 328–32.

Table 24.5 Initial antibiotic therapy of hospital- or nursing-home-acquired pneumonia

Non-severe	Severe	At risk of *Pseudomonas* infection (ITU-acquired or bronchiectasis/cystic fibrosis or immunocompromised)
Preferred: Amoxycillin/clavulanate 625 mg 8-hly PO or 1.2 g 8-hly IV	*Preferred:* Cefotaxime 1 g 8-hly IV or Ceftriaxone 2 g daily IV *and* Erythromycin 0.5–1.0 g 6-hly IV or clarithromycin 0.5 g 12-hly IV *and* Rifampicin 600 mg 12-hly PO or IV	*Preferred:* Antipseudomonal penicillin (azlocillin or piperacillin) *and* Erythromycin 0.5–1.0 g 6-hly IV or Clarithromycin 0.5 g 12-hly IV *and* Aminoglycoside (gentamicin or netilmicin)
Alternative: Clarithromycin 250–500 mg 12-hly PO or Sparfloxacin 200–400 mg daily PO or Cefuroxime 750 mg 8-hly IV	*Alternative:* Meropenem 0.5 g 8-hly IV *and* Erythromycin 0.5–1.0 g 6-hly IV or Clarithromycin 0.5 g 12-hly IV *and* Rifampicin 600 mg 12-hly PO or IV	*Alternative:* Meropenem 0.5 g 8-hly IV *and* Erythromycin 0.5–1.0 g 6-hly IV or clarithromycin 0.5 g 12-hly IV *and* Aminoglycoside (gentamicin or netilmicin)

Problems

The patient is no better despite 48 h of antibiotic therapy

Address the following points:

1 Review the clinical, microbiological and radiological findings. Are you confident the diagnosis is pneumonia, and that the patient's current antibiotic therapy is appropriate for the possible pathogens?

• Re-examine the patient, and check for signs of metastatic infection, such as septic arthritis, pericarditis or endocarditis.

• Repeat the chest X-ray. Are there any new findings such as cavitation or pleural effusion? If pleural fluid is now present, this should be aspirated and sent for Gram stain and culture. If the fluid is cloudy rather than mildly turbid, drain completely and treat as empyema (discuss with a chest physician). A pH < 7 also favours empyema rather than a parapneumonic effusion.

2 Consider underlying airways or lung disease, such as chronic obstructive pulmonary disease, bronchiectasis, bronchial carcinoma and inhaled foreign body.

3 Consider pulmonary tuberculosis. Send sputum for Ziehl–Neelsen stain. If no sputum is being produced, consider fibreoptic bronchoscopy. A Mantoux skin test (0.1 mL or 1 in 10 000 intradermally) may be performed, but interpretation can be difficult—a strongly positive test is good evidence of active infection, but a negative reaction can occur in the presence of active infection.

4 Consider HIV/AIDS. If HIV infection is possible, test for HIV antibodies, with the patient's informed consent.

5 Consider non-infective causes of chest X-ray shadowing, such as pulmonary infarction, pulmonary oedema or bronchial carcinoma (**Table 24.2**).

6 Consider broadening your antibiotic therapy, in case the organism is unusual or resistant.

7 Ask advice from a chest physician. Fibreoptic bronchoscopy (Table 24.6) may be indicated.

The postoperative patient: pneumonia or pulmonary embolism?

Acute dyspnoea and fever are features of both. Pneumonia is favoured by an initial fever > 39°C, white cell count > 15×10^9/L and purulent

Table 24.6 Indications for fibreoptic bronchoscopy in the patient with pneumonia

Early bronchoscopy
Suspected foreign body inhalation
No organism identified from blood or sputum and patient not responding to initial
    antibiotic therapy (especially in immunocompromised patient or if tuberculosis is
    suspected)
Cavitating pneumonia with negative sputum microscopy and culture
Lobar or segmental collapse with significant hypoxia

Late bronchoscopy
Persistent (>1 week) segmental or lobar collapse
Slow resolution of symptoms and signs (chest X-ray shadowing may take up to 6
    weeks to clear completely)
Recurrent pneumonia at the same site

sputum. If you remain uncertain, treat for both conditions until a ventilation/perfusion scan can be done. See p. 183 for further management of pulmonary embolism.

Appendix

Aspiration (inhalation) pneumonia
• Is a consequence of material from the stomach or upper respiratory tract entering the lower airways (Table 24.7).
• Suspect aspiration if pneumonia develops in patients with disordered swallowing or after a period of reduced consciousness, or if anaerobic infection is found. Common clinical settings for aspiration pneumonia are cardiopulmonary resuscitation; stroke; poisoning with alcohol or psychotropic drugs; and diabetic ketoacidosis.
• If aspiration occurred when the patient was supine, the pneumonia typically involves the superior segments of the lower lobes and pos-

Table 24.7 Characteristics of different forms of aspiration pneumonia

Inoculum	Pulmonary sequelae	Clinical features	Therapy
Acid	Chemical pneumonitis	Acute dyspnoea, tachypnoea, possible cyanosis, bronchospasm, fever, pink frothy sputum, infiltrates in one or both lower lobes, hypoxaemia	Positive-pressure breathing, IV fluids, tracheal suction
Oropharyngeal bacteria	Bacterial infection	Usually insidious onset; cough, fever, purulent sputum, infiltrate involving dependent pulmonary segment or lobe, with or without cavitation	Antibiotic therapy
Inert fluids	Mechanical obstruction, reflex airway closure	Acute dyspnoea, cyanosis, pulmonary oedema	Tracheal suction, intermittent positive-pressure breathing with oxygen, bronchodilator
Particulate matter	Mechanical obstruction	Dependent on level of obstruction, ranging from acute apnoea to chronic cough with or without recurrent infections	Extraction of particulate matter, antibiotic therapy

Reference: Bartlett JG et al. Community-acquired pneumonia in adults: guidelines for management. *Clinical Infectious Diseases* 1998; **26:** 811–38.

Pneumonia

terior segments of the upper lobes; if aspiration occurred in the upright position, one or both lower lobes may be involved.

• Antibiotic therapy needs to cover a broad range of aerobic and anaerobic bacteria. Options for initial treatment (before culture results are known) are amoxycillin/clavulanate or a fluoroquinolone plus clindamycin or metronidazole.

• If you suspect aspiration pneumonia, discuss with a chest physician as to whether bronchoscopy should be done to remove particulate matter from the airways.

25 Pneumothorax

Consider the diagnosis in any patient with:
- sudden breathlessness or chest pain, particularly in young, otherwise fit adults and following invasive procedures, e.g. subclavian vein puncture, lung biopsy, chest aspiration;
- acute exacerbations of chronic obstructive pulmonary disease (or rarely asthma): pneumothorax may be painless and contribute to respiratory failure;
- hypoxia or an increase in inflation pressure if mechanically ventilated: asymmetry of chest expansion is a useful clue.

Priorities

If the patient has signs of a pneumothorax and there is imminent cardiorespiratory arrest, treat as tension pneumothorax:
- Insert the largest cannula to hand into the 2nd intercostal space in the mid-clavicular line on the side with absent or reduced breath sounds. If air rushes out, leave the cannula in place until a chest drain is inserted.
- Insert an intercostal drain immediately (p. 455).

Further management

1 Obtain a chest X-ray
Do not mistake an emphysematous bulla for a small pneumothorax. Points in favour of a bulla are:
- adhesions between the lung and the parietal pleura;
- a scallop-shaped edge to the cavity;
- faint markings over the lucency caused by the lung enfolding the bulla;
- the presence of other bullae.

If you suspected a pneumothorax, but the chest X-ray appears normal, recheck the lung apices and the right border of the heart. In the supine patient look for:
• unusually sharp appearance of the cardiac border or diaphragm with increased transradiancy of the adjacent parts of the thorax and abdomen;
• a vertical line parallel to the chest wall (caused by retraction of the middle lobe from the chest wall);
• a diagonal line from the heart to the costophrenic angle.

2 Assess the respiratory status of the patient

Check oxygen saturation. Check arterial blood gases in severely breathless patients, those with underlying chronic lung disease, and if Sao_2 is < 92%.

3 Management options (Fig. 25.1)

If the pneumothorax is left alone or managed by needle aspiration (Table 25.1):
• Advise the patient to return to hospital if breathlessness recurs, and to avoid air travel until the chest X-ray is normal.
• Arrange a further chest X-ray with clinical review in 7–10 days.

Table 25.1 Needle aspiration of a small pneumothorax

1 Identify the 3rd–4th intercostal space in the mid-axillary line
2 Infiltrate with lignocaine down to and around the pleura over the pneumothorax
3 Connect a 21 G (green) needle to a three-way tap and a 60 mL syringe
4 With the patient semirecumbent, insert the needle into the pleural space. Withdraw air and expel it via the three-way tap
5 Obtain a chest X-ray to confirm resolution of the pneumothorax

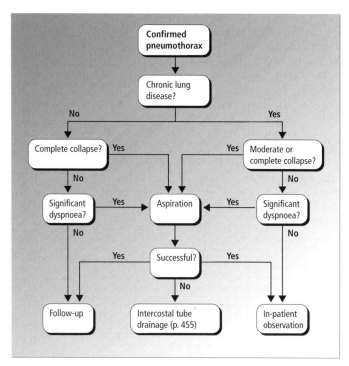

Fig. 25.1 Management of pneumothorax. Degree of collapse: small, rim of air around lung; moderate, lung collapsed halfway towards heart border; complete, airless lung separated from diaphragm.

Needle aspiration: see Table 25.1. Intercostal tube drainage: see p. 455.

Reference: Miller AC, Harvey JE. Guidelines for the management of spontaneous pneumothorax. *British Medical Journal* 1993; **307**: 114–16.

4 Surgical advice should be sought

• if there are bilateral pneumothoraces;

• the lung fails to re-expand on intercostal tube drainage;

• there is a history of one or more previous pneumothoraces on the same side as the current episode;

• there is a history of pneumothorax on the other side.

5 If the patient is over 30 or has other respiratory symptoms

The pneumothorax may be secondary to underlying lung disease
(Table 25.2): ask the opinion of a chest physician.

• Chronic obstructive pulmonary disease and *Pneumocystis carinii*
pneumonia related to HIV infection are the most common causes of
secondary pneumothorax.

Table 25.2 Causes of pneumothorax

Spontaneous
Primary
   No clinical lung disease
   Typically occurs in tall thin males aged 10–30
   Rare in patients over 40

Secondary
   Airways disease (COPD, cystic fibrosis, acute severe asthma)
   Infectious lung disease (*Pneumocystis carinii* pneumonia; necrotizing pneumonia
     caused by anaerobic, Gram-negative bacteria or *Staphylococcus*)
   Interstitial lung disease (e.g. sarcoidosis)
   Connective tissue disease (e.g. rheumatoid arthritis, Marfan syndrome)
   Malignancy (bronchial carcinoma or sarcoma)
   Thoracic endometriosis

Traumatic (due to penetrating or blunt chest trauma)

Iatrogenic
Transthoracic needle aspiration
Subclavian vein puncture
Thoracocentesis and pleural biopsy
Barotrauma related to mechanical ventilation

Reference: Sahn SA, Heffner JE. Spontaneous pneumothorax. *New England Journal
of Medicine* 2000; **342**: 868–74.

26 Haemoptysis

• Every patient presenting with haemoptysis should have the cause established (Table 26.1). If the diagnosis is not clear, refer to a chest physician for further investigation.

• **Haemoptysis can be distinguished from haematemesis** by its colour and pH: haemoptysis is bright red and alkaline; haematemesis is brown and acid. **Bleeding from the nasopharynx** may be confused with haemoptysis: if in doubt, ask the advice of an ENT surgeon.

Priorities

Patients with massive haemoptysis (>1000 mL in 24 h)
There is a risk of death from drowning or exsanguination.

1 Call an anaesthetist: endotracheal intubation may be needed to allow suctioning of the airway and adequate ventilation. Meanwhile, lay the patient head down and give high-flow oxygen.

2 Put in a large-bore venous cannula and take blood for urgent cross-match and other investigation (Table 26.2).

3 Contact a thoracic surgeon for advice on further management. Bleeding may occasionally be stopped through a rigid bronchoscope, but usually requires resection of the bleeding segment or lobe.

Other patients

1 Investigation is given in Table 26.2. Further management is directed by the likely diagnosis.

2 It may not be necessary to admit the patient if the diagnosis is clear (e.g. bronchial carcinoma, bronchiectasis) and the patient is stable. Ask advice from a chest physician if you are in doubt. If you discharge the patient, make sure that early chest follow-up is arranged.

Table 26.1 Causes of haemoptysis

Cause	Comment
Bronchial carcinoma	Persistent blood-streaking of mucoid sputum; weight loss
Tuberculosis	Blood-streaking of purulent sputum; weight loss; fever
Bronchiectasis	Blood-streaking of copious purulent sputum; chronic sputum production; previous episodes of haemoptysis occurring over months or years
Acute bronchitis	Blood-streaking of mucopurulent sputum
Pneumonia	'Rusty' sputum; acute illness with fever and breathlessness; signs of consolidation
Lung abscess	Blood-streaking of purulent sputum; fever; pleuritic chest pain
Pulmonary infarction	Gross blood not mixed with sputum; pleuritic chest pain and breathlessness; at risk of deep-vein thrombosis
Pulmonary oedema	Frothy blood-tinged sputum; severe breathlessness; associated cardiac disease
Lung contusion	Preceding chest trauma
Mycetoma	Fungal ball on chest X-ray; previous pulmonary tuberculosis
Vascular malformation	Recurrent haemoptysis; Osler–Weber–Rendu syndrome with multiple telangiectasia
Bronchial adenoma	Recurrent haemoptysis in an otherwise well woman
Bleeding tendency	Haemoptysis following persistent coughing; bleeding from other sites
Pulmonary vasculitis	Wegener's granulomatosis (upper and lower respiratory tract involvement, ANCA +ve; Goodpasture syndrome (pulmonary and renal involvement, antiglomerular basement membrane antibodies +ve)
Eisenmenger syndrome	Cyanosis and clubbing
Other causes of pulmonary hypertension	Mitral stenosis; primary pulmonary hypertension

Table 26.2 Investigation of the patient with haemoptysis

Massive haemoptysis
Full blood count
Clotting screen
Urgent cross-match 6 units
Creatinine, sodium and potassium
Arterial blood gases
Chest X-ray when stable

Other patients
Chest X-ray
Arterial blood gases (if pleuritic chest pain or breathlessness, or $Sao_2 < 90\%$)
ECG
Sputum for Gram and Ziehl–Neelsen stains, culture and cytology
Full blood count
ESR and C-reactive protein
Anti-neutrophil cytoplasmic antibodies
Clotting screen if bleeding tendency suspected
Creatinine, sodium and potassium
Urinalysis

Further investigation
Bronchoscopy
Computed tomography of thorax
Echocardiography (to look for evidence of pulmonary hypertension and its causes)
Bronchial angiography (to identify site of bleeding; embolization may be indicated)

Haemoptysis

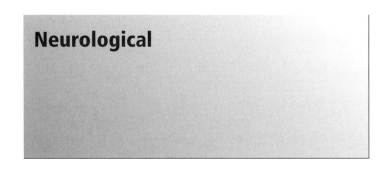

Neurological

27 Stroke

• The working diagnosis of stroke is based on the sudden or rapid onset of a focal neurological deficit likely to be due to vascular disease.

• Completed stroke is arbitrarily distinguished from transient ischaemic attack (Chapter 28) by the persistence of symptoms for > 24 h.

• About 80% of strokes are due to cerebral infarction. Headache, vomiting and coma at onset are more common in haemorrhagic stroke, but accurate differentiation requires computed tomography (CT). Establishing whether the stroke is due to infarction or haemorrhage is important as a guide to further management, including thrombolysis, and secondary prevention.

Priorities

1 If the patient is unconscious

Initial resuscitation is as for coma from any cause (Chapter 6). **Check blood glucose to exclude hyper- or hypoglycaemia.** Other investigations needed urgently are given in Table 27.1.

2 Is this a stroke and not some other illness which may mimic stroke?

Important features on history or examination are:

• History of trauma or alcohol abuse (? extradural or subdural haematoma (Appendix)).

• Progressive onset over days (? subdural haematoma, tumour).

• Fever (? brain abscess, meningitis, encephalitis, cerebral malaria, endocarditis, cerebral lupus).

• Neck stiffness (? meningitis, subarachnoid haemorrhage).

• Severe hypertension (diastolic pressure >120 mmHg) and papil-

Table 27.1 Urgent investigation of the patient with stroke

Blood glucose
Full blood count
INR if taking warfarin
Sickle solubility test if possible sickle cell disease (p. 409)
Creatinine and electrolytes
Blood culture (x 2) if febrile or endocarditis suspected
ECG (? atrial fibrillation, left ventricular hypertrophy, myocardial infarction)
Cranial CT (see text)
Echocardiography if suspected endocarditis, myxoma or aortic dissection

loedema with retinal haemorrhages and exudates (? hypertensive encephalopathy).

3 Is thrombolysis with alteplase indicated?

This treatment should only be considered in specialist centres. In practice, thrombolysis will be appropriate in few cases.

Indications are:
• Treatment within 3h of the onset of symptoms is possible (i.e. including the time needed to obtain a CT scan).
• Dense hemiparesis or other major neurological deficit.

Contraindications are:
• Cerebral haemorrhage.
• Early ischaemic signs on CT (a marker for risk of haemorrhagic transformation of a cerebral infarct).
• Severe hypertension and other major contraindications to thrombolysis (p. 141).

4 Where is the stroke?

The findings on examination are a guide (Table 27.2).

5 Is an urgent CT scan needed?

CT should be done urgently if:
• Thrombolysis is being considered.
• There is evidence of head injury.

Table 27.2 Clinical features of stroke according to site

Cerebral hemisphere
Higher cerebral dysfunction (e.g. dysphasia)
Homonymous visual field defect
Ipsilateral motor and/or sensory deficit

Brainstem
Ipsilateral cranial nerve palsy with contralateral motor and/or sensory deficit
Bilateral motor and/or sensory deficit
Disorder of conjugate eye movement
Cerebellar dysfunction

Lacunar infarction*
Pure motor hemiparesis
Pure sensory stroke
Ataxic hemiparesis (cerebellar and upper motor neuron signs in the same limbs)
Conscious level, higher cerebral functions and visual fields are normal

* Lacunar infarction is due to occlusion of a single perforating artery in the basal
ganglia or pons by lipo-hyalinosis or microatheroma.

- The patient is taking warfarin or has a bleeding tendency.
- The conscious level is deteriorating (if neurosurgical intervention to evacuate a haematoma or relieve obstructive hydrocephalus would be considered).
- Meningitis, encephalitis or brain abscess are possible diagnoses.
- The diagnosis of stroke is uncertain.

For other patients with suspected stroke, CT should be done within 48 h.

6 Does the stroke have a potentially treatable cause?

Further investigation is given in Table 27.3 and Fig. 27.1. Important diagnoses to consider are:

- Subarachnoid haemorrhage (Chapter 29).
- Cerebellar haematoma (see Appendix).
- Embolism from the heart (see Appendix).

Table 27.3 Further investigation after stroke (see also Fig. 27.1)

ESR (if raised, consider vasculitis, endocarditis, myxoma)
Cholesterol and triglycerides in patients aged < 50
Urinalysis (if abnormal, consider vasculitis or endocarditis)
Cranial CT (if not already done)
Chest X-ray (? cardiac enlargement)
Echocardiography if indicated (Table 27.4)

• Carotid or vertebral artery dissection (consider if there was preceding neck trauma (which may have been minor) or if ischaemic stroke is associated with ipsilateral craniocervical headache, Horner syndrome or pulsatile tinnitus; if suspected, discuss further management with a neurologist).
• Vaso-occlusive crisis of sickle cell disease (Chapter 51).
• Vasculitis (e.g. cranial arteritis, systemic lupus erythematosus).

Further management

Many therapies to improve the outcome in stroke have been tried, but none is of proved benefit except management in a stroke unit, aspirin and thrombolysis. Patients not admitted directly to a stroke unit should be transferred there for further management and rehabilitation when medically stable.

1 Aspirin for ischaemic stroke
Give 300 mg daily (orally, via nasogastric tube or rectally) for the first 14 days (International Stroke Trial regimen), then 75–150 mg daily.

2 Careful management of fluid balance
• The aim should be to avoid either dehydration (which may cause haemoconcentration and worsen cerebral blood flow) or fluid overload (possibly worsening cerebral oedema)).

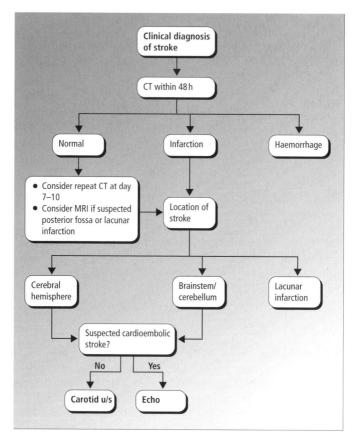

Fig. 27.1 Imaging after ischaemic stroke. CT, computed tomography; carotid u/s, duplex scan of carotid arteries; echo, echocardiography.

• If the patient is conscious, check if a small volume of water can be swallowed safely with the patient sitting upright. If so, fluids can be given by mouth.

• If the conscious level is depressed, if voluntary cough is weak or absent, or if water cannot be swallowed safely, oral fluids should not be given. Start an IV or subcutaneous infusion (usually 2 L in 24 h) or insert a fine-bore nasogastric tube.

• Use normal saline in the first 24 h. Dextrose should be avoided as a high blood glucose level may worsen prognosis.

3 Feeding
If the patient is unable to swallow safely by 4 days after the stroke, place a fine-bore nasogastric tube to allow feeding. If swallowing has not recovered by 2 weeks after the stroke, feeding via a percutaneous gastrostomy tube may be preferable.

4 When to treat hypertension?
• Acute treatment (within the first week) is not indicated unless there is hypertensive encephalopathy, aortic dissection or intracerebral haemorrhage with severe hypertension (systolic pressure > 230 mmHg or diastolic > 140 mmHg).

• If indicated, use intravenous labetolol or nitroprusside (p. 162) so that the dose can be titrated carefully.

• If the patient has been taking antihypertensive therapy, this should be continued.

5 Anticoagulation
• Deep vein thrombosis is a common complication. The incidence can be reduced by early mobilization and graded compression stockings. Low-dose subcutaneous heparin may result in haemorrhagic transformation of a cerebral infarct and should not routinely be used. Patients with cerebral infarction who have had a previous DVT or pulmonary embolism, or who are morbidly obese (BMI > 40) should be considered for prophylactic heparin.

• Patients in atrial fibrillation have to be considered individually. Atrial fibrillation is often a marker for stroke rather than its direct cause and occurs in 10–15% of patients with cerebral haemorrhage. If there is no haemorrhage on CT and the risk of further ischaemic stroke is very high (e.g. mitral stenosis or hypertrophic cardiomyopathy), start heparin by infusion (p. 404). In other patients start aspirin immediately and change to warfarin at 14 days.

• Patients with stroke due to internal carotid artery dissection should receive heparin by infusion (p. 404).

6 Glucose
• Hyperglycaemia is an adverse risk factor but the threshold for and benefits of treatment are not established.
• An insulin sliding scale if the blood glucose >15 mmol/L is a reasonable approach (p. 322) pending the results of current trials.

7 Fever
• In patients febrile at presentation, always consider brain abscess, meningitis or endocarditis.
• Fever beginning 12–48 h after presentation may be due to the stroke itself, aspiration pneumonia (in patients with a reduced conscious level or disordered swallowing) (p. 214), urinary tract infection or venous thromboembolism.
• Examine the patient, send blood and urine for culture, and obtain a chest X-ray.
• If you suspect aspiration pneumonia, options for initial treatment (before culture results are known) are amoxycillin/clavulanate or a fluoroquinolone plus clindamycin or metronidazole.
• Measures to reduce body temperature (paracetamol, fan) may help reduce neuronal damage.

8 Other supportive therapy
• Give a stool softener to prevent constipation and faecal impaction.
• Urinary incontinence is common but often temporary. Exclude faecal impaction and urinary tract infection. A urinary catheter (or penile sheath) should be used to prevent skin maceration.
• Start physiotherapy within 1–2 days to prevent contractures and pressure ulceration, and encourage recovery of function.
• Patients with language disorders should be referred for speech therapy.

9 Further investigation
Further investigation to establish the cause of the stroke is given in Tables 27.3 and 27.4 and in Fig. 27.1.

Stroke

Table 27.4 Criteria for requesting echocardiography after ischaemic stroke or transient ischaemic attack

Urgent transthoracic or transoesophageal echocardiography
Possible endocarditis
Possible aortic dissection (Chapter 15)
Possible atrial myxoma (signs of mitral valve disease; high ESR)

Routine transthoracic echocardiography
Pansystolic murmur
Any diastolic murmur
Atrial fibrillation (if age < 70, to determine cause of AF)
Other major ECG abnormality (e.g. Q waves indicative of previous myocardial
    infarction, LV hypertrophy with strain pattern (? hypertrophic cardiomyopathy),
    complete left bundle branch block (? dilated cardiomyopathy))
Significant cardiac enlargement on chest X-ray (e.g. CTR > 0.6)

Routine transoesophageal echocardiography
Possible endocarditis but normal transthoracic study
Mechanical cardiac valve prosthesis (to exclude thrombus and vegetations)
Age < 50 with unexplained stroke (may be indicated in patients > 50 with
    unexplained stroke: discuss with a stroke physician)

Secondary prevention

The following measures reduce the risk of further ischaemic stroke:
• Warfarin if in atrial fibrillation or aspirin 75–150 mg daily if in sinus rhythm or warfarin contraindicated for patients with ischaemic stroke.
• Treat hypertension after about 10 days. Target BP is 140/85 mmHg or below.
• Stop cigarette smoking.
• Control diabetes.
• Consider statin therapy of hypercholesterolaemia especially if there is other arterial disease. There is, as yet, no consensus on thresholds for drug treatment in stroke alone.

• Consider for carotid endarterectomy if there is a severe stenosis of the extracranial portion of the ipsilateral internal carotid artery in patients who have had a minor ischaemic stroke or TIA. The presence of a carotid bruit is unfortunately neither a specific nor a sensitive sign of a severe stenosis. Carotid duplex scanning is the best non-invasive method of screening.

Appendix

1 Chronic subdural haematoma
Risk factors
Risk factors (which may often be absent)
• Previous head injury (within 1 year).
• Alcohol abuse.
• Anticoagulant therapy.

Clinical features
• Headache.
• Reduced conscious level relatively common and sometimes fluctuating.
• Hemiparesis.
• Visual field defect and hemisensory loss are rare.
• Papilloedema (in 30% of cases).

2 Cerebellar stroke
Risk factors
• Age > 50 (M > F).
• Previous hypertension.

Clinical features
• Headache (usually occipital).
• Dizziness, vertigo, nausea and vomiting.
• Nystagmus and gaze paresis.
• Truncal ataxia (may be unable to stand).
• Limb ataxia (less common).

3 Embolism from the heart
Embolism from the heart accounts for around 15–20% of ischaemic strokes, and should be suspected in the following circumstances:

Stroke

• Sudden neurological deficit, maximal at onset (but this is not specific for cardiac embolism).

• Valsalva manoeuvre (yawning, coughing, straining) at onset.

• Dysphasia or hemianopia without other neurological deficit.

• Single cortical or sub-corticol branch territory infarct on cranial CT or MRI.

• Previous cerebral infarcts in other arterial territories or peripheral embolism.

• Fever at presentation (? endocarditis).

• Preceding systemic illness (? endocarditis, myxoma).

• Clinical cardiac abnormality (e.g. pansystolic murmur, mid-diastolic murmur, signs of heart failure).

• Replacement heart valve especially mechanical in the mitral position.

• Recent anterior myocardial infarct.

• Atrial fibrillation.

• Other major ECG abnormality (e.g. Q waves indicative of previous myocardial infarction, LV hypertrophy with strain pattern (? hypertrophic cardiomyopathy), complete left bundle branch block (? dilated cardiomyopathy)).

• Significant cardiac enlargement on chest X-ray.

Criteria for requesting echocardiography are given in Table 27.4.

28 Transient ischaemic attack

Transient ischaemic attack (TIA) is defined as a focal cerebral or monocular deficit of presumed vascular origin which fully resolves clinically within 24 h.

Priorities

Your clinical assessment and investigation (Fig. 28.1, Table 28.1) are directed at answering three questions.

1 Was this a TIA?
• The symptoms of TIA are of sudden onset, lack prodromal features such as nausea or palpitation, reach their peak within seconds and usually last for less than 15 min.
• TIAs usually cause loss of function. 'Positive' symptoms such as limb movement, paraesthesiae or hallucinations are more likely to be due to epilepsy or migraine.
• Presyncope or syncope is rare as a result of TIA unless associated with other focal neurological symptoms.
• Other causes of transient neurological and visual symptoms are given in Table 28.2.

2 Which arterial territory was affected: carotid or vertebrobasilar? (Table 28.3)
• A carotid bruit is not a sensitive or specific sign of severe carotid stenosis.
• Carotid ultrasound is indicated in patients who have had a carotid territory TIA and would be candidates for endarterectomy.

3 Does the TIA have a potentially treatable cause?
Always consider:

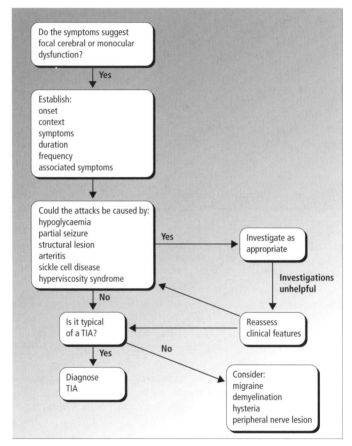

Fig. 28.1 Diagnosis of transient ischaemic attack. From Dennis M. *Hospital Update*. Dec 1991: 978.

1 **Embolism from the heart**, possible in the presence of:
  • Replacement heart valve, especially a mechanical valve in the mitral position.
  • Clinical cardiac abnormality (e.g. pansystolic murmur, mid-diastolic murmur, signs of heart failure).

Table 28.1 Investigation of the patient with suspected TIA

All patients
Full blood count
ESR
Creatinine, sodium and potassium
Blood glucose
Cholesterol
Urinalysis
ECG (? atrial fibrillation, left ventricular hypertrophy, myocardial infarction)
Chest X-ray (? lung neoplasm, cardiac enlargement)

Selected patients
CT scan if there is doubt about the diagnosis
Carotid duplex scanning if amaurosis fugax or carotid territory TIA (Table 28.3)
Echocardiography if carotid ultrasound normal and clinical or ECG evidence of
    cardiac disease (see Table 27.4)

- Atrial fibrillation.
- Recent anterior myocardial infarction.
- Other major ECG abnormality (e.g. Q waves indicative of previous myocardial infarction, LV hypertrophy with strain pattern (? hypertrophic cardiomyopathy), complete left bundle branch block (? dilated cardiomyopathy)).
- Significant cardiac enlargement on chest X-ray (e.g. CTR >0.6).

2 **Arteritis**, suggested by
- High ESR.
- Headache or systemic symptoms.

3 **Haematological disease**
- Hyperviscosity syndrome.
- Sickle cell disease.

Table 28.2 Causes of transient neurological or visual symptoms

Neurological
Arterial disease: atheroembolism or arteritis
Embolism from the heart
Haematological disease: hyperviscosity syndrome, sickle cell disease
Migraine
Focal seizure
Structural brain lesions causing epilepsy, e.g. subdural haematoma
Peripheral nerve lesions
Multiple sclerosis
Transient global amnesia
Labyrinthine disorders
Psychological disorders including hyperventilation
Metabolic disorders, e.g. hypoglycaemia

Visual
Arterial disease: atheroembolism or arteritis (especially giant cell)
Embolism from the heart
Haematological disease: hyperviscosity syndrome, sickle cell disease
Migraine
Glaucoma
Raised intracranial pressure
Retinal detachment
Retinal/vitreous haemorrhage
Malignant hypertension
Retinal vein thrombosis
Orbital tumour
Psychological disorders including hyperventilation

Transient ischaemic attack

Further management

• Further management of definite TIA is the same as for minor ischaemic stroke (Chapter 27). Deficits lasting longer than 1 h are likely to be associated with minor cerebral infarction on CT scanning. If

Table 28.3 Symptoms of carotid and vertebrobasilar TIA

Symptom	Carotid TIA	Vertebrobasilar TIA
Dysphasia	Yes	No
Loss of vision in one eye only	Yes	No
Loss of vision in both eyes	No	Yes
Hemianopia	Yes	Yes
Diplopia	No	Yes
Dysarthria	Yes	Yes
Loss of balance	Yes	Yes
Unilateral motor loss	Yes	Yes
Unilateral sensory loss	Yes	Yes

symptoms lasted > 24 h, CT should be done to exclude cerebral haemorrhage before aspirin is started.

• If the diagnosis is unclear, refer the patient to a neurologist (or an ophthalmologist if the patient has had only amaurosis fugax).

Transient ischaemic attack

29 Subarachnoid haemorrhage

Consider the diagnosis in any patient with:
- severe headache of sudden onset; or
- stroke with neck stiffness; or
- coma.

Priorities

1 **If the patient is comatose**: see Chapter 6 for initial management.

2 **If the patient is not comatose**, give pethidine (1 mg/kg) IM (plus an antiemetic, e.g. metoclopramide 10 mg IM) to relieve the headache. The clinical features (Table 29.1) will usually allow you to distinguish subarachnoid haemorrhage from other causes of headache (Chapter 9).

3 **If the diagnosis is suspected**, request computed tomography (CT). This is most sensitive within 12 h of onset.

4 **Lumbar puncture should be done if the CT scan is negative or equivocal** (Table 29.2).

Lumbar puncture:
- Should not be performed in patients with focal neurological signs or reduced conscious level who may have an intracerebral haematoma.
- Should be performed if CT is normal or equivocal in patients with a suggestive history (as minor bleeds may not be detected on CT).
- Should be performed >12 h after the onset of headache, unless meningitis is suspected, in order to confirm or exclude xanthochromia (the most reliable method of differentiating between SAH and a traumatic tap).

5 **If subarachnoid haemorrhage is confirmed, discuss further management with a neurosurgeon.** Rupture of a berry aneurysm is the commonest cause (Table 29.3), and obliteration of the aneurysm by

Table 29.1 Clinical features of aneurysmal subarachnoid haemorrhage

History

Onset of headache: abrupt, maximal at onset, 'thunderclap' headache

Severity of headache: usually 'worst of life' or very severe

Qualitative characteristics: first headache ever of this intensity, unique or different in
    patients with prior headaches

Associated symptoms: transient loss of consciousness, diplopia, fit, focal
    neurological symptoms*

Background

Cigarette smoking

Hypertension

Alcohol consumption (especially after recent binge)

Personal or family history of subarachnoid haemorrhage*

Polycystic kidney disease*

Heritable connective tissue diseases: Ehlers–Danlos syndrome type IV,
    pseudoxanthoma elasticum, fibromuscular dysplasia*

Sickle cell disease, alpha$_1$-antitrypsin deficiency

Examination

Retinal or subhyaloid haemorrhages (retinal haemorrhages with curved lower and
    straight upper borders)*

Neck stiffness*

Focal neurological signs

Low-grade fever

* Patients with these features are at very high risk of having an intracranial
aneurysm. Ask advice on management from a neurologist, even if CT/LP are
negative.

Reference: Edlow JA, Caplan LR. Avoiding pitfalls in the diagnosis of subarachnoid
hemorrhage. *New England Journal of Medicine* 2000; **342**: 29–36.

Subarachnoid haemorrhage

Table 29.2 Urgent investigation in suspected subarachnoid haemorrhage

Computed tomography (CT)
Blood in subarachnoid spaces
May show intracerebral haematoma

Lumbar puncture
Raised opening pressure
Uniformly blood-stained CSF
Xanthochromia of the supernatant (always found from 12 h to 2 weeks after the
    bleed; centrifuge the CSF and examine the supernatant by spectrophotometry if
    available; if not, compare against a white background with a control tube filled
    with water)

Table 29.3 Causes of subarachnoid haemorrhage

Rupture of saccular ('berry') aneurysm of circle of Willis
Bleeding from arteriovenous malformation
Primary intracerebral haemorrhage with rupture of the haematoma into the
    subarachnoid space
Bleeding tendency
Bleeding from intracranial tumours, notably metastatic melanoma
Trauma (most common in the elderly with occipital skull fracture)
Unknown cause (i.e. cerebral angiography normal and no other cause identified)

surgical clipping or interventional radiology prevents rebleeding. The optimum timing of surgery remains controversial.

Further management (before aneurysm surgery)

• Bed rest, preferably in a darkened side-room.
• Drug treatment to reduce anxiety may be helpful (e.g. diazepam 2–10 mg 8-hly PO).
• Analgesia as required (e.g. codeine phosphate 30–60 mg 4-hly PO). Start a stool softener to prevent constipation.
• Ensure an adequate fluid intake (3 L/day, giving some IV if needed).
• Treatment with the calcium antagonist nimodipine 60 mg 4-hly by mouth or nasogastric tube (or by IV infusion via a central line: 1 mg/h initially, increased after 2 h to 2 mg/h if no significant fall in BP) reduces cerebral infarction and improves the outcome after subarachnoid haemorrhage. Nimodipine should be continued for 21 days. Other therapies (e.g. with antifibrinolytic drugs) are not of proved benefit.

Problems

Hypertension
• First ensure that adequate analgesia has been given.
• If sustained and severe (systolic BP >200 mmHg, diastolic BP >110 mmHg) cautious treatment should be given.
• In patients not receiving nimodipine, start nifedipine initally 10 mg 8-hly PO. Add a beta-blocker if not contraindicated, e.g. metoprolol initally 50 mg 12-hly PO. In patients unable to take a beta-blocker, an alpha-blocker can be used, e.g. prazosin initially 1 mg 12-hly PO.

Neurological deterioration
• Check plasma sodium and urea: hyponatraemia may occur due to sodium depletion and/or inappropriate ADH secretion.
• Obtain a CT scan and discuss further management with a neurosurgeon. The possibilities are:

- Recurrent haemorrhage—peak incidence in the first 2 weeks (10% of patients).
- Vasospasm causing cerebral ischaemia or infarction—peak incidence between day 5 and day 14 (25% of patients).
- Communicating hydrocephalus—from 1 to 8 weeks after the haemorrhage (15–20% of patients).

30 Bacterial meningitis

• Consider the diagnosis in any febrile patient with headache, neck stiffness or a reduced conscious level.

• Disorders which can mimic meningitis include subarachnoid haemorrhage (Chapter 29), viral encephalitis (Appendix), brain abscess, subdural empyema and cerebral malaria (p. 396).

Priorities

1 If the clinical picture suggests meningitis (Table 30.1), and the patient has a reduced conscious level or focal neurological signs or a petechial/purpuric rash (? meningococcal infection), take blood cultures (× 2) and start antibiotic therapy immediately (Table 30.2).

2 In patients with a reduced conscious level or focal neurological signs, CT must be done before lumbar puncture to exclude an intracranial mass lesion: if found, ask advice on further management from a neurosurgeon.

3 If there are no contraindications to **lumbar puncture** (see p. 461), this should be done without delay.

• Measure and record the opening pressure.

• If the CSF opening pressure is > 40 cm, i.e. severe cerebral oedema, give mannitol 0.5 g/kg IV over 10 min plus dexamethasone 12 mg IV. Discuss further management with a neurologist.

• Send CSF for cell count; protein concentration; glucose (fluoride tube); Gram stain (plus Ziehl–Neelsen stain and India ink preparation if immunocompromised, to check for tuberculous or cryptococcal meningitis (see Appendix)).

• If the CSF is cloudy, i.e. pyogenic bacterial meningitis, start antibiotic therapy (Table 30.2).

• Blood-stained CSF may be due to a traumatic tap or subarachnoid haemorrhage. Collect 3 consecutive tubes and check the red cell

Bacterial meningitis

Table 30.1 Clinical features of bacterial meningitis

Prodrome of <48 h

Meningeal irritation: headache, neck stiffness, vomiting, photophobia

Reduced conscious level

Fits

Cranial nerve palsies

Focal signs (if bacterial meningitis is complicated by cerebral venous sinus thrombosis or arteritis)

Table 30.2 Initial antibiotic therapy for suspected bacterial meningitis in adults

	Previously healthy adult under 50	Previously healthy adult over 50 or immunocompromised
If lumbar puncture has not been done, or if Gram stain of the CSF indicates probable pneumococcal infection	Cefotaxime 2–4 g 8-hly IV and Vancomycin 60 mg/kg daily IV in 4 divided doses	Cefotaxime 2–4 g 8-hly IV and Ampicillin 200–400 mg/kg daily IV in 4 divided doses and Vancomycin 60 mg/kg daily IV in 4 divided doses
If Gram stain of the CSF does not suggest pneumococcal infection	Ceftriaxone 80 mg/kg every 12 h for first 3 doses then 80 mg/kg once daily IV. Maximum 4 g single dose	

NB: Intrathecal antibiotics are unnecessary and potentially dangerous.

Table 30.3 Urgent investigation in suspected meningitis

Lumbar puncture if not contraindicated
Blood culture (x 2)
Full blood count
Blood glucose (for comparison with CSF glucose)
Creatinine, sodium and potassium
Chest X-ray (? pneumonia or lung abscess)
Skull X-ray if suspected sinus infection (nasal discharge, sinus tenderness) or skull
    fracture
CT if suspected intracranial mass lesion or skull X-ray abnormal

count in the first and third. Check for xanthochromia in the supernatant (see p. 244). Xanthochromia is detectable from 12 h to 2 weeks
after subarachnoid haemorrhage. See Chapter 29 for further management of subarachnoid haemorrhage.

4 **Other urgent investigations** in suspected meningitis are given in
Table 30.3.

Further management

1 If organisms are seen on Gram stain of the CSF, bacterial meningitis is confirmed. The cell count will usually be high with a polymorphonuclear leucocytosis but may be low in overwhelming infection.

• Modify or start antibiotic therapy (Table 30.2). Ask advice from a
microbiologist or infectious diseases specialist on the exact antibiotic
regimen and duration of treatment.

• Adjunctive corticosteroid therapy is probably of benefit in these
patients with a high concentration of bacteria in the CSF. Give
dexamethasone 0.15 mg/kg 6-hly IV for 4 days.

2 If no organisms are seen on Gram stain, management is directed by
the clinical picture and CSF formula (Table 30.4).

• Normal cell count, i.e. meningitis excluded. Consider other infectious diseases which may give rise to meningism (e.g. tonsillitis,
viral hepatitis).

Bacterial meningitis

Table 30.4 CSF formulae in meningitis

	Pyogenic	Viral	Tuberculous	Cryptococcal
Cell count/mm^3	>1000	<500	<500	<150
Predominant cell type	Polymorphs	Lymphocytes	Lymphocytes	Lymphocytes
Protein conc. (g/L)	>1.5	0.5–1.0	1.0–5.0	0.5–1.0
CSF:blood glucose	<50%	>50%	<50%	<50%

The values given are typical, but many exceptions occur.

Antibiotic therapy substantially changes the CSF formula in pyogenic bacterial meningitis, leading to a fall in cell count, increased proportion of lymphocytes and fall in protein level. However, the low CSF glucose level usually persists.

- High polymorph count. This is typical of pyogenic bacterial meningitis but may occur early in the course of viral meningitis. If the patient has a reduced conscious level and/or CSF glucose is low, start antibiotic therapy. If the patient is alert, the CSF glucose is normal and there are no other features to suggest bacterial infection, hold off antibiotic therapy and repeat the LP in 12 h. By this time an increasing proportion of the cells will be lymphocytes in viral meningitis.
- High lymphocyte count. This may be seen in many diseases (Table 30.5). Distinguishing between viral and partially treated pyogenic bacterial meningitis can be difficult. If in doubt, start antibiotic therapy, awaiting the results of culture of blood and CSF. If tuberculous or cryptococcal meningitis is possible on clinical grounds (see Appendix) or on the results of CSF examination, ask for a Ziehl–Neelsen stain and India ink preparation.

3 Supportive treatment of bacterial meningitis includes:
- Analgesia as required (e.g. paracetamol, NSAID or codeine).
- Control of fits (see Chapter 33).

Bacterial meningitis

Table 30.5 Causes of meningitis with a high CSF lymphocyte count*

Viral meningitis
Partially treated pyogenic bacterial meningitis
Other bacterial infections—tuberculosis (Appendix), leptospirosis, brucellosis, syphilis
Fungal (cryptococcal) infection (Appendix)
Parameningeal infection—brain abscess or subdural empyema
Neoplastic infiltration

* Viral encephalitis (Appendix) may give a similar CSF picture.

- Attention to fluid balance. Losses are increased due to fever. Aim for an intake of 2–3 L/day, supplementing oral with IV fluids if needed. Check creatinine and electrolytes initially daily. Hyponatraemia may occur due to inappropriate ADH secretion.

4 Contacts of patients with meningococcal meningitis should be identified. Rifampicin should be given to family members and other close contacts (600 mg or 10 mg/kg twice daily for 2 days).

5 The district community medicine specialist should be informed about confirmed cases of meningitis.

Appendix

Tuberculous meningitis

- At risk: immigrants from India, Pakistan and Africa; recent contact with TB; previous pulmonary TB; alcoholics; IV drug abusers; immunocompromised.
- Suggestive clinical features: subacute onset; cranial nerve palsies; retinal tubercles (pathognomonic but rarely seen); hyponatraemia.
- The chest X-ray is often normal.
- The CSF usually shows a high lymphocyte count with a high protein concentration (Table 30.4). Acid-fast bacilli may not be seen on Ziehl–Neelsen stain.

• CT scan commonly shows hydrocephalus (and may also show cerebral infarction due to arteritis or tuberculoma).
• Treatment: combination chemotherapy with isoniazid, rifampicin, pyrazinamide and streptomycin plus pyridoxine to avoid neuropathy.
• Seek expert advice if the diagnosis is suspected.

Cryptococcal meningitis
• At risk: immunocompromised (organ transplant, lymphoma, steroid therapy, AIDS).
• Suggestive clinical features: insidious onset; neck stiffness absent or mild; papular or nodular skin lesions.
• The CSF usually shows a high lymphocyte count with a raised protein concentration (Table 30.4). Cryptococci may be seen on Gram stain as large Gram-positive cocci. India ink preparation is positive in 60%.
• The diagnosis may also be confirmed by CSF culture or serological tests for cryptococcal antigen on CSF or blood.
• Treatment: amphotericin plus flucytosine.
• Seek expert advice if the diagnosis is suspected.

Viral encephalitis
• May be due to many viruses: herpes simplex virus is the most important as it may cause severe cerebral damage, which can be limited by early treatment with acyclovir.
• Suggestive clinical features: febrile illness, headache, personality change, abnormal behaviour, alteration in conscious level, fits, focal neurological signs.
• The CSF may be normal or may show a high lymphocyte count ($50–500/mm^3$). There may be predominance of polymorphs in the early phase. Red cells are often present in herpes simplex encephalitis. The protein concentration may be increased, up to $2.5\,g/L$. CSF glucose is usually normal but may be low.
• Save samples of CSF and serum for later assay, and repeat LP in 10 days: a fourfold rise in CSF viral antibody titre is diagnostic.
• CT scan may show generalized brain swelling with loss of cortical sulci and small ventricles, but may be normal. In herpes simplex encephalitis there may be areas of low attenuation in the temporal and/or frontal lobes.

Bacterial meningitis

• Electroencephalography (EEG) is usually abnormal in two-thirds of cases, with a spike and slow wave pattern localized to the area of brain involved.

• Seek expert advice if viral encephalitis is suspected. For suspected herpes simplex encephalitis, start acyclovir 10 mg/kg by slow IV infusion over 1 h, 8-hly for 10 days (reduce dose in renal failure).

Bacterial meningitis

31 Spinal cord compression

Consider the diagnosis in any patient with:
- thoracic or lumbar spine pain; or
- weak legs but normal arms; or
- urinary or faecal incontinence.

Early diagnosis and treatment are crucial to preserving cord function.

Priorities

1 The working diagnosis of cord compression is based on the clinical features, which may be mild in the early stages. Details of the innervation of muscle and skin are given on pp. 491–5. Characteristic symptoms and signs are:
- Spinal or radicular pain.
- Leg stiffness or clumsy gait.
- Urinary hesistancy or frequency (painless retention is a late sign).
- Tendon reflexes depressed at the level of the compression and increased below it.
- Bilateral upper motor neurone signs in the legs.
- Impaired sensation with a sensory level.
- Reduced anal tone.

2 Look for a cause. Cord compression is usually due to extradural disease (Table 31.1).

3 If you suspect cord compression is due to malignancy (the commonest cause), start high-dose dexamethasone (10–100 mg IV, followed by 4–24 mg IV 6-hly; use the maximum doses in patients with severe or rapidly progressive signs, and lower doses if the signs are mild or equivocal).

Table 31.1 Causes of non-traumatic extradural spinal cord compression

Cause	Comment
Malignancy	Most commonly carcinoma of breast, bronchus or prostate
	Compression is at thoracic level in 70%, lumbar in 20% and cervical in 10%
Spinal extradural abscess	Severe back pain; local spinal tenderness; systemic illness with fever
Extradural haematoma	Rare complication of warfarin anticoagulation
Prolapse of cervical or thoracic intervertebral disc	Spinal pain accompanied by root pain
Atlanto-axial subluxation	Complication of rheumatoid arthritis

Table 31.2 Urgent investigation in suspected spinal cord compression

AP and lateral X-rays of the spine (look for loss of pedicles, vertebral body destruction, spondylolisthesis, soft tissue mass)
Magnetic resonance imaging of the spine
Chest X-ray (look for primary or secondary tumour, or evidence of tuberculosis)
Full blood count
ESR, C-reactive protein
Blood culture
Creatinine, sodium and potassium

4 Arrange urgent magnetic resonance imaging (MRI) of the spine and other investigations (Table 31.2). If MRI confirms cord compression, discuss further management with a neurosurgeon. If MRI is not available, discuss alternative imaging with a radiologist.

32 Guillain–Barré syndrome

Consider the diagnosis in any patient with:
• paraesthesiae in the fingers and toes;
• weakness of the arms and legs.

Respiratory failure (which may rapidly progress to respiratory arrest) and autonomic instability are the major complications.

Priorities

1 Make the diagnosis from the clinical features (Table 32.1): generalized areflexia is the clue (found in 75% of patients at presentation and 90% with fully developed illness).

• Exclude severe hypokalaemia (plasma potassium < 2.5 mmol/L), which may cause paralysis.

• Causes of acute neuromuscular paralysis other than Guillain–Barré syndrome are rare and can be excluded on clinical grounds or by later investigation (Table 32.2 and Table 32.3).

• Spinal cord compression (Chapter 31) is the most important differential diagnosis, and must be excluded (by MRI scan of the spine) if there is spinal pain, a sensory level, marked sphincter disturbance or upper motor neurone signs.

2 Measure the vital capacity with a spirometer. Predicted normal values are given on p. 489. As a rule of thumb, vital capacity (ml) is $25 \times$ height (cm) in men and $20 \times$ height (cm) in women.

• If no spirometer is available, the breath-holding time in full inspiration is a guide to the vital capacity (normal > 30 s), provided there is no coexisting respiratory disease.

• Arterial blood gases can remain normal despite a severely reduced vital capacity. Pulse oximetry or an arterial sample is not a substitute for measuring vital capacity.

Table 32.1 Diagnostic criteria for Guillain–Barré syndrome

Features required for the diagnosis
Progressive symmetrical weakness in both arms and both legs
Areflexia

Features strongly supporting the diagnosis
Progression of symptoms over days to 4 weeks
Relative symmetry of symptoms
Mild sensory symptoms or signs
Cranial nerve involvement, especially bilateral weakness of facial muscles
Recovery beginning 2–4 weeks after progression ceases
Autonomic dysfunction
Absence of fever at onset
High concentration of protein in cerebrospinal fluid, with fewer than 50/mm^3 cells
Typical electrodiagnostic features

Features excluding the diagnosis
Diagnosis of botulism, myasthenia, poliomyelitis or toxic neuropathy
Abnormal porphyrin metabolism
Recent diphtheria
Purely sensory syndrome, without weakness

Reference: Hahn A F. Guillain–Barré syndrome. *Lancet* 1998; **352**: 635-641.

Guillain–Barré syndrome

3 Transfer to ITU:
• Patients whose vital capacity is < 80% predicted (falling towards 20 mL/kg body weight).
• Patients who are unable to walk.
Discuss their further management with an anaesthetist and a neurologist. Ventilation may be necessary: see *Problems* below.
4 Arrange continuous ECG monitoring for patients at high risk of cardiac arrhythmia as shown by signs of autonomic dysfunction (e.g. pupils fluctuating rapidly in size, significant sweating, piloerection, abnormal response to Valsalva).

Table 32.2 Investigation in suspected Guillain–Barré syndrome (GBS)

Potassium, sodium, magnesium, calcium, phosphate and creatinine

Full blood count

ESR and C-reactive protein (if high, consider fulminant mononeuritis multiplex, which can mimic GBS)

Liver function tests

Anti-nuclear antibodies and anti-neutrophil cytoplasmic antibodies

Chest X-ray

ECG

CSF protein and cell count

Electrophysiological tests (if the diagnosis is not certain)

Urine for porphobilinogen

Stool culture for *Campylobacter jejuni* (the commonest recognized cause of GBS in the UK) and poliomyelitis

5 Admit other patients to a general ward for observation and further investigation.

Further management

1 Confirm the diagnosis by CSF examination, which typically shows:
- normal opening pressure;
- raised protein (> 0.55 g/L after the first week of illness);
- normal cell count or mild lymphocytic pleocytosis (usually < 20 lymphocytes/mm^3; > 50 makes Guillain–Barré syndrome unlikely, and other diagnoses should be considered).

2 Electrophysiological tests may be needed if there is doubt about the diagnosis. These may be normal in the first week. Discuss with a neurologist.

3 Measure vital capacity (4-hly–daily, depending on initial value) until the weakness has reached a plateau. Pulse oximetry is not a substitute.

4 If the patient cannot walk or is not improving, discuss with a neurologist treatment with:
  • high-dose IV immunoglobulin (0.4 g/kg body weight daily for 5 consecutive days); or
  • plasma exchange.
5 Supportive management consists of:
  • Bed rest.
  • Physiotherapy to prevent contractures.
  • Ventilation for respiratory failure (see *Problems*).
  • Feeding by nasogastric tube (or parenteral nutrition) if lower cranial nerve involvement interferes with swallowing.
  • Heparin 5000 units SC 12-hly if unable to walk.
  • Aspirin or paracetamol for myalgia and arthralgia and/or tricyclic antidepressants.
  • Stool softener to prevent constipation.
  • Fluid restriction if hyponatraemia occurs (due to inappropriate ADH secretion).

Problems

Respiratory failure
• Patients whose vital capacity falls below 80% predicted should be transferred to the ITU with facilities for endotracheal intubation to hand.
• Measure vital capacity 4-hly. As a general rule, ventilation is required if the vital capacity falls below 25–30% predicted.

Arrhythmias
• Transient arrhythmias (supraventricular tachycardia or bradycardia) without haemodynamic compromise require no treatment.
• Severe prolonged bradycardias may occur and are treated with temporary pacing.

Abnormalities of blood pressure
• Sustained severe hypertension (diastolic BP > 120 mmHg) should be treated with labetalol by infusion (p. 158).
• If hypotension does not respond to IV fluids (guided by measurement of CVP), treat with dopamine or noradrenaline infusion (pp. 481–5).

Guillain–Barré syndrome

Table 32.3 Causes of acute paralysis

Site of lesion	Causes
Brain	Stroke
	Mass lesion with brainstem compression
	Encephalitis
	Sedative drugs
	Status epilepticus
Spinal cord	Cord compression
	Transverse myelitis
	Anterior spinal artery occlusion
	Haematomyelia
	Poliomyelitis
	Rabies
Peripheral nerve	Guillain–Barré syndrome
	Critical illness polyneuropathy
	Toxins
	Acute intermittent porphyria
	Vasculitis, e.g. SLE
	Diphtheria
Neuromuscular junction	Myasthenia gravis
	Eaton–Lambert syndrome
	Botulism
	Toxins
Muscle	Hypokalaemia
	Hypophosphataemia
	Rhabdomyolysis

33 Epilepsy

Four topics are discussed:
1 Generalized tonic–clonic status epilepticus.
2 What to do after a first generalized tonic–clonic fit.
3 What to do after a generalized fit in a patient with known epilepsy.
4 Management of fits related to alcohol withdrawal.

Generalized tonic–clonic status epilepticus

• Defined as a generalized tonic–clonic fit lasting more than 30 min or repeated fits without recovery of normal alertness in between.
• Prompt treatment is needed to reduce cerebral damage and metabolic complications (hypoglycaemia, lactic acidosis and hyperpyrexia), and prevent mortality.

Priorities

1 Airway, breathing and circulation
• Clear the airway. Remove false teeth if loose and aspirate the pharynx, larynx and trachea with a suction catheter.
• Put the patient in the lateral semiprone position.
• Give oxygen.
• Attach an ECG monitor.
• Get IV access.
• Send blood for urgent investigation (Table 33.1).

2 Exclude hypoglycaemia
Check blood glucose immediately by stick test. If blood glucose is < 5 mmol/L, give dextrose 25 g IV (50 mL of dextrose 50% solution), via a large vein. In chronic alcoholics, there is a remote risk of precipitating Wernicke's encephalopathy by a glucose load; prevent this by giving thiamine 100 mg IV before or shortly after the dextrose.

Table 33.1 Investigation in status epilepticus or after a first fit

Urgent
Blood glucose
Sodium, potassium, calcium, magnesium and creatinine
Arterial blood gases and pH (not required after first fit)

Later
Anticonvulsant levels (if on therapy)
Full blood count
Serum (10 mL) and urine sample (50 mL) at 4°C for toxicology screen if poisoning
  suspected or cause of fit unclear
Blood culture (x 2) if febrile
Liver function tests
Chest X-ray
CT scan*
Lumbar puncture (after CT) if suspected meningitis or encephalitis
ECG (look for long QT interval, conduction abnormality (e.g. left bundle branch
  block), Q waves indicative of previous myocardial infarction: if present, consider
  arrhythmia rather than fit)
EEG

* CT scan should be performed urgently after control of status epilepticus or after a
first fit if any of the following features is present: focal neurological deficit; reduced
conscious level; fever; recent head injury; persistent headache; known malignancy;
warfarin anticoagulation; AIDS. For patients after a first fit who are fully recovered
and have no abnormal signs, CT can be done at a later date.

3 Give diazepam
Give **diazepam** 10–20 mg IV at a rate of <2.5 mg/min (faster injection
rates carry the risk of sudden apnoea) or **lorazepam** (which is less
likely to cause respiratory suppression) 2–4 mg IV over 5–10 min (Table
33.2). If fitting continues, give further doses, to a maximum of
diazepam 40 mg or lorazepam 8 mg.

Table 33.2 Drug therapy for generalized convulsive status epilepticus

Drug	Comments
First line	
Diazepam	10–20 mg IV at a rate of <2.5 mg/min. Risk of sudden apnoea with faster injection. Dose should not be repeated more than twice, or to a total dose >40 mg, because of the risks of respiratory depression and hypotension. Second-line therapy should be started if control is not achieved within
or	total dose of 40 mg
Lorazepam	2–4 mg IV. Dose can be repeated once after 20 min. Ampoules contain lorazepam 4 mg in 1 mL. Dilute 1 : 1 with water for injection. Longer duration of action and less likely to cause sudden hypotension or respiratory arrest than diazepam
Second line	
Phenytoin	Loading dose: 15 mg/kg IV. Infusion rate should not exceed 50 mg/min. For average-sized adult, give 1000 mg over
or	20 min. Maintenance dose of 100 mg 6–8-hly IV
Phenobarbitone	Loading dose: 10 mg/kg to a maximum of 1000 mg, given at 100 mg/min. Maintenance dose 1–4 mg/kg/day given IV, IM or PO
Third line (refractory status)	
Thiopentone	100–250 mg IV bolus, then 50 mg bolus every 3 min until burst suppression on EEG. Maintenance dose 2–5 mg/kg/h
or	
Propofol	2 mg/kg IV bolus, then repeat bolus if necessary. Maintenance dose 5–10 mg/kg/h

Epilepsy

4 What is the likely cause of fitting? (Table 33.3)
- Obtain the history from all available sources, and make a systematic examination of the patient. Check the blood results.
- Correct severe hyponatraemia (plasma sodium < 120 mmol/L) with hypertonic saline (p. 341).

Table 33.3 Causes of tonic-clonic status epilepticus

In a patient known to have epilepsy
Poor compliance with therapy, therapy recently reduced or stopped, or altered drug
   pharmacokinetics
Intercurrent infection
Alcohol withdrawal

In a patient not known to have epilepsy
Stroke, especially haemorrhagic stroke
Encephalitis
Brain tumour
Brain abscess
Arteriovenous malformation
Meningitis
Acute head injury
Metabolic disorder: cerebral anoxia from cardiac arrest, acute renal failure,
   hyponatraemia, hypocalcaemia, hypomagnesaemia, hepatic encephalopathy
Poisoning: alcohol, tricyclics, phenothiazines, theophylline, cocaine, amphetamines,
   MDMA ('ecstasy'), heroin
Cerebral vasculitis
Hypertensive encephalopathy

• Correct severe hypocalcaemia (plasma total calcium < 1.5 mmol/L)
with calcium gluconate 1 g IV (10 mL of 10% solution) (p. 352).
• Give dexamethasone 10 mg IV if the patient is known to have a brain
tumour or active vasculitis.

Further management
If fitting continues
• Transfer the patient to the ITU and discuss management with an
anaesthetist and neurologist.
• Consider the possibility of **pseudoseizures** (Table 33.4), which are
not uncommon. Diagnosis may require EEG.

Table 33.4 Characteristics of pseudoseizures

Asynchronous bilateral movements of the limbs, asymmetrical clonic contractions, pelvic thrusting and side-to-side movements of the head, often intensified by restraint

Gaze aversion, resistance to passive limb movement or eye-opening, prevention of the hand falling on to the face

Incontinence, tongue biting and injury rare

Normal tendon reflexes, plantar responses, blink, corneal and eyelash reflexes

Absence of metabolic complications (normal plasma prolactin level)

No post-ictal confusion (drowsiness may be due to diazepam given to treat suspected fit)

• Unless the patient is known to be taking phenytoin with good compliance, give **phenytoin** IV (Table 33.2). Monitor the ECG during infusion as phenytoin may cause arrhythmias (and may also cause hypotension if given too quickly).

• If the patient is taking phenytoin, give **phenobarbitone** IV (contraindicated in acute intermittent porphyria) (Table 33.2).

If there is refractory status epilepticus

If fitting continues for > 60 min despite phenytoin or phenobarbitone IV:

• The patient should be intubated and ventilated.

• **Thiopentone** or **propofol** (Table 33.2) should be given, preferably with EEG monitoring.

Once fitting has stopped

• Determine the cause (Table 33.3).

• Ask advice from a neurologist on further management.

• If patient is known to have epilepsy, restart any antiepileptic medication stopped within the last 3 weeks.

Epilepsy

After a first generalized tonic–clonic fit

1 Was it a fit? (Table 33.5)

Distinguishing between a fit and syncope requires a detailed history, taken from the patient and any eye-witnesses. Points to cover include the following.

Background
• Any previous similar attacks.
• Previous significant head injury (i.e. with skull fracture or loss of consciousness).
• Birth injury, febrile convulsions in childhood, meningitis or encephalitis.
• Family history of epilepsy.
• Cardiac disease (? previous myocardial infarction, hypertrophic or dilated cardiomyopathy, long QT interval (at risk of ventricular tachycardia)).
• Drug therapy.
• Alcohol or substance abuse.
• Sleep deprivation.

Before the attack
• Prodromal symptoms: were these cardiovascular (e.g. dizziness, palpitation, chest pain) or focal neurological (aura)?
• Circumstances, e.g. exercising, standing, sitting or lying, asleep.
• Precipitants, e.g. coughing, micturition, head-turning.

The attack
• Were there any focal neurological features at the onset: sustained deviation of the head or eyes or unilateral jerking of the limbs? (Bilateral 'twitching' is common in syncope.)
• Was there a cry (may occur in tonic phase of fit)?
• Duration of fit.
• Associated tongue biting, urinary incontinence or injury.
• Facial colour changes (pallor common in syncope, uncommon with a fit).
• Abnormal pulse (must be assessed in relation to the reliability of the witness).

Epilepsy

Table 33.5 Features differentiating a generalized fit from vasovagal and cardiac syncope (Stokes–Adams attack).

Generalized fit	Vasovagal syncope	Cardiac syncope	(Stokes–Adams attack)
Occurrence when sitting or lying	Common	Rare	Common
Occurrence during sleep	Common	Does not occur	May occur
Prodromal symptoms	May occur, with focal neurological symptoms, automatisms or hallucinations	Typical, with dizziness, sweating, nausea, blurring of vision, disturbance of hearing, yawning	Often none Palpitation may precede syncope in tachyarrhythmias
Focal neurological features at onset	May occur (and signify focal cerebral lesion)	Never occur	Never occur
Tonic–clonic movements	Characteristic, occur within 30 s of onset	May occur after 30 s of syncope (secondary anoxic seizure)	May occur after 30 s of syncope (secondary anoxic seizure)
Facial colour	Flush or cyanosis at onset	Pallor at onset and after syncope	Pallor at onset, flush on recovery
Tongue biting	Common	Rare	Rare
Urinary incontinence	Common	Uncommon	May occur
Injury	May occur	Uncommon	May occur
Post-ictal confusion	Common	Uncommon	Uncommon

After the attack
Immediately well or delayed recovery with confusion or headache?

2 Is there an underlying cause?
• Are there any focal neurological signs? Like an aura preceding the fit, these indicate a structural cause.
• Was there headache (suggesting subarachnoid haemorrhage)?
• Does the patient have an infectious or metabolic disease requiring urgent treatment, e.g. bacterial meningitis, acute renal failure?
• Confusion, dysphasia and frontal release suggest encephalitis.

3 If the patient is well
• Discharge if fully recovered and supervision by an adult for the next 24 h can be arranged.
• Advise the patient not to drive.
• Out-patient investigation (EEG and CT if indicated) and follow-up by a neurologist should be arranged.
• Whether anticonvulsant therapy should be started after a first fit is controversial: find out the policy in your area.

After a generalized fit in a patient with known epilepsy

• Take blood for anticonvulsant levels.
• If the current history deviates from the usual pattern of seizures, consider intercurrent infection, alcohol abuse or poor compliance with therapy.
• Discharge (with out-patient follow-up arranged) if the patient is fully recovered and has no evidence of acute illness. Advise the patient not to drive.

Fits related to alcohol withdrawal

• Alcohol withdrawal fits—'rum fits'—consist of 1–6 tonic–clonic fits without focal features which begin within 48 h of stopping drinking (although may occur up to 7 days after stopping drinking if the patient has been taking benzodiazepines). They are usually brief and self-limiting.

- CT scan is not needed if:
  - (a) a clear history of alcohol withdrawal is obtained;
  - (b) the fits have no focal features;
  - (c) there is no evidence of head injury;
  - (d) there are no more than 6 fits;
  - (e) the fits do not occur over a period > 6 h;
  - (f) post-ictal confusion is brief.
- Management of alcohol withdrawal is given on p. 91.

Epilepsy

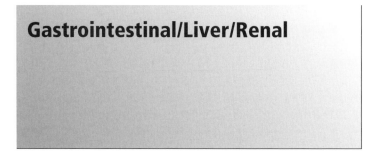

Gastrointestinal/Liver/Renal

34 Acute upper gastrointestinal haemorrhage

- This usually presents with **haematemesis or melaena** but should be considered in any patient with syncope (especially with associated anaemia), unexplained hypotension or hepatic encephalopathy (Chapter 37).
- A good outcome requires vigorous resuscitation of the patient and close collaboration between medical and surgical teams. Contact promptly a gastroenterologist or surgeon (depending on your local protocol) to discuss the management of patients admitted with major bleeding.
- Management is summarized in Fig. 34.1.

Priorities

1 Make a rapid clinical assessment
To include:
- an estimate of the volume of blood lost, based on the pulse rate, blood pressure and skin perfusion (Table 34.1). Bear in mind that the cardiovascular responses to blood loss are affected by rate of bleeding, age, associated cardiovascular disease and therapy (e.g. beta-blockers);
- any previous gastrointestinal bleeding and its cause;
- current and recent drug therapy (ask specifically about non-steroidal anti-inflammatory drugs (NSAIDs), aspirin and other antiplatelet agents, and warfarin);
- usual and recent alcohol intake;
- whether vomiting preceded the first haematemesis (suggesting Mallory–Weiss tear);
- known liver disease or signs of chronic liver disease;
- other medical problems, in particular cardiac disorders.

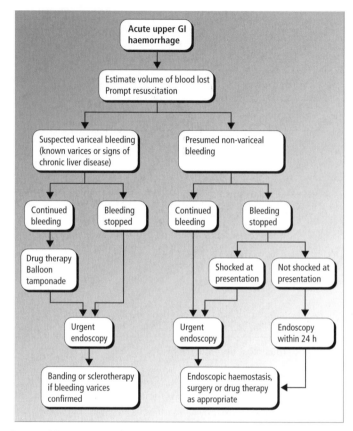

Fig. 34.1 Management of upper GI haemorrhage.

2 Put in a large-bore IV cannula

For example, grey Venflon. Take 20 mL of blood for urgent investigations (Table 34.2).

3 If there is hypovolaemic shock

Systolic blood pressure < 90 mmHg with cold extremities:

• Give oxygen and attach an ECG monitor.
• Rapidly transfuse colloid until the systolic blood pressure is around

Table 34.1 Upper GI haemorrhage: estimating the volume of blood loss

Major bleed (>1500 mL; >30% of blood volume)
Pulse >120/min
Systolic BP <120 mmHg (note this is influenced by age and usual blood pressure)
Cool or cold extremities with slow or absent capillary refill
Tachypnoea (respiratory rate >20/min)
Abnormal mental state: agitation, confusion, reduced conscious level

Minor bleed (<750 mL; <15% of blood volume)
Pulse <100/min
Systolic BP >120 mmHg, with postural fall <20 mmHg from lying to sitting
Normal perfusion of extremities
Normal respiratory rate
Normal mental state

Table 34.2 Urgent investigation in upper GI haemorrhage

Full blood count
Group and save serum: cross-match at least 4 units of whole blood if there is shock, significant blood loss or Hb <10 g/dl
Prothrombin time (if liver disease is suspected)
Urea, creatinine, sodium and potassium
ECG if age >50 or known cardiac disease

100 mmHg. If, despite 1000 mL of colloid, systolic BP is still <90 mmHg, use grouped but not cross-matched blood. Save a sample of the transfused blood for a retrospective cross-match.

• Put in a central line, and adjust the infusion rate to maintain the central venous pressure around +5 cm water.

• Put in a urinary catheter to monitor the urine output.

• Start transfusing blood as soon as it is available via a second IV cannula.

• Correct clotting abnormalities. If the prothrombin time is >1.5 × control, give vitamin K 10 mg IV (not IM) and 2 units of fresh frozen plasma. If the platelet count is < 50×10^{12}/L, give platelet concentrate. Recheck the platelet count if >4 units of blood have been transfused.

• Contact the on-call gastroenterology or surgical team for advice, and to arrange urgent endoscopy.

4 In patients without shock

Patients without shock but with evidence of significant blood loss (syncope in association with bleeding; clinical signs of blood loss > 750 mL) or haemoglobin < 10 g/dL:

• Start an infusion of colloid.

• Transfuse blood when it is available.

• Correct clotting abnormalities (see above).

• Put in a central line if age > 60 or suspected variceal bleeding.

• Contact the on-call gastroenterology or surgical team to discuss the timing of endoscopy.

5 No hypovolaemia

If there are no signs of hypovolaemia, either heparinize the venous cannula or start a slow infusion of normal saline to keep it patent.

6 Patients with suspected bleeding oesophageal varices

These constitute a special group. The mortality of variceal bleeding is around 50%. Urgent endoscopy is required to define the source of bleeding. Therapeutic endoscopy (injection sclerotherapy or banding) is the best treatment of bleeding varices. Management is summarized below:

• Ask for help from a gastroenterologist.

• Correct hypovolaemia and clotting abnormalities. Give blood as soon as it is available, to minimize the sodium load from colloid or saline infusions.

• Give terlipressin (causes less myocardial ischaemia than vasopressin, and is more effective than octreotide): 2 mg IV followed by 1–2 mg every 4–6 h until bleeding is controlled, for up to 72 h.

• If bleeding continues, insert a Sengstaken–Blakemore tube (Chapter 61).

• Arrange urgent endoscopy with a view to injection sclerotherapy or banding of varices. To prevent inhalation, this is best done with a cuffed endotracheal tube placed.

• Other supportive measures include omeprazole 40 mg daily orally or via gastric channel of Sengstaken tube or IV to prevent stress ulceration, and lactulose initially 30 mL 3-hly to prevent encephalopathy (p. 297).

Further management

1 Blood transfusion
This should be given until a normal blood volume has been restored as shown by:
• pulse rate <100/min;
• systolic blood pressure >110 mmHg;
• warm extremities;
• urine output >30 mL/h (0.5 mL/kg/h).

If the initial haemoglobin was < 10 g/dL (indicating either prolonged acute or previous chronic loss), continue transfusion until the haemoglobin is around 12 g/dL. As a rough guide, each unit of blood restores about 1 g/dL to the haemoglobin count.

Check the haemoglobin daily for the first 3 days and again before discharge. If the final haemoglobin is less than 12 g/dL, give ferrous sulphate 200 mg 12-hly for 1 month.

2 Allowed to eat or nil by mouth?
• Patients shocked on admission or with evidence of significant blood loss should not eat until endoscopy has been performed, in case urgent surgery is needed.

• Patients without signs of hypovolaemia can eat (but should remain nil by mouth for 6 h before endoscopy).

3 Acute drug therapy?
There is no firm evidence to support the use of antifibrinolytic therapy or drugs to inhibit gastric acid secretion in patients with acute upper gastrointestinal bleeding with the exception of patients who have had endoscopic haemostasis for bleeding peptic ulcers (see below).

Acute upper GI haemorrhage

4 Emergency endoscopy

This is needed for patients with:

- shock on admission (but not before adequate resuscitation);
- continued bleeding or rebleeding;
- signs of chronic liver disease or known varices.

In such patients it may be more practical to perform endoscopy in the operating theatre with the patient prepared for surgery.

Other patients should if possible be endoscoped within 24 h of admission.

Management after endoscopy

Peptic ulcer

- Bleeding from a peptic ulcer usually stops spontaneously.
- The mortality is highest in patients over 60 who continue to bleed or rebleed, and may be reduced by endoscopic haemostasis or surgery (Table 34.3). Treatment with IV omeprazole reduces the risk of rebleeding after endoscopic haemostasis.

Table 34.3 Indications for surgery in bleeding peptic ulcer

Age > 60

Continued bleeding (requiring > 4 units of blood/colloid over 24 h after initial restoration of blood volume); or:

One episode of rebleeding (with fall in blood pressure); or:

Endoscopy shows active bleeding from the ulcer or signs of recent bleeding (adherent clot, visible vessel) and endoscopic haemostasis not possible

Age < 60

Continued bleeding (requiring > 8 units of blood/colloid over 24 h after initial restoration of blood volume); or:

Two episodes of rebleeding (with fall in blood pressure); or:

Endoscopy shows active bleeding from the ulcer or signs of recent bleeding (adherent clot, visible vessel) and endoscopic haemostasis not possible

Acute upper GI haemorrhage

• Drug treatment to heal the ulcer (e.g. proton pump inhibitor or H2-receptor antagonist) should be given. In elderly patients, long-term treatment with a gastric antisecretory drug may be advisable to prevent recurrent bleeding.

• Treatment to eradicate *Helicobacter pylori* should be given; nearly all duodenal ulcers and most gastric ulcers not due to NSAIDs are associated with *H. pylori* infection.

• Patients with gastric ulcers (some of which are malignant) should have endoscopy repeated at 6–8 weeks.

Erosive gastritis

There are two groups of patients:

1 Previously well patients in whom erosive gastritis is related to aspirin, NSAIDs or alcohol. Bleeding usually stops quickly and no specific treatment is needed.

2 Critically ill patients with stress ulceration, in whom the mortality is high. Treatment consists of:

  • Omeprazole 40 mg daily IV.

  • Correction of clotting abnormalities (see above).

  • As a last resort, if bleeding is catastrophic, surgery with partial gastric resection can be performed but carries a high mortality.

Mallory–Weiss tear

Bleeding usually stops spontaneously and rebleeding is rare. If bleeding continues, the options are:

• Surgery with oversewing of the bleeding point.

• Tamponade using a Sengstaken–Blakemore tube.

• Interventional radiology: either selective infusion of vasopressin into the left gastric artery or embolization.

Oesophagitis and oesophageal ulcer

Give a proton pump inhibitor for 4 weeks, followed by a further 4–8 weeks' treatment if not fully healed.

Acute upper GI haemorrhage

Table 34.4 Small bowel and proximal colonic sources of melaena

Adenomatous polyp
Arteriovenous malformation
Meckel's diverticulum
Angiodysplasia of colon
Inflammatory bowel disease
Haemobilia
Aorto-enteric fistula

Problems

Suspected upper GI haemorrhage with 'negative' endoscopy

In a significant proportion of patients, a first endoscopy does not reveal a source of bleeding.

• Discuss repeating the endoscopy especially if blood or food obscured the views obtained or the patient has chronic liver disease (as varices which have recently bled may not be visible).

• Patients who presented with melaena only should be investigated for a small bowel or proximal colonic source of bleeding (Table 34.4) if no upper gastrointestinal source is found. A normal blood urea suggests a colonic cause of melaena, except in patients with chronic liver disease.

• Visceral angiography can be useful after two negative endoscopies, but only if done when the patient is actively bleeding.

35 Acute diarrhoea

Acute diarrhoea is usually due to intestinal infections or an adverse effect of medications. When it begins in hospital, *Clostridium difficile* (Appendix) is the commonest cause.

Priorities

1 The setting and clinical features (Table 35.1)
These provide important clues to the diagnosis. You need to establish:
• The mode of onset of diarrhoea (abrupt, subacute or gradual) and its duration.
• The frequency and nature of the stools (watery or containing blood and mucus; bloody stools are a common feature of shigellosis, salmonellosis, severe campylobacter enteritis and ulcerative colitis, and are rare (5%) in *C. difficile* infection).
• If others in the same household or who have shared the same food have also developed diarrhoea.
• If other symptoms (malaise, fever, vomiting, abdominal pain) have been prominent.
• If there has been travel abroad in the past 6 months.
• If there have been previous significant gastrointestinal symptoms or known GI diagnosis.
• What medications (in particular antibiotics) have been taken in the 6 weeks before the onset of diarrhoea.
• What other medical problems the patient has.

2 Examination
The examination is directed at determining:
• The severity of the illness and the degree of volume depletion (mental state, temperature, pulse, blood pressure lying and sitting).

Table 35.1 Important causes of acute diarrhoea by setting

Cause	Clinical features	Diagnosis/treatment (if indicated)
Community acquired:		
Campylobacter enteritis (*C. jejuni*)	Incubation period 2–6 days. Associated fever and abdominal pain. Diarrhoea initially watery, later may contain blood and mucus. Usually self-limiting, lasting 2–5 days. May be followed after 1–3 weeks by Guillain–Barré syndrome (p. 256)	Culture of C. jejuni from stool Ciprofloxacin 500 mg 12-hly PO for 5 days or Erythromycin 500 mg 12-hly PO for 5 days
Non-typhoid salmonellosis (*Salmonella* species)	Incubation period 1–2 days. Associated fever, vomiting and abdominal pain. Diarrhoea may become bloody if colon involved. Usually self-limiting. More severe in immunosuppressed	Culture of *Salmonella* species from stool Ciprofloxacin 500 mg 12-hly PO for 5 days or Trimethoprim 200 mg 12-hly PO for 5 days
Escherichia coli O157:H7 (enterohaemorrhagic *E. coli*)	Incubation period 1–3 days. Associated vomiting and abdominal pain. May have low-grade fever. Watery diarrhoea which may become bloody. May be complicated by haemolytic uraemic syndrome from 2–14 (mean 7) days after onset of illness	Culture of E. coli O157 from stool (using sorbitol MacConkey agar; missed by standard culture) Serological tests Supportive treatment: antibiotic therapy unhelpful

Acute diarrhoea

Clostridium difficile colitis	Typically causes diarrhoea in hospital, but may occur in community. See Appendix	See Appendix
Ulcerative colitis	May present with acute diarrhoea, usually bloody. Vomiting does not occur, and abdominal pain is not a prominent feature	Exclusion of infective causes of diarrhoea and typical histological appearances on rectal biopsy IV and rectal steroid
Faecal impaction with overflow diarrhoea	At risk of faecal impaction. No vomiting or systemic illness	Rectal examination discloses hard impacted faeces Laxatives/enemas
Hospital acquired: *Clostridium difficile* colitis	See Appendix	See Appendix
Drugs	Many drugs may cause diarrhoea, including chemotherapeutic agents, proton pump inhibitors and laxatives in excess	Diarrhoea resolves after treatment completed or with withdrawal of the causative drug
Recent travel abroad: Giardiasis (*Giardia lamblia*)	Widespread distribution. Explosive onset of watery diarrhoea 1–3 weeks after exposure	Identification of cysts or trophozoites in stool or jejunal or biopsy Metronidazole 400 mg 8-hly for 5 days
Amoebic dysentery (*Entamoeba histolytica*)	Mexico, South America, South Asia, West and South-East Africa. Diarrhoea may be severe with blood and mucus	Identification of cysts in stools Metronidazole 800 mg 8-hly for 5 days

Continued p. 284

Table 35.1 *Continued*

Cause	Clinical features	Diagnosis / Treatment (if indicated)
Schistosomiasis (*S. mansoni* and *japonicum*)	*S. mansoni*: South America and Middle East; *S. japonicum*: China and the Philippines. Diarrhoea onset 2–6 weeks or longer after exposure	Identification of ova in stool Praziquantel (seek expert advice)
Shigellosis (*Shigella* species)	Incubation period 1–2 days. Associated fever and abdominal pain. Diarrhoea may be watery or bloody.	Culture of *Shigella* species from stool Ciprofloxacin 500mg 12-hly PO for 5 days or Trimethoprim 200mg 12-hly PO for 5 days
Non-typhoid salmonellosis	See Community-acquired diarrhoea	See Community-acquired diarrhoea
HIV positive or immunosuppressed. In addition to the above causes of acute diarrhoea, other pathogens may be responsible:		
Cryptosporidiosis (*Cryptosporidium* species)	Subacute onset. Associated abdominal pain. Severe diarrhoea.	Identification of oocysts in stool Seek expert advice on treatment
Isosporiasis (*Isospora belli*)	Incubation period 1 week. Associated fever, abdominal pain. Diarrhoea with fatty stools	Identification of oocysts in stool, duodenal aspirate or jejunal biopsy
Cytomegalovirus	Diarrhoea may be accompanied by systemic illness and hepatitis	Serological tests for CMV Seek expert advice on treatment

Table 35.2 Investigation of acute diarrhoea

Stool microscopy and culture
Test for *Clostridium difficile* toxin in stool
Full blood count
ESR and C-reactive protein
Creatinine, sodium and potassium
Albumin and liver function tests
Blood culture if febrile
Sigmoidoscopy if bloody diarrhoea
Abdominal X-ray if marked distension or tenderness (to check for toxic megacolon)

Acute diarrhoea

• Signs of toxic megacolon (marked abdominal distension and tenderness), which may complicate many forms of infective colitis (including *C. difficile*) as well as colitis due to inflammatory bowel disease.
• Extra-abdominal features which may help make the diagnosis (check for rash and arthropathy).

3 Investigations
Investigations that are needed urgently are given in Table 35.2.

If the patient is ill
If the patient has impaired consciousness level, severe volume depletion, marked abdominal distension or tenderness, you should:
• Start vigorous fluid resuscitation, initially via a peripheral IV line and correct hypokalaemia (p. 346).
• Start antibiotic therapy to cover the likely pathogens: ciprofloxacin 400 mg 12-hly IV and metronidazole 500 mg 8-hly IV will be appropriate for community-acquired diarrhoea in immunocompetent patients.
• Obtain an abdominal X-ray to check for segmental or total colonic distension indicative of toxic megacolon.
• Seek urgent help from a gastroenterologist.

• Nurse the patient with standard isolation technique in a single room until the diagnosis is established.

If the patient is well
Further management will be determined by the results of microscopy and culture of the stool, and other investigations.
• If the patient has severe diarrhoea (4 or more bowel motions daily) and infection is the working diagnosis, it is reasonable to start treatment for the likely pathogen while awaiting results e.g. ciprofloxacin 500 mg 12-hly PO (for 1–5 days) for community-acquired diarrhoea and metronidazole 400 mg 8-hly PO (for 7–10 days) for hospital-acquired diarrhoea.
• Anti-motility drugs such as loperamide can be given to most patients for symptomatic relief, but are contraindicated in patients with shigellosis or dysentery (bloody stools and fever).

Appendix

Clostridium difficile **colitis**
• Is an acute colitis due to toxins (A and B) produced by *Clostridium difficile*.
• Is largely a complication of antibiotic therapy (in particular, ampicillin, amoxycillin, cephalosporins and clindamycin). Diarrhoea usually begins within 4–10 days of treatment, but may not appear for 4–6 weeks. The elderly are more susceptible.
• Is the commonest cause of acute diarrhoea acquired in hospital.
• Presentations range from mild self-limiting watery diarrhoea to (rarely) acute fulminating toxic megacolon. Low-grade fever and abdominal tenderness are common.
• Diagnosis is based on detection of *C. difficile* toxins A and B in the stool. In severe colitis, sigmoidoscopy may show adherent yellow plaques (2–10 mm in diameter), but although the rectum and sigmoid colon are usually involved, in 10% of cases, colitis is confined to the more proximal colon.

Management
• Supportive measures and isolation of the patient to reduce the risk of spread.

• Stop antibiotic therapy if possible. In patients with mild diarrhoea (1–2 bowel motions daily), symptoms may resolve within 1–2 weeks without further treatment.

• If antibiotic therapy needs to be continued, or if the patient has moderate–severe diarrhoea (3 or more bowel motions daily), give metronidazole 400 mg 8-hly PO for 7–10 days.

• Around 20% of patients will have a relapse after completing a course of metronidazole, due to germination of residual spores within the colon, reinfection with *C. difficile* or further antibiotic treatment: give either a further course of metronidazole or vancomycin 125 mg 6-hly PO for 7–10 days.

• If the patient is severely ill and unable to take oral medication, metronidazole can be given IV 500 mg 8-hly (IV vancomycin should not be used as significant excretion into the gut does not occur).

Acute diarrhoea

36 Acute abdominal pain

• Acute abdominal pain is usually due to surgical pathology.

• Unless acute abdominal pain clearly has a 'medical' cause (see Appendix), you should seek a surgical opinion without delay.

Priorities

1 If the patient has severe abdominal pain and is shocked (systolic BP < 90 mmHg with cold skin), the likely diagnosis is generalized peritonitis, mesenteric infarction or severe pancreatitis (Tables 36.4–36.6). The patient will need:

• Vigorous fluid resuscitation, initially via a peripheral IV line and then guided by measurement of the CVP (see Chapter 3), with monitoring of the urine output—put in a urinary catheter.

• Antibiotic therapy: start cefotaxime 1–2 g 6-hly IV + metronidazole 500 mg 8-hly IV.

• An urgent surgical opinion.

2 Your history needs to establish the characteristics of the abdominal pain, and the patient's other medical problems:

• When and how did the pain start—gradually or abruptly?

• Where is the pain felt, and has it moved since its onset (Table 36.1)?

• How severe is the pain?

• Has there been vomiting, and when did vomiting begin in relation to the onset of the pain?

• Has the patient had previous abdominal surgery and if so what for?

3 As well as a careful examination of the abdomen (Table 36.2), you should:

• Check the temperature, pulse, JVP and blood pressure.

• Listen to the heart and over the lung bases.

Table 36.1 Site of abdominal pain*

Organ involved	Site and radiation of visceral pain*	Common pathology
Stomach	Epigastric; occasional radiation to back, esp. left subscapular region	Peptic ulcer Carcinoma
Duodenum	Epigastric; radiation to back, esp. right subscapular region	Peptic ulcer
Gallbladder	Right upper quadrant or epigastric; radiation to right subscapular or midthoracic region	Cholecystitis Biliary colic
Pancreas	Epigastric; radiation to thoracic or left lumbar region	Pancreatitis due to gallstones or alcohol
Small intestine	Periumbilical	Obstruction due to hernia or adhesions
Appendix	Periumbilical	Appendicitis
Large intestine	Depends on site of lesion; sigmoid pain may radiate to sacral region	Obstruction due to tumour

* Visceral pain arising from the gut, biliary tract or pancreas is poorly localised to the body surface. In contrast, the pain of peritoneal irritation (due to inflammation or infection) is well-localised (unless there is generalised peritonitis) and constant, and associated with abdominal tenderness.

Acute abdominal pain

Table 36.2 Examination of the abdomen

Abdominal distension?

Presence of abdominal scars? If present, check what operations have been done;
  adhesions from previous surgery may cause obstruction

Tenderness: localized or generalized?

Palpable organs or masses?

Hernial orifices (inguinal, femoral and umbilical)

Femoral pulses

Bowel sounds

Check for jaundice Rectal examination

- Give oxygen if the patient has severe pain, is breathless, or if oxygen saturation by pulse oximetry is <90%.
- Put in an IV cannula and take blood for urgent investigations (Table 36.3).
- Relieve severe pain with diamorphine 2.5–5 mg (or morphine 5–10 mg IV) plus an antiemetic, e.g. prochlorperazine 12.5 mg IV.
- Start an infusion of colloid 500 mL over 15–30 min if systolic BP is < 90 mmHg.

4 Further management will be determined by the results of investigations and assessment by a surgeon. 'Medical' causes of abdominal pain are summarized in the Appendix (Fig. 36.1).

Table 36.3 Investigation of acute abdominal pain

Full blood count (white cell count >16 x 10^9/L seen in severe pancreatitis and mesenteric ischaemia; white cell count may be low in overwhelming bacterial sepsis; low platelet count may reflect disseminated intravascular coagulation, p. 104)

Clotting screen if purpura or jaundice, prolonged oozing from puncture sites or low platelet count

Group and save

Creatinine, sodium and potassium

Blood glucose

Serum amylase (raised in pancreatitis, perforated ulcer, mesenteric ischaemia and severe sepsis)

Other tests to confirm or exclude pancreatitis if indicated (serum lipase; urine dipstick test for trypsinogen-2 (which has a high negative predictive value))

Liver function tests

Arterial gases and pH if hypotensive or oxygen saturation <90% (metabolic acidosis seen in generalized peritonitis, mesenteric infarction and severe pancreatitis)

Blood culture if febrile or suspected peritonitis

Urine microscopy and culture

ECG if age > 60 or known cardiac disease or unexplained upper abdominal pain

Chest X-ray (looking for free gas under the diaphragm, indicating perforation, and evidence of basal pneumonia)

Abdominal X-ray (supine and erect or lateral decubitus) (looking for evidence of obstruction of large and/or small bowel; ischaemic bowel (dilated and thickened loops of small bowel); cholangitis (gas in biliary tree); radiodense gall stones; radiodense urinary tract stones)

Acute abdominal pain

Appendix

Table 36.4 Causes of generalized peritonitis

Perforation of viscus

Mesenteric vascular occlusion leading to intestinal infarction (Table 36.5)

Inflammatory conditions (most commonly appendicitis, cholecystitis, diverticulitis, pancreatitis (Table 36.6))

Late intestinal obstruction (most commonly due to large bowel tumour, adhesions, hernia or volvulus)

Table 36.5 Causes of acute mesenteric vascular occlusion

Thrombosis complicating atherosclerotic disease of the mesenteric arteries, polycythaemia, sickle cell disease, cryoglobulinaemia and amyloidosis

Embolism from the heart (e.g. atrial fibrillation, endocarditis)

Aortic dissection (p. 156)

Vasculitis

Table 36.6 Causes of pancreatitis

Common
Gallstones
Alcohol abuse

Less common
Endoscopic retrograde cholangiopancreatography (ERCP)
Hyperlipidaemia
Drugs
Pancreas divisum
Abdominal trauma

Table 36.7 Management of acute pancreatitis

Recognition of clinically severe acute pancreatitis
Ranson score of 3 or more: score 1 for each feature
   Present on admission:
      Age >55; white cell count >16 x 10^9/L; blood glucose >11 mmol/L; serum LDH
         >350 IU/L; serum AST >250 IU/L;
   During first 48 hours:
      Fall in haematocrit >10%; increase in blood urea >1.8 mmol/L; plasma calcium
         <2 mmol/L; PaO_2 < 8 kPa; base deficit >4 mmol/L; fluid sequestration > 6 l
APACHE II score of 8 or more
Organ failure (shock, renal failure, respiratory failure)
Substantial pancreatic necrosis (at least 30% glandular necrosis on contrast-
   enhanced CT)

Intensive care unit management for clinically severe acute pancreatitis
Supportive care
Antibiotic therapy with imipenem-cilastatin for radiographically documented
   pancreatic necrosis
ERCP/ sphincterotomy for patients with gallstone pancreatitis in whom biliary
   obstruction is suspected on the basis of raised bilirubin and clinical cholangitis
Nutritional support (enteral feeding by nasoenteric tube beyond the ligament of
   Treitz, in the absence of substantial ileus)

Identification of infected necrosis
CT or ultrasound guided fine-needle aspiration

Debridement of infected necrosis
Operative management
Alternative techniques (percutaneous or endoscopic) if available

Reference: Baron TH, Morgan DE. Acute necrotizing pancreatitis. *New England Journal of Medicine* 1999; **340**, 1412–7.

Acute abdominal pain

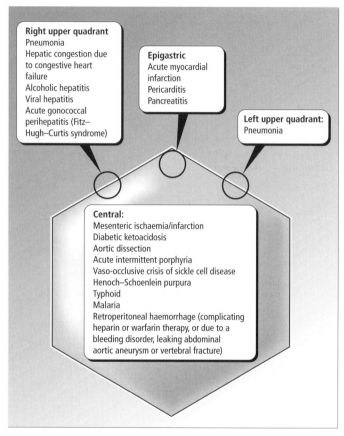

Fig. 36.1 'Medical' causes of acute abdominal pain.

37 Acute liver failure

Consider acute liver failure in any patient with:
- jaundice *and*
- abnormal behaviour or reduced conscious level *or*
- asterixis ('liver flap') or hepatic fetor.

Acute liver failure is usually due to decompensated chronic liver disease (Table 37.1). Fulminant hepatic failure is uncommon: in the UK, paracetamol poisoning (p. 119) accounts for around 50% of cases and viral hepatitis for around 40%. Other causes are given in Table 37.5.

Priorities

1 **Check the blood glucose**.
   - If < 3.5 mmol/L, give 50 mL of 50% dextrose IV.
   - Start an IV infusion of 10% dextrose (initially 1 L 12-hly) in all cases because of the high risk of hypoglycaemia. Use a large peripheral vein as it can cause thrombophlebitis.
   - Recheck blood glucose 1–4-hly.
2 **Other investigations needed urgently** are given in Table 37.2.
   - A prolonged prothrombin time (which is not corrected by vitamin K 10 mg IV) confirms the diagnosis.
3 **If there is grade 3 or 4 coma** (Table 37.3), transfer the patient to the ITU for further management, which will include elective endotracheal intubation and ventilation.
4 **Obtain advice on management** from a gastroenterologist:
   - if you suspect fulminant hepatic failure; or
   - the patient has decompensated chronic liver disease with encephalopathy more severe than grade 2.
5 **If acute liver failure is due to paracetamol poisoning** and the patient has not already received acetylcysteine, this should be given

Table 37.1 Causes of decompensation in chronic liver disease

Acute gastrointestinal haemorrhage
Drugs: diuretics, hypnotics, sedatives and narcotic analgesics
Hypokalaemia and hypoglycaemia
Intercurrent infection, especially bacterial peritonitis
Alcoholic binge
Acute viral hepatitis
Major surgery and anaesthesia
Constipation

Table 37.2 Urgent investigation in suspected liver failure

Prothrombin time
Full blood count (including platelets)
Urea*, creatinine, sodium and potassium
Blood glucose
Paracetamol level
Arterial blood gases and pH
Blood culture
Urine microscopy and culture
Microscopy and culture of ascites if present (inoculate blood culture bottles with a
   specimen of ascites)
Chest X-ray

For later analysis (if suspected fulminant hepatic failure)
Liver function tests
Markers of viral hepatitis
Plasma ceruloplasmin in patients aged < 50 (to exclude Wilson's disease)
Serum (10 mL) and urine (50 mL) for toxicological analysis if needed

* Urea may be low because of reduced hepatic synthesis; if markedly elevated with
a normal creatinine, suspect upper gastrointestinal haemorrhage.

Table 37.3 Grading of hepatic encephalopathy

Grade 1	Mildly drowsy with impaired concentration and psychomotor function
Grade 2	Confused, but able to answer questions
Grade 3	Very drowsy and able to respond only to simple commands; incoherent and agitated
Grade 4	Unrousable: 4a, responsive to painful stimuli; 4b, unresponsive

using the standard regimen (p. 122), as it has been shown to improve outcome, even when given > 24 h after ingestion.

Further management of decompensated chronic liver disease

1 Look for and treat precipitants (Table 37.1)
• Spontaneous bacterial peritonitis is common and may not be accompanied by abdominal tenderness. If there is ascites, aspirate 10 mL for microscopy and culture (inoculate blood culture bottles). Assume peritonitis is present if ascitic fluid shows >250 white blood cells/mm^3, of which >75% are polymorphs, and treat with a combination of amoxycillin, gentamicin and metronidazole.
• Start empirical antibiotic therapy with cefotaxime and gentamicin if there is fever, even in the absence of focal signs of infection, after taking blood cultures.

2 Start a liver failure regimen
• **Reduce the intestinal nitrogenous load**: stop dietary protein and start lactulose 30 mL 3-hly until diarrhoea begins, then reduce to 30 mL 12-hly. Give magnesium sulphate enemata 80 mL of a 50% solution 12-hly (useful even in the absence of gastrointestinal bleeding). Neomycin may be helpful, although its contribution is controversial: it works faster than lactulose, but has potential toxicity.
• **Parenteral nutrition** should be considered: it should be started early to prevent a hypercatabolic state.

• **Reduce the risk of gastric stress ulceration.** Give prophylaxis with omeprazole, ranitidine or sucralfate.

• **Maintain blood glucose >3.5mmol/L.** Give dextrose 10% by IV infusion initially 1 L 12-hly. Check blood glucose 1–4-hly and immediately if conscious level deteriorates.

• **Fluid and electrolyte balance.** The diet should be low in sodium. Give potassium supplements to maintain a plasma level >3.5mmol/L. If IV fluid is needed, use albumin solution or dextrose 5% or 10%. Avoid saline. Treat ascites with spironolactone combined with a loop diuretic if necessary, aiming for weight loss of 0.5kg/day. If ascites is refractory to diuretic therapy, use paracentesis with IV infusion of salt-poor albumin.

• **Drugs.** Give vitamin K 10mg IV (not intramuscularly) and folic acid 15mg PO once daily. Avoid sedatives and opiates. Other drugs that are contraindicated are listed in the *British National Formulary*.

Further management of acute liver failure before transfer

Ask for help
Ask for help from your local gastroenterologist/hepatologist or discuss management with the regional liver unit.

Monitoring and general care
• Nurse the patient with 20° head-up tilt in a quiet area of an ITU or high-dependency unit, avoiding unnecessary disturbance.

• Monitor the conscious level 1–4-hly, pulse and blood pressure 1–4-hly and temperature 8-hly.

• Check blood glucose 1–4-hly and immediately if the conscious level deteriorates.

• Monitor blood oxygen saturation by pulse oximeter and give oxygen by mask to maintain $Sao_2 > 90\%$.

• Give platelet concentrate before placing central venous and arterial lines if the platelet count is $< 50 \times 10^{12}/L$. Avoid giving fresh frozen plasma unless there is active bleeding, as this affects coagulation tests—the best prognostic marker—for several days.

• If encephalopathy is grade 2 or more or if systolic BP is <90mmHg, put in a pulmonary artery catheter (as the central venous pressure may

Table 37.4 Major complications of acute liver failure

Complication	Management
Cerebral oedema	See text
Hypotension	Correct hypovolaemia (aim for wedge pressure 12–15 mmHg) with blood or 4.5% human albumin solution. Use adrenaline or noradrenaline infusion (p. 481–3) to maintain mean arterial pressure > 60 mmHg
Oliguria/renal failure	Correct hypovolaemia. Consider dopamine infusion at 2.5 μg/kg/min. Avoid high-dose frusemide. Start renal replacement therapy if anuric or oliguric with plasma creatinine > 400 μmol/L
Hypoglycaemia	Give dextrose 10% IV 1 L 12-hly. Check blood glucose 1–4-hly and give stat doses of dextrose 25 g IV if < 3.5 mmol/L
Coagulopathy	Give vitamin K 10 mg IV daily. Give platelet transfusion if count < 50×10^{12}/L. Give fresh frozen plasma only if there is active bleeding
Gastric stress ulceration	Prophylaxis with omeprazole, ranitidine or sucralfate
Hypoxaemia	Many possible causes: inhalation pneumonia, infection, pulmonary oedema, atelectasis, intrapulmonary haemorrhage. Increase inspired oxygen. Ventilate with positive end expiratory pressure if Sao_2 remains < 90%
Infection	Daily culture of blood, sputum and urine. Early treatment of presumed infection with broad-spectrum antibiotic therapy. Consider antifungal therapy with amphotericin if fever with negative blood cultures

Acute liver failure

Table 37.5 Principal causes of fulminant hepatic failure

Cause	Agent responsible
Viral hepatitis	Hepatitis A, B, C, D or E virus
	Herpes simplex virus (usually associated with immunosuppressive therapy)
Drug related	Paracetamol poisoning (p. 119)
	Idiosyncratic reactions
Toxins	Carbon tetrachloride
	Amanita phalloides
	Phosphorus
Vascular	Ischaemia due to cardiac disease
	Veno-occlusive disease
	Budd–Chiari syndrome
	Heatstroke
Others	Wilson's disease
	Acute fatty liver of pregnancy
	Reye's syndrome
	Malignant infiltration, especially lymphoma
	Overwhelming sepsis

Acute liver failure

not be an adequate guide to left ventricular filling pressure), a radial arterial line and urinary catheter.

• Give blood if haemoglobin is <10 g/dL. Fluid therapy should be with albumin solution or dextrose 5% or 10%. Saline should not be used.

• If encephalopathy progresses to grade 3 or 4, arrange elective endotracheal intubation and ventilation.

• Put in a nasogastric tube for gastric drainage if the patient is vomiting or is ventilated.

Management of complications

• Management of complications is summarized in Table 37.4. Cerebral oedema occurs in 75–80% of patients with grade 4 encephalopathy and is often fatal. It may result in paroxysmal hypertension, dilated pupils, sustained ankle clonus and sometimes decerebrate posturing (papilloedema is usually absent). If these occur:

• Give mannitol 20% 100–200 mL (0.5 g/kg) IV over 10 min, provided urine output is >30 mL/h and pulmonary artery wedge pressure is <15 mmHg. Check plasma osmolality: further mannitol may be given until plasma osmolality is 320 mosmol/kg.

• Hyperventilate to an arterial $P\text{co}_2$ of 4.0 kPa (30 mmHg).

• If there is no response to these measures, give thiopentone 125–250 mg IV over 15 min, followed by an infusion of 50–250 mg/h for up to 4 h.

Acute liver failure

38 Acute renal failure

Acute renal failure is diagnosed by:
- a rapidly rising plasma urea or creatinine; or
- a urine output of <400 mL/day or <30 mL/h for 3 consecutive hours: this is not an invariable feature and non-oliguric renal failure occurs in 50% of cases.

Causes of acute renal failure (ARF) are given in Fig. 38.1 and in the Appendix; pre-renal causes account for around 70% of cases.

Priorities

You need to answer three questions:
1 Is the patient at imminent risk of cardiorespiratory arrest from severe hyperkalaemia or pulmonary oedema?
2 What is the likely cause of renal failure?
3 Are there any correctable factors?

1 Does the patient have severe hyperkalaemia or pulmonary oedema?
These are the immediate life-threatening complications of acute renal failure. Severe hyperkalaemia may be asymptomatic until cardiac arrest.

Severe hyperkalaemia
- Check plasma potassium if this has not already been done.
- Attach an ECG.

If the plasma potassium is >7 mmol/L or the ECG has abnormalities associated with hyperkalaemia (widening of the QRS complex, loss of the P wave, peaking of the T wave or a sine wave pattern) and plasma potassium is > 6.0 mmol/L:

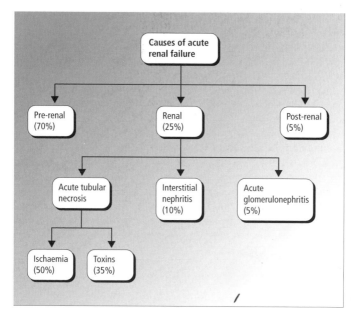

Fig. 38.1 Causes of acute renal failure (percentage frequency).

- Give 10 mL of calcium chloride 10% IV over 5 min. This can be repeated every 5 min up to a total dose of 40 mL.
- Give 25 g of dextrose (50 mL of dextrose 50%) with 10 U of soluble insulin IV over 30 min. This will usually reduce plasma potassium for several hours. Check blood glucose after dextrose/insulin has been given to exclude rebound hypoglycaemia.
- If hyperkalaemia is associated with a severe metabolic acidosis (arterial pH < 7.2), give sodium bicarbonate 50 mmol (50 mL of 8.4% solution) IV over 30 min. This concentration of bicarbonate is irritant to veins and should preferably be given via a central line. Bicarbonate should not be given if alveolar ventilation is impaired (raised $Paco_2$).
- Stop potassium supplements or any drugs (e.g. ACE inhibitors, potassium-retaining diuretics) which may be contributing to hyperkalaemia.

- Start calcium resonium (15 g 8-hly PO or 30 g by retention enema).
- Recheck plasma potassium after 2–4 h.

If renal function is not improving despite vigorous management of correctable factors (see below), renal replacement therapy will be needed for recurrent hyperkalaemia:

- Haemodialysis: discuss transfer to your regional renal unit.
- Haemofiltration: discuss this with your ITU if the patient is not suitable for transfer.
- Peritoneal dialysis (if transfer for haemodialysis or local haemofiltration is not possible) (see Chapter 60).

Severe pulmonary oedema

This is clinically obvious, with breathlessness, widespread lung crackles and wheeze, and hypoxaemia. A chest X-ray will show alveolar shadowing. Pulmonary oedema in acute renal failure may be exacerbated by cardiac disease, and investigation should include an ECG and echocardiogram (Chapter 17).

- Sit the patient up and give oxygen 35–60% by mask, aiming for an oxygen saturation of > 90%. If this is not achieved, consider using a continuous positive airways pressure system. Intubation and mechanical ventilation may be indicated if there is refractory hypoxaemia: discuss this with an ITU physician.
- Give diamorphine 2.5–5 mg (or morphine 5–10 mg) by slow IV injection to relieve distress.
- Start an infusion of frusemide 100 mg over 60 min by syringe pump. If there is no significant diuresis (<500 mL in 4 h) in response to this, renal replacement therapy will be needed.
- Venesection of 100–200 mL of blood should be considered for severe pulmonary oedema while awaiting haemodialysis or haemofiltration.

2 What is the likely cause of renal failure?

- Most causes of acute renal failure can be diagnosed from the clinical assessment, examination of the urine and ultrasound of the urinary tract.
- Other investigations needed are given in Table 38.1.
- Acute renal failure developing in hospital is often due to a combination of factors, most commonly hypovolaemia, hypotension, sepsis and nephrotoxic drugs.

Table 38.1 Investigation in acute renal failure

Urgent

Creatinine, urea, sodium, potassium and calcium

Blood glucose

Arterial gases and pH

Full blood count

Clotting screen if the patient has purpura or jaundice, or the blood film shows
haemolysis or a low platelet count

Urine stick test for glucose, blood and protein

Urine microscopy

ECG

Chest X-ray

Ultrasound of the kidneys and urinary tract if the diagnosis is not clear from clinical
assessment and examination of the urine

Later

Full biochemical profile, including urate

Creatine kinase if suspected rhabdomyolysis (urine stick test positive for blood, but
no RBC on microscopy)

ESR and C-reactive protein

Culture of blood and urine

Serum and urine protein electrophoresis

Serum complement and other immunological tests (antinuclear antibodies,
antineutrophil cytoplasmic antibodies, antiglomerular basement membrane
antibodies) if suspected acute glomerulonephritis

Ultrasound of kidneys and urinary tract if not already done

Echocardiography if clinical cardiac abnormality, major ECG abnormality or positive
blood culture (? endocarditis)

Acute renal failure

Clinical assessment

Points to cover include:

1 History (including review of the notes, and drug, observation and
fluid balance charts).

• Has there been anuria, oliguria or polyuria? Anuria is seen in
severe hypotension or complete urinary tract obstruction. It is more

rarely due to bilateral renal artery occlusion (e.g. with aortic dissection), renal cortical necrosis or necrotizing glomerular disease.

• Has the blood pressure been normal, high or low and, if low, for how long?

• Is hypovolaemia likely? Has there been haemorrhage, vomiting, diarrhoea, recent surgery or the use of diuretics?

• Is sepsis possible? What are the results of recent blood, urine and other cultures?

• Is there a past history of renal or urinary tract disease? Are there previous biochemistry results to establish when renal function was last normal? Over how long has renal function been deteriorating?

• Is there known cardiac disease with heart failure, hypertension or peripheral arterial disease (commonly associated with atherosclerotic renal artery stenosis) (p. 163)?

• Is there liver disease (associated with the hepatorenal syndrome)?

• Is there diabetes or other multisystem disorder which might involve the kidneys? Don't forget endocarditis and myeloma as causes of renal failure.

• Has renal failure followed cardiac catheterization via the femoral artery (raising the possibility of renal atheroembolism)?

• Has the patient been exposed to any nephrotoxic drugs (including contrast media) or poisons? Consider occupational exposure to toxins.

2 Physical examination

• Conscious level, temperature, pulse, blood pressure, respiratory rate, oxygen saturation.

• Signs of fluid depletion (tachycardia, low JVP with flat neck veins, hypotension or postural hypotension) or fluid overload (high JVP, triple cardiac rhythm, hypertension, lung crackles, pleural effusions, ascites, peripheral oedema).

• Presence of a pericardial rub (uraemic pericarditis is an indication for renal replacement therapy).

• Abdomen (check for palpable kidneys or bladder) and rectal examination (to assess the prostate and to check for a pelvic mass).

• Peripheral pulses.

• Purpura (ARF with purpura may be due to sepsis complicated by disseminated intravascular coagulation; meningococcal sepsis; thrombotic thrombocytopenic purpura; haemolytic uraemic syndrome; Henoch–Schoenlein purpura and other vasculitides).

• Jaundice (ARF with jaundice may be due to hepatorenal syndrome; paracetamol poisoning; severe congestive heart failure; severe sepsis; leptospirosis; incompatible blood transfusion; haemolytic–uraemic syndrome).

Examination of the urine
• A specimen of urine should be tested for glucose, blood and protein and sent for urgent microscopy and culture.
• If urine has not been passed in the previous 6 h or the patient is hypotensive, a bladder catheter should be placed to obtain a specimen and to monitor urine output.
• Findings on urinalysis and urine microscopy in acute renal failure are summarized in Table 38.2. Measurement of urine biochemistry is of little practical use.

Ultrasound of the urinary tract
• If the diagnosis is not clear from clinical assessment and examination of the urine, arrange urgent ultrasound of the urinary tract to exclude obstruction, and assess renal size.
• Acute renal failure beginning in hospital is rarely due to urinary tract obstruction, once bladder outflow obstruction has been excluded by catheterization.
• The hallmark of obstruction is dilatation of the urinary tract above the obstruction, although this is not an invariable feature.

3 Are there any correctable factors?
In every patient with acute renal failure, you need to address systematically those causes of renal impairment which are potentially correctable:
• Hypovolaemia.
• Hypotension.
• Heart failure.
• Systemic sepsis.
• Urinary tract infection (especially of a single kidney).
• Accelerated-phase hypertension.
• Hypercalcaemia.
• Urinary tract obstruction.
• Nephrotoxic drugs and toxins (including endogenous toxins such as free haemoglobin (intravascular haemolysis), free myoglobin (rhabdomyolysis) and light chains (myeloma)).

Acute renal failure

Table 38.2 Urinalysis and urine microscopy in acute renal failure

*Red cells, red cell casts, proteinuria (2+ or more)**
Acute glomerulonephritis
Acute vasculitis

Stick test positive for blood, but no red cells on microscopy
Rhabdomyolysis

Tubular cell casts, granular casts, tubular casts
Acute tubular necrosis

Normal or near normal
Pre-renal causes
Urinary tract obstruction
Some cases of acute tubular necrosis (more commonly in nephrotoxic or non-oliguric ATN)
Hypercalcaemia
Tubular obstruction (myeloma, acute uric acid nephropathy, acyclovir, methotrexate, ethylene glycol poisoning)
Renal atheroembolism (consider in the elderly patient with renal failure and skin lesions (especially livedo reticularis) or after cardiac catheterization)

* In patients with a bladder catheter, red and white cells in the urine may be due to the catheter itself.

Correcting hypovolaemia and hypotension

Prompt and vigorous correction of hypovolaemia and hypotension will often reverse pre-renal failure and prevent progression to ischaemic acute tubular necrosis.

• If there is clinically obvious hypovolaemia, give IV fluid (blood, colloid or saline as appropriate to the cause of hypovolaemia). A CVP line may be helpful (to avoid over-replacement of fluid), but the patient should be resuscitated first before this is placed.

• If the evidence for hypovolaemia is less certain, but there are no clinical signs of fluid overload, give a fluid challenge, ideally with monitoring of the CVP, especially if the JVP is difficult to assess. How

to give a fluid challenge is described on p. 43. Target CVP is 5–10 cm water, measured from a mid-axillary line zero reference point.
• If the systolic BP remains <90 mmHg despite correction or exclusion of hypovolaemia, search for and treat other causes of hypotension, of which sepsis is the most likely (p. 100). If the BP remains low, inotropic–vasopressor therapy will be needed (p. 42).

Further management

Your patient can now be placed in one of four groups.

Pre-renal failure, now corrected, with improving renal function
Management is that of the underlying disorder, taking care to avoid hypovolaemia and nephrotoxic drugs.

Suspected pre-renal or nephrotoxic renal failure with no improvement despite correction of hypovolaemia or hypotension.
• It is likely the patient now has ischaemic acute tubular necrosis. The management of established acute renal failure is summarized in the Appendix.
• Treatment with high-dose frusemide or dopamine has been advocated in this situation, with the aim of preventing progression to acute tubular necrosis or converting oliguric to non-oliguric renal failure. There is no clear evidence to support this approach, and adverse effects may outweigh any benefits.
• Indications for renal replacement therapy are given in Table 38.3.
• Contact your renal unit early about patients with acute renal failure, before the plasma creatinine is over 400 μmol/L.
• Preserve forearm veins as these may be needed for the creation of an arteriovenous fistula, if long-term dialysis is needed. Where possible, IV infusions should be given into central veins.

Suspected urinary tract obstruction
Ask advice from a urologist. Percutaneous nephrostomy drainage may be indicated.

Possible intrinsic renal disease or renal failure unexplained
Ask advice from a nephrologist. A renal biopsy may be needed to establish the diagnosis.

Acute renal failure

Table 38.3 Indications for renal replacement therapy

Refractory hyperkalaemia

Refractory pulmonary oedema

Severe metabolic acidosis

Uraemic pericarditis

Uraemic encephalopathy

Uraemic bleeeding

Plasma creatinine > 500–700 μmol/L and/or plasma urea > 25–30 mmol/L, unless there is clear evidence that renal function is recovering

Appendix

Appendix 1 Causes of acute renal failure
See Table 38.4.

Appendix 2 Management of the patient with established acute tubular necrosis (before renal replacement therapy is instituted)

1 *Fluid balance*

• Restrict the daily fluid intake to 500 mL plus the previous day's measured losses (urine, nasogastric drainage, etc.), allowing more if the patient is febrile (500 mL for each °C of fever).

• The patient's fluid status should be assessed twice daily (by weighing and fluid balance chart) and the next 12 hours' fluids adjusted appropriately.

2 *Diet*

• Aim for an energy content >2000 kcal/day (8400 kJ/day).

• Restrict sodium and potassium content to <50 mmol/day.

• Restrict protein content to 20–40 g/day.

• Restrict dietary phosphate to <800 mg/day.

• Consider enteral or parenteral nutrition if renal failure is prolonged or the patient is hypercatabolic.

Table 38.4 Clinical features, typical findings on examination of the urine and confirmatory tests for diagnosis of the major causes of acute renal failure

Cause of acute renal failure	Suggestive clinical features	Typical urinalysis	Confirmatory tests
Pre-renal azotaemia (~70%)	Evidence of volume depletion (thirst, postural hypotension and tachycardia, low JVP, dry mucous membranes, weight loss, fluid output > input), or decreased 'effective' circulatory volume (e.g., heart failure, liver failure); NSAIDs or ACEI	Hyaline casts, FeNa < 1%, UNa < 10, SG > 1.018	Occasionally requires invasive haemodynamic monitoring; rapid resolution of ARF on restoration of renal perfusion
Intrinsic renal azotaemia (~25%) *Diseases involving large renal vessels*			
Renal artery thrombosis	History of atrial fibrillation or recent myocardial infarct, nausea, vomiting, flank or abdominal pain	Mild proteinuria, occasionally red cells	Elevated LDH with normal transaminases, renal arteriogram
Atheroembolism	Usually age > 50 years, recent manipulation of aorta, retinal plaques, subcutaneous nodules, palpable purpura, livedo reticularis, vasculopathy, hypertension	Often normal, eosinophiluria, rarely casts	Eosinophilia, hypocomplementaemia, skin biopsy, renal biopsy

Continued p. 312

Acute renal failure

Table 38.4 Continued

Cause of acute renal failure	Suggestive clinical features	Typical urinalysis	Confirmatory tests
Renal vein thrombosis	Evidence of nephrotic syndrome or pulmonary embolism, flank pain	Proteinuria, haematuria	Inferior vena cavagram and selective renal venogram
Diseases of small vessels and glomeruli			
Glomerulonephritis/vasculitis	Compatible clinical history (e.g. recent infection) or evidence of multisystem diseases (sinusitis), lung haemorrhage, rash, or skin ulcers, arthralgias)	Red cell or granular casts, dysmorphic red cells, proteinuria	C3 level, ANCA, anti-GBM Ab, ANA, ASO, anti-DNAse cryoglobulins, renal biopsy
HUS/TTP	Compatible clinical history (e.g. recent gastrointestinal infection, cyclosporin, anovulants), fever, pallor, ecchymoses, neurological abnormalities	May be normal, red cells, mild proteinuria, rarely red cell/granular casts	Anaemia, thrombocytopenia, schistocytes on blood smear, increased LDH, renal biopsy
Malignant hypertension	Severe hypertension with headaches, cardiac failure, retinopathy, neurological dysfunction, papilloedema	Red cells, red cell casts, proteinuria	LVH by echocardiography/ECG, resolution with control of blood pressure
*Acute tubular necrosis (ATN) due to ischaemia or toxins**			
Ischaemia	Recent haemorrhage, hypotension (e.g. cardiac arrest, pancreatitis), major surgery or burns	'Muddy brown' granular or epithelial cell casts, FeNa >1%, UNa >20, SG 1.010	Clinical assessment and urinalysis usually sufficient for diagnosis

Exogenous toxins	Recent radiocontrast study, nephrotoxic antibiotics or anticancer agents often coexistent with volume depletion, sepsis or chronic renal insufficiency	'Muddy brown' granular or tubular epithelial cell casts, FeNa >1%, UNa > 20, SG 1.010	Clinical assessment of urinalysis usually sufficient for diagnosis
Endogenous toxins	(1) History suggestive of rhabdomyolysis (seizures, coma, ethanol abuse, trauma)	Urine supernatant tests positive for haem	Hyperkalaemia, hyperphosphataemia, hypocalcaemia, increased circulating myoglobin, CPK MM, and uric acid
	(2) History suggestive of haemolysis (blood transfusion)	Urine supernatant pink and positive for haem	Hyperkalaemia, hyperphosphataemia, hypocalcaemia, hyperuricaemia, pink plasma positive for haemoglobin
	(3) History suggestive of (a) tumour lysis (recent chemotherapy), (b) myeloma (bone pain), or (c) ethylene glycol ingestion	Urate crystals (a), dipstick-negative proteinuria (b), oxalate crystals (c)	Hyperuricaemia, hyperkalaemia, hyperphosphataemia (a); circulating or urinary paraprotein (b); toxicology screen, acidosis, osmolal gap (c)

Continued p. 314

Acute renal failure

Acute renal failure

Table 38.4 *Continued*

Cause of acute renal failure	Suggestive clinical features	Typical urinalysis	Confirmatory tests
Acute diseases of the tubulointerstitium			
Allergic interstitial nephritis	Recent ingestion of drug, and fever, rash or arthralgias	White cell casts, white cells (often eosinophils), red cells, proteinuria (occasionally nephrotic)	Systemic eosinophilia, skin biopsy of rash (leucocytoclastic vasculitis), renal biopsy
Acute bilateral pyelonephritis	Flank pain and tenderness, toxic, febrile	Leucocytes, proteinuria, red cells, bacteria	Urine and blood cultures
Postrenal azotaemia (5%)	Abdominal or flank pain, palpable bladder	Frequently normal, haematuria without casts or proteinuria	Plain film, renal ultrasound, IVP, retrograde or anterograde pyelography, computed tomography

* Denotes major cause of acute intrinsic renal azotaemia. NSAIDs = non-steroidal anti-inflammatory drugs, ACEI = angiotensin-converting enzyme inhibitor, SG = specific gravity (mmol/kg), FeNa = fractional excretion of sodium (%), UNa = urinary sodium, concentration (mmol/L), LDH = lactate dehydrogenase, ANCA = antineutrohil cytoplasmic antibody, anti-GBM Ab = antiglomerular basement membrane antibody, ANA = antinuclear antibody, ASO = antistreptolysin-O antibody, LVH = left ventricular hypertrophy, ECG = electrocardiography, HUS/TTP = haemolytic–uraemic syndrome/thrombotic thrombocytopenic purpura, IVP = intravenous pyelogram, JVP = jugular venous pressure, CPK = creatine phosphokinase.

Reference: Brady HR, Singer GG. Acute renal failure. *Lancet* 1995; **346**, 1533–40.

3 Potassium
- Stop potassium supplements and potassium-retaining drugs.
- Restrict dietary potassium intake to <50 mmol/day.
- If plasma potassium rises above 5 mmol/L despite dietary restriction, start calcium resonium, which may be given orally (15 g 8-hly PO) or by retention enema (30 g).

4 Infection
- Patients with ARF are vulnerable to infection, especially pneumonia and urinary tract infection.
- Urinary catheters and vascular lines should be removed wherever possible.
- If the patient develops fever or unexplained hypotension, search for a focus of infection, send blood and urine for culture and start antibiotic therapy to cover both Gram-positive and negative organisms (e.g. amoxycillin 500 mg 8-hly IV plus flucloxacillin 500 mg 6-hly IV, or a third-generation cephalosporin).

5 Gastrointestinal bleeding
- Gastrointestinal bleeding occurs in 10–30% of patients with ARF.
- Start prophylactic therapy with a proton pump inhibitor or H2-receptor antagonist.

6 Drugs
- Avoid potentially nephrotoxic drugs, such as NSAIDs, ACE inhibitors and nephrotoxic antibiotics.
- Make sure all drug dosages are adjusted appropriately: consult the section on drug therapy in renal impairment in the *British National Formulary*.

Acute renal failure

Endocrine/Metabolic

39 Overview of diabetes

- Urine should be tested for glucose in all hospital patients.
- Blood glucose must be tested in any patient with glycosuria, any ill patient with diabetes, and any patient with a clinical state in which derangements of blood glucose must be excluded (Table 39.1).

Hypoglycaemia

1 If the patient is drowsy or fitting (this may sometimes occur with mild hypoglycaemia, especially in young diabetic patients):
   - give 50 mL of 50% dextrose IV via a large vein or glucagon 1 mg IV/IM/SC;
   - recheck blood glucose after 5 min and again after 30 min.
2 Consider the possible causes (Table 39.2).
3 If hypoglycaemia recurs or is likely to recur (e.g. liver disease, sepsis, sulphonylurea excess):
   - start 10% dextrose at 1 L 12-hly via a central or large peripheral vein;
   - adjust the rate to keep the blood glucose level at 5–10 mmol/L;
   - after excess sulphonylurea therapy, maintain the glucose infusion for 24 h, then tail off, but check blood glucose routinely for 3 days.
4 If hypoglycaemia is only partially responsive to 10% dextrose infusion:
   - give 20 or 30% dextrose via a central vein;
   - if the cause is intentional insulin overdose, consider local excision of the injection site.

Glycosuria on routine testing

- Check the blood glucose either fasting or 2 h after a meal.
- Diabetes is diagnosed by a fasting venous plasma level >7 mmol/L

Table 39.1 Clinical states in which derangements of blood glucose must be excluded

Clinical state

Coma or reduced conscious level
Acute confusional state
Fits
Suspected stroke
Salicylate poisoning
Metabolic acidosis
Severe hyponatraemia
Sepsis syndrome
Liver failure
Hypothermia
Parenteral nutrition
Steroid treatment
Acute myocardial infarction
After cardiac arrest

Table 39.2 Causes of hypoglycaemia

Common
Excess insulin
Sulphonylureas—more common with chlorpropamide and glibenclamide than with tolbutamide or glipizide
Alcoholic binge
Severe liver disease
Sepsis syndrome

Others
Insulinoma
Hypopituitarism
Adrenal insufficiency
Salicylate poisoning

or a level 2 h after a meal of >11 mmol/L. Two abnormal levels are required to make the diagnosis in an asymptomatic patient.

Blood glucose >11 mmol/L

1 Check the urine or plasma for ketones. If 2+ or greater and the patient is unwell (particularly if there is vomiting), measure venous bicarbonate. Avoid unnecessary arterial blood sampling.

2 Assess the conscious level and state of hydration.

3 The patient can now be placed in one of three groups (Table 39.3).

4 Further management is as follows:
  • Diabetic ketoacidosis (DKA): see Chapter 40.
  • Hyperosmolar non-ketotic hyperglycaemia (HONK): see Chapter 41.
  • Poorly controlled insulin-treated diabetes: modify the insulin regimen, or treat with an insulin infusion (Table 39.4) if there is significant intercurrent illness (e.g. sepsis, myocardial infarction).
  • Poorly controlled non-insulin-dependent diabetes: if the patient has acute myocardial infarction or other significant intercurrent illness, treat with an insulin infusion (Table 39.4).
  • Newly diagnosed diabetes: see next section.

Table 39.3 Categorization of patients with blood glucose > 11 mmol/L

Diagnosis	Blood glucose (mmol/L)	Venous bicarbonate (mmol/L)	Degree of ketonuria	Dehydration	Drowsiness
DKA	>11	<15	+++	++	++
HONK	>30	>15	+	++++	+++
Diabetes*	>11	>15	− to ++	−/+	−

DKA, diabetic ketoacidosis.

HONK, hyperosmolar non-ketotic hyperglycaemia.

*Either poorly controlled or newly diagnosed.

Overview of diabetes

Table 39.4 Continuous insulin infusion using a syringe pump

1 Make 50 U of soluble insulin up to 50 ml with normal saline (i.e. 1 U/ml). Flush 10 ml of the solution through the line before connecting to the patient (as some insulin will be adsorbed on to the plastic)

2 Check blood glucose and start the infusion at the appropriate rate (see below)

3 Dextrose 5% should be infused concurrently at an appropriate rate e.g. 1 L 12-hly IV (500 ml 12-hly after myocardial infarction)

4 Check blood glucose after 1 h and then at least 2-hly. Adjust the insulin infusion rate as needed, aiming to keep blood glucose between 5–10 mmol/L

Blood glucose (mmol/L)	Insulin infusion rate (U/h)
<5	Stop insulin. Check blood glucose every 15 min and restart infusion at 1 U/h when blood glucose is >7 mmol/L
5–7	1
7–10	2
10–15	3
15–20	4
>20	6 and review scale

If blood glucose is repeatedly <5 mmol/L, reduce the insulin infusion rates by 0.5–1 U/h; if repeatedly over 15 mmol/L, increase the rates by 2–4 U/h

Newly diagnosed diabetes

- Management depends on the clinical state, ketone level and blood glucose (Table 39.5).
- Patients who are unwell or vomiting should be treated with a continuous insulin infusion (Table 39.4).
- Provided the patient is well and not vomiting, insulin therapy may be started at home with the help of a specialist nurse: ask advice from

Table 39.5 Management of newly diagnosed diabetes (blood glucose > 11 mmol/L)

Clinical state	Blood glucose	Urinary ketones	Management
Well	>11	++	Insulin*
Well	11–20	–/+	Diet
Well	>20	–/+	Oral hypoglycaemic
Acute myocardial infarction	>11	May be – to +++	Insulin
Other intercurrent illness	11–15	+	Check laboratory glucose in 2 h: start insulin if >15 mmol/L
	>15	+/++	Insulin

*The patient has insulin-dependent diabetes with mild ketoacidosis caught early before major fluid loss has occurred. Insulin can be given as an IV infusion (Table 39.4) or as a four-times daily SC regimen: ask advice from a diabetologist.

a diabetologist. If expert advice is not immediately available, admit the patient and treat with soluble insulin SC: start with 4–6 U 6-hly SC and increase the dose as necessary to keep preprandial/22.00 h blood glucose in the range 5–15 mmol/L.

Management of diabetes/hyperglycaemia after acute myocardial infarction

Known diabetes or blood glucose >11 mmol/L

1 Confirm initial stick test result with laboratory measurement of blood glucose, and check HbA1c.

2 If blood glucose is >11 mmol/L, start an insulin infusion (Table 39.4) and continue insulin by infusion for 24 h or until there is stability of the blood glucose and cardiovascular system, whichever is the longer.

While the patient is receiving insulin by infusion, also give dextrose 5% 500 mL 12-hly IV.

3 If blood glucose is <11 mmol/L in a patient with known diabetes, continue usual treatment and monitor blood glucose preprandially and at 22.00 h. If blood glucose rises above 11 mmol/L, start an insulin infusion (Table 39.4).

4 After insulin has been given by infusion for 24 h, transfer to SC insulin.

Management after insulin infusion discontinued

1 Estimate the daily insulin requirement from the total dose given by infusion over the previous 24 h. Give one-third as intermediate-acting (isophane) insulin SC at 22.00 h. Divide the remaining two-thirds into 3 and give as short-acting (soluble) insulin SC before meals.

2 Monitor blood glucose preprandially and at 22.00 h, and adjust doses of insulin as needed.

3 Ask advice from a diabetologist on long-term management. In general:

- Insulin treated, with good control (HbA1c <7.5%): return to usual regimen.
- Insulin treated, with poor control (HbA1c >7.5%): review regimen.
- Oral therapy with good control (HbA1c <7.5%): return to usual therapy.
- Oral therapy with poor control (HbA1c >7.5%): transfer to insulin.
- Previously undiagnosed: individualized management.

Perioperative management of diabetes

The perioperative management of the diabetic patient is determined by:

- the nature of the surgery (minor surgery is defined as a procedure after which the patient may be expected to eat and drink within 4 h; all other procedures are classed as major);
- whether the patient has insulin-treated or non-insulin-treated diabetes;
- the quality of preoperative diabetic control (Table 39.6). Good control is defined as a random blood glucose on admission of

Table 39.6 Preoperative assessment of the diabetic patient

Laboratory measurement of blood glucose and HbA1c on admission
Blood glucose by stick test before meals and at 22.00 h
Creatinine, sodium and potassium
Urinalysis
ECG
Clinical assessment for diabetic complications which may affect surgical risk and
    perioperative management: ischaemic heart disease, renal failure, autonomic or
    peripheral neuropathy, proliferative retinopathy

<10 mmol/L. If this is >15 mmol/L, consider postponing non-urgent procedures so that control can be improved: seek expert advice from a diabetologist.

Insulin-treated diabetes

Minor surgery
This protocol is only suitable for patients whose random blood glucose is <10 mmol/L on admission, are first on a morning list and are expected to be eating by lunchtime. Manage other patients as for major surgery.

Preoperative. Give usual medication.

Day of operation

1 Omit usual morning insulin if blood glucose is <7 mmol/L. Give half of usual morning insulin if blood glucose is >7 mmol/L.

2 Check blood glucose by stick test:

- 1 h preoperatively, i.e. at time of premedication;
- at least once during the procedure;
- 2-hly postoperatively until the patient is eating/drinking;
- then preprandially and at 22.00 h until discharge.

3 Restart usual insulin regimen with lunch (give half of the usual morning dose as soluble insulin before lunch if the patient is on a twice-daily regimen).

4 If blood glucose is >10 mmol/L on 2 consecutive readings perioperatively, set up an insulin infusion (Table 39.4).

Major surgery

Preoperative. Give usual medication.

Day of operation

1 Omit usual SC insulin.

2 Start an insulin infusion (Table 39.4).

3 Start an infusion of dextrose 5%, 1 L 12-hly IV.

4 Check blood glucose by stick test:
- initally hourly, then 2-hly once stable;
- at least once during surgery;
- each hour if surgery takes longer than 1 h;
- at least once in the recovery area;
- 2-hly postoperatively until the patient is eating/drinking;
- then preprandially and at 22.00 h until discharge.

Postoperative

- Continue insulin infusion until the patient is able to eat and drink.
- Continue dextrose 5% 1 L 12-hly IV, plus additional fluids if needed.
- When the patient can eat and drink, take down the insulin and dextrose infusions and restart SC insulin.
- The usual SC insulin regimen may need to be modified until a full diet is resumed: control may initially be easier using a regimen of short-acting (soluble) insulin given before meals and intermediate-acting (isophane or zinc suspension) insulin at bedtime.

Diabetes treated with oral hypoglycaemic agents

Minor surgery

This protocol is only suitable for patients whose random blood glucose is <10 mmol/L. Manage other patients as for major surgery.

Preoperative. Give usual medication.

Day of operation

1 Omit usual oral hypoglycaemic therapy.

2 Check blood glucose by stick test:
- 1 h preoperatively, i.e. at time of premedication;
- at least once during the procedure;
- 2-hly postoperatively until the patient is eating/drinking;
- then preprandially and at 22.00 h until discharge.

Major surgery

Preoperative. Give usual medication.

Day of operation

1 Omit oral hypoglycaemic therapy.

2 Start an insulin infusion (Table 39.4).

3 Start an infusion of dextrose 5%, 1 L 12-hly IV.

4 Check blood glucose by stick test:
   - initially hourly, then 2-hly once stable;
   - at least once during surgery;
   - each hour if surgery takes longer than one hour;
   - at least once in the recovery area;
   - 2-hly postoperatively until eating/drinking;
   - then preprandially and at 22.00 h until discharge.

Postoperative

- Continue insulin infusion until the patient is able to eat and drink.
- Continue dextrose 5% 1 L 12-hly IV, plus additional fluids if needed.
- When the patient can eat and drink, take down the insulin and dextrose infusions and restart usual oral hypoglycaemic therapy.

40 Diabetic ketoacidosis

• Diabetic ketoacidosis (DKA) is defined by a metabolic acidosis (venous bicarbonate <15 mmol/L or arterial pH <7.3) associated with ketonaemia and a blood glucose >11 mmol/L.
• Consider ketoacidosis in any ill diabetic, particularly if there is vomiting or tachypnoea (which may be misdiagnosed as primary hyperventilation), and in any patient with unexplained confusional state, coma, abdominal pain or metabolic acidosis.
• Causes of DKA are given in Table 40.1.
• The management of patients with DKA should be discussed with a diabetologist, and follow-up in a diabetic clinic arranged.

Priorities

1 If DKA is suspected, check blood glucose by laboratory test, as plasma ketones may interfere with the accuracy of stick tests. A value of less than 10 mmol/L excludes the diagnosis. If blood glucose is over 11 mmol/L, DKA is possible, and you should check venous bicarbonate or arterial pH to confirm or exclude the diagnosis. Other investigations required urgently are given in Table 40.2.
2 If blood glucose is >30 mmol/L but there is no acidosis or significant ketonaemia, suspect hyperosmolar non-ketotic hyperglycaemia (HONK). The treatment of HONK is similar to that of DKA, but there are important differences: see Chapter 41.
3 If DKA is confirmed, start fluid and electrolyte replacement (Table 40.3) via a peripheral IV line.

   • The fluid deficit of patients with DKA is usually 6–10 L. Give 3 L of **normal saline** in the first 4 h (1 L/h for the first 2 h, 500 mL/h for the next 2 h), then individualized fluid replacement, guided by clinical condition, urine output, measurement of the JVP or CVP and blood glucose (see *Further management*).

Table 40.1 Causes of diabetic ketoacidosis

In patients with known insulin-dependent diabetes:
Inappropriate reduction in insulin therapy
Infection
Surgery
Myocardial infarction
Emotional stress

Presentation of insulin-dependent diabetes

Table 40.2 Urgent investigation in suspected diabetic ketoacidosis

Blood glucose (laboratory measurement)
Ketones (stick test of plasma or urine with Ketostix)
Venous plasma bicarbonate
Creatinine, sodium and potassium
Arterial blood gases and pH
Full blood count (high white count may be due to acidosis, rather than infection)
Blood culture (by separate venepuncture)
Urine stick test, microscopy and culture
Chest X-ray
ECG

Diabetic ketoacidosis

- Patients with DKA who are hypotensive on admission (systolic BP<90 mmHg) should have volume resuscitation initially with colloid: 500 mL over 15 min, followed by 500 mL over 30 min, then normal saline as above, guided by measurement of the CVP (p. 43).
- Give no **potassium** in the first litre of normal saline whilst awaiting the plasma level. On average, 20 mmol is added to each litre of

Table 40.3 Fluid and electrolyte replacement in diabetic ketoacidosis

1 *Your fluid regimen must take account of:*
the likely fluid deficit
the BP, CVP and urine output
coexisting renal or cardiac disease

2 *Start fluid replacement via a peripheral IV line:*
if systolic BP is <90 mmHg, give colloid 500 mL over 15 min, followed by a further
    500 mL over 30 min if BP remains low
if systolic BP is >90 mmHg, give normal saline 1 L over 1 h without added potassium

3 *Then put in a CVP line if appropriate* (see pp. 329 & 332)

4 *Give further normal saline (with potassium added according to the plasma level
    —see Table 40.4)* 1 L over 1 h then 1 L over 2 h
then individualized to the patient, e.g. 1 L 4- to 8-hly until the fluid deficit has been
    corrected, as shown by warm extremities with a normal pulse and blood pressure
    and normal creatinine

5 When blood glucose is <15 mmol/L, change to dextrose (with potassium added
    according to the plasma level—see Table 40.4)
use 10% dextrose 1 L 8-hly if significant metabolic correction is still needed
    (persisting acidosis)
otherwise use 5% dextrose 1 L 8-hly
give concurrent normal saline (without potassium added) if still hypovolaemic

Table 40.4 Potassium replacement in diabetic ketoacidosis

Plasma potassium (mmol/L)	Potassium added (mmol/L)
<3	40
3–4	30
4–5	20
>5	None

Check plasma potassium on admission, after 2 h and then 4-hly until the rate of
    fluid infusion is 8-hly or slower

Table 40.5 Insulin infusion in diabetic ketoacidosis using a syringe pump

1 Give 10 U soluble insulin IV stat while the infusion is being prepared
2 Make 50 U of soluble insulin up to 50 mL with normal saline (i.e. 1 U/mL). Flush 10 mL of the solution through the line before connecting to the patient (as some insulin will be adsorbed on to the plastic)
3 Start the infusion at 6 U/ h. Check blood glucose by hourly stick test and 2-hly laboratory measurement, and adjust the infusion rate as below. Blood glucose will usually fall by around 5 mmol/L/h
4 If there is no fall in blood glucose after 2 h, confirm that the pump is working and the IV line connected properly and double the infusion rate
Recheck blood glucose after a further 2 h and double the insulin infusion rate again if necessary

Blood glucose (mmol/L)	Insulin infusion rate (U/h)	IV fluid
<5	Stop insulin. Check blood glucose every 15 min and restart infusion at 1 U/h when blood glucose is >7 mmol/L	Dextrose*
5–7	1	Dextrose*
7–10	2	Dextrose*
10–15	3	Dextrose*
15–20	4	N/saline
>20	6	N/saline
	Call doctor to review scale	

If blood glucose is repeatedly <5 mmol/L, reduce the insulin infusion rates by 0.5–1 U/h; if repeatedly over 15 mmol/L, increase the rates by 2–4 U/h.

* Use 10% dextrose 1 L 8-hly if significant metabolic correction is still needed (persisting acidosis), otherwise use 5% dextrose 1 L 8-hly. Give concurrent normal saline (without potassium added) if still hypovolaemic.

Diabetic ketoacidosis

fluid, but titrate according to the plasma level (Table 40.4): hypokalaemia is a potential cause of death in treating DKA.
4 Give **insulin** 10 units IV while an insulin infusion is being prepared (Table 40.5), and then infuse according to a sliding scale.

• Monitor blood glucose hourly.
• If blood glucose does not fall, check that the pump is working and the infusion connected.
• If no technical problem is found, increase the insulin infusion rate by 2–4 U/h.

5 **Supportive management** includes the following:
  • **Nasogastric drainage** if the patient is too drowsy to answer questions or there is a gastric succussion splash: pass a nasogastric tube, aspirate the stomach and leave on continuous drainage. Inhalation of vomit is a potentially fatal complication of DKA.
  • **Bladder catheterization** if no urine has been passed after 4 h or the patient is incontinent, but not otherwise.
  • **Continuous ECG monitoring** if the patient has cardiac disease or hypo- or hyperkalaemia.
  • **Oxygen** (35% or more, as needed) if oxygen saturation is <92%, or Pao_2 is <10 kPa.

6 **Arrange to transfer the patient to the ITU** or high-dependency unit.

Further management

1 Monitoring progress
A schedule is given in Table 40.6. Fluid balance, clinical observations and biochemical results should be recorded together on a flow chart.

2 Fluid and electrolyte replacement
• A standard regimen is given in Table 40.4 and 40.5, but must be adapted to the individual patient. The infusion rate must take into account urinary losses of salt and water, which will remain high until the blood glucose is below the renal threshold (around 10 mmol/L).
• Put in a **CVP line** to guide fluid replacement if plasma creatinine is >200 μmol/L or the patient has cardiac disease. Reduce the infusion rate if the CVP rises > +10 cm water.
• **Bicarbonate** should only be given if arterial pH is <7.0 and systolic BP is <90 mmHg despite fluid replacement. Give 50 mL of 8.4% sodium bicarbonate over 30 min and recheck arterial pH, giving further doses if needed to increase arterial pH > 7.0.

Diabetic ketoacidosis

Table 40.6 Diabetic ketoacidosis: monitoring progress in the first 24 h

Check hourly
Conscious level (e.g. Glasgow Coma Scale: p. 72) until fully conscious
Blood pressure and pulse rate until stable and then 4-hly
CVP until the infusion rate is 1L 8-hly or less
Blood glucose by stick test
Urine output

Check 2-hly
Blood glucose by laboratory measurement until < 20 mmol/L, then check 4-hly

Check 4-hly
Plasma potassium until the infusion rate is 1L 8-hly or less
Venous bicarbonate until > 15 mmol/L and then monitor ketogenesis from the urine
ketone level

3 Infection and DKA

• Infection is a common precipitant and complication of ketoacidosis and may not cause fever. Check carefully for a focus of infection, including an examination of the feet and perineum.

• If there is soft tissue infection of the feet, treat with coamoxiclav plus metronidazole IV (if allergic to penicillin, use clindamycin plus a fluoroquinolone or aztreonam IV), and obtain a surgical opinion.

• Rhinocerebral mucormycosis is a fungal infection of the paranasal sinuses particularly associated with DKA, and should be suspected in patients with headache, ocular or facial pain. Seek an urgent ENT opinion. Treatment is with surgical debridement and amphotericin IV.

• A case can be made for giving antibiotic therapy to all patients in whom a non-infective precipitant cannot be identified. In the absence of an obvious focus of infection, give cefotaxime plus gentamicin IV.

Table 40.7 Establishing an SC insulin regimen

1 Estimate the daily insulin requirement from double the total dose given by infusion over the last 12 h
2 Give one-third of the total daily dose as intermediate-acting (isophane) insulin SC at 22.00 h. Divide the remaining two-thirds into 3 and give as short-acting (soluble) insulin SC before meals
3 Check blood glucose before meals and at 22.00 h, and adjust doses of insulin as needed, aiming for levels of 4–7 mmol/L
4 Ask advice from a diabetologist on a suitable long-term regimen

4 Thromboprophylaxis

Give heparin 5000 units 8-hly SC until the patient is well enough to walk.

5 Changeover from infusion to subcutaneous insulin

• Continue insulin by infusion until ketoacidosis has resolved (plasma bicarbonate >20 mmol/L, urinary ketones negative or only 1+) and the patient is well enough to eat and drink.
• Start with short-acting (soluble) insulin three times daily before meals and intermediate-acting (isophane or zinc suspension) insulin at bedtime. Base the total daily dose on double the total dose of insulin given over the last 12 h.
• Continue the insulin infusion for one hour after the first SC dose.
• Check blood glucose 6-hly and give top-up soluble insulin injections if it rises above 15 mmol/L.
• When insulin requirements are stable, change newly diagnosed diabetic patients to a twice-daily insulin regimen (Table 40.7). Put known diabetic patients back onto their usual regimen.

Diabetic ketoacidosis

41 Hyperosmolar non-ketotic hyperglycaemia

Consider the diagnosis in any patient with hyperglycaemia where dehydration and drowsiness are prominent.

Hyperosmolar non-ketotic hyperglycaemia (HONK) is differentiated from diabetic ketoacidosis by:

- blood glucose > 30 mmol/L, but no ketoacidosis (venous bicarbonate > 15 mmol/L, arterial pH > 7.3) and
- plasma osmolality > 350 mosmol/kg (normal range 285–295 mosmol/kg). This can be measured directly or calculated from the formula: plasma osmolality = [2 (Na + K) + urea + glucose].

Management

This is the same as for diabetic ketoacidosis (Chapter 40), with the differences noted below:

1 Dextrose–saline (dextrose 4%, sodium chloride 0.18% (sodium 30 mmol/L)) should be used for fluid replacement in place of normal saline if plasma sodium is > 145 mmol/L after volume resuscitation.

2 Insulin sensitivity is greater in the absence of severe acidosis.

3 The risk of thromboembolism is high. Unless contraindicated (e.g. recent stroke), give full-dose low-molecular-weight heparin or unfractionated heparin by IV infusion (p. 404).

4 Total body potassium is lower and the plasma level more variable as treatment begins. Check the level 30 min after starting insulin and then 2-hly.

5 Most patients can subsequently be maintained on oral hypoglycaemic therapy (or even managed by diet alone), although recovery of endogenous insulin production may be delayed.

- Continue insulin (SC regimen; Table 40.7, p. 334) unless the total daily requirement falls below 20 U, when an oral hypoglycaemic can be tried.

6 Arrange early follow-up with a diabetologist to review therapy.

42 Electrolyte disorders

Sodium

Derangements of plasma sodium concentration (Table 42.1) are usually due to disordered water handling by the kidney. Defective concentration of the urine, without an adequate intake of water, results in hypernatraemia, whilst defective dilution of the urine (often due to non-osmotic release of antidiuretic hormone) results in hyponatraemia. Thiazide diuretics are one of the commonest causes of hyponatraemia.

Hypernatraemia (Fig. 42.1)

Hypernatraemia may result in muscle weakness, confusional state and coma.

Principles of management
• Treat the underlying disorder.
• Your choice of fluid depends on the volume status of the patient.
• Avoid rapid correction or overcorrection of hypernatraemia, which may result in cerebral oedema: aim for a rate of decrease of plasma sodium of no more than 1 mmol/L/h, and no more than 10 mmol/L/day, with a target plasma sodium of 145 mmol/L.

Hypovolaemic hypernatraemia
• If the patient has hypotension with signs of low cardiac output, give normal saline IV until systolic BP is >110 mmHg.
• Then give half-normal (0.45%) saline or 5% dextrose IV, or water PO, until the water deficit is corrected.

Table 42.1 Classification of plasma sodium concentration

Plasma sodium concentration (mmol/L)	Classification
>155	Severe hypernatraemia
150–155	Moderate hypernatraemia
143–149	Mild hypernatraemia
138–142	Normal range
130–137	Mild hyponatraemia
124–129	Moderate hyponatraemia
<125	Severe hyponatraemia

Electrolyte disorders

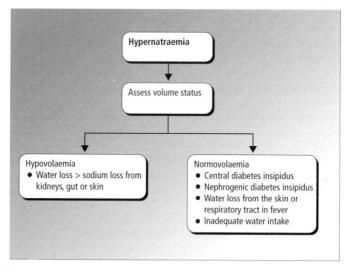

Fig. 42.1 Diagnosis of patients with hypernatraemia. Management depends on the volume status of the patient.

Normovolaemic hypernatraemia
- Correct the water deficit with 5% dextrose IV or water PO.
- If the patient has central diabetes insipidus, give vasopressin.

Hypervolaemic hypernatraemia
- This is rare, and is only seen when hypertonic solutions, e.g. sodium bicarbonate, are given for the treatment of metabolic acidosis or hyperkalaemia.
- Discontinue the infusion. Use a loop diuretic (or dialysis) to remove excess sodium.

Hyponatraemia (Fig. 42.2)

Hyponatraemia may result in headache, nausea, vomiting, muscle weakness and confusional state. Coma, respiratory failure and seizures may occur with severe hyponatraemia, reflecting cerebral oedema, especially when this has developed rapidly.

Principles of management
- Always check blood glucose, so that you don't miss hyperglycaemia: hyponatraemia may occur in severe hyperglycaemia due to osmotic shift of water from the intracellular space. Plasma osmolality is normal or high, and treatment with hypertonic saline is inappropriate and may be fatal.
- Rapid correction of hypo-osmolar hyponatraemia is only indicated if this is the cause of severe neurological abnormalities (coma, major seizures); it may result in osmotic demyelination of pontine neurones, especially if the brain has adapted to hyponatraemia. The risk of osmotic demyelination is increased in patients with liver failure, malnutrition and potassium depletion, and elderly women taking thiazide diuretics.

Hyponatraemia with severe neurological abnormalities
1 If the patient is comatose, start resuscitation along standard lines. Fits should be treated with diazepam or lorazepam IV (p. 263). Transfer the patient to the ITU for supportive care: endotracheal intubation and mechanical ventilation may be needed to treat respiratory failure.

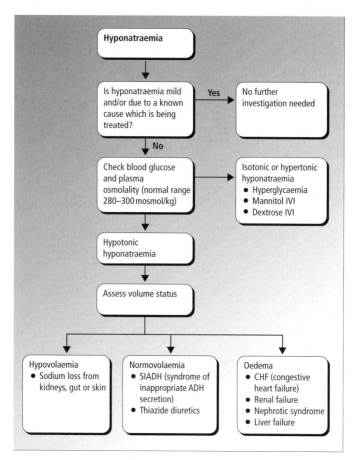

Fig. 42.2 Diagnosis of hyponatraemia.

Table 42.2 Hyponatraemia with severe neurological symptoms: targets and treatment

Rate of development of hyponatraemia and volume status	Target/treatment
Acute hyponatraemia (developing in < 48 h)	Target: increase plasma sodium by 2 mmol/L/h until symptoms resolve or it has reached 130 mmol/L
Administration of hypotonic fluids after surgery	Hypertonic saline IV (Table 42.3) plus loop diuretic IV
Chronic hyponatraemia	Target: increase plasma sodium by no more than 1 mmol/L/h and no more than 10–15 mmol/L in 24 h, until symptoms resolve or it has reached 130 mmol/L
1 Volume-depleted	Isotonic saline IV guided by measurement of central venous pressure
2 Normovolaemic with normal cardiac function	Hypertonic saline IV (Table 42.3)
3 Volume-overloaded (oedematous) or with impaired cardiac function	Hypertonic saline IV (Table 42.3) plus loop diuretic IV or Haemofiltration/dialysis

2 Assess the patient's fluid status from the fluid charts, blood pressure, JVP and the presence or absence of peripheral and pulmonary oedema. Check previous biochemical results. Is cardiac, renal and liver function normal? How quickly has hyponatraemia developed?

3 If severe hyponatraemia is confirmed (plasma sodium <120 mmol/L), and hyperglycaemia excluded, your choice of treatment depends on the volume and cardiac status of the patient, and how rapidly hyponatraemia has developed (over < 48 h or >48 h) (Tables 42.2 and 42.3).

Electrolyte disorders

Table 42.3 Hyponatraemia with severe neurological symptoms: hypertonic saline regimen

1 Estimate the patient's total body water volume (litres) (roughly 50% of body weight)

2 Subtract the patient's plasma sodium from 130: this number is the required correction of plasma sodium in mmol/L, and the number of hours over which plasma sodium should be corrected in patients with chronic hyponatraemia

3 Multiply the total body water volume (litres) by the required correction of plasma sodium (mmol/L). This gives the number of mmol of sodium needed to correct the patient's plasma sodium to 130 mmol/L

4 Divide the number of mmol of sodium needed for correction by 514 (the number of mmol of sodium in 1 L of 514 mM sodium chloride). Multiply by 1000 to give the number of mL of 514 mM sodium chloride needed to correct plasma sodium to 130 mmol/L

5 Divide the number of mL of 514 mM sodium chloride to be given by the number of hours needed for correction of the plasma sodium. This gives the infusion rate in mL/h. Hypertonic saline should be given by a volumetric pump

6 Give a loop diuretic IV (or consider haemofiltration/dialysis in severe renal failure) if the patient is oedematous or has impaired cardiac function

7 Monitor CVP, blood pressure, conscious level and urine output hourly. Check plasma sodium 2-hly, and modify the infusion rate as appropriate

Acute hyponatraemia (due to administration of hypotonic fluids after surgery): aim for an increase in plasma sodium of 2 mmol/L/h until symptoms resolve or plasma sodium reaches 130 mmol/L

Chronic hyponatraemia: aim for an increase in plasma sodium of no more than 1 mmol/L and no more than 10–15 mmol/L in 24 h, until symptoms resolve or plasma sodium reaches 130 mmol/L

Hyponatraemia without severe neurological symptoms

If the patient has no symptoms attributable to hyponatraemia or is only mildly symptomatic (e.g. headache, nausea, lethargy), hypertonic saline should not be given. Management depends principally on the patient's fluid status:

Table 42.4 Criteria for the syndrome of inappropriate ADH secretion (SIADH)

Plasma sodium concentration <130 mmol/L and plasma osmolality <275
  mosmol/kg
Urine sodium concentration >20 mmol/L and urine osmolality greater than
  plasma osmolality
No oedema and no signs of hypovolaemia
Normal renal, thyroid and adrenal function (checked by Synacthen test, p. 367)
The patient is not taking diuretics or purgatives

Hypovolaemic hyponatraemia

• Give normal saline IV (with potassium supplements if required) until the volume deficit has been corrected.

• In asymptomatic patients in whom hyponatraemia is due to diuretic therapy, withdrawal of the diuretic and a normal diet is usually sufficient to correct plasma sodium to normal.

Normovolaemic hyponatraemia

• Causes include hypothyroidism (p. 373), adrenal insufficiency (p. 364), treatment with thiazide diuretics and the syndrome of inappropriate ADH secretion (SIADH) (Tables 42.4 and 42.5).

• Management depends on the cause. In patients with SIADH, plasma sodium can be increased by fluid restriction (to 800 mL/day), treatment with demeclocycline (which inhibits the renal response to ADH), or a loop diuretic (e.g. frusemide 40 mg daily PO) combined with a high sodium diet (2–3 g NaCl daily).

Oedematous hyponatraemia

• The combination of hyponatraemia and oedema can occur in congestive heart failure, liver failure, renal failure (acute or chronic) and the nephrotic syndrome.

• Correction of the hyponatraemia (if indicated) requires treatment of the underlying disease. Management is often difficult and expert advice should be sought.

Electrolyte disorders

Table 42.5 Causes of osmotically inappropriate secretion of antidiuretic hormone (SIADH)

Malignant disease
Small cell carcinoma of bronchus, thymoma, lymphoma, sarcoma, mesothelioma, carcinoma of pancreas and duodenum

Chest disorders
Pneumonia, tuberculosis, empyema, asthma, pneumothorax, positive-pressure ventilation

Neurological disorders
Meningitis, encephalitis, head injury, brain tumour, cerebral abscess, subarachnoid haemorrhage, Guillain–Barré syndrome, acute intermittent porphyria

Drugs
Antidepressants, carbamazepine, cytotoxics, MDMA ('ecstasy'), opioids, oxytocin, phenothiazines, thiazides

Others
Postoperative state
Adrenal insufficiency
Idiopathic
HIV infection

Potassium

Derangements of plasma potassium concentration (Table 42.6) may be an acute effect of drugs, or result from disordered renal plasma potassium handling, release of potassium from damaged cells or excessive gut loss of potassium.

Electrolyte disorders

Table 42.6 Classification of plasma potassium concentration

Plasma potassium concentration (mmol/L)	Classification
> 6.0	Severe hyperkalaemia
5.6–6.0	Moderate hyperkalaemia
5.1–5.5	Mild hyperkalaemia
3.5–5.0	Normal range
3.0–3.4	Mild hypokalaemia
2.5–2.9	Moderate hypokalaemia
< 2.5	Severe hypokalaemia

Hyperkalaemia (Fig. 42.3)

Principles of management
• Hyperkalaemia must be excluded in any patient with oligoanuria or acute renal failure. Severe hyperkalaemia may be asymptomatic until it results in cardiac arrest.
• Stop drugs which may be contributing to hyperkalaemia, and reduce the dietary intake of potassium.
• To increase excretion of potassium, the options are to improve renal function, start renal replacement therapy, or use an ion-exchange resin such as calcium resonium to bind potassium in the gut.

Severe hyperkalaemia with ECG abnormalities
If the plasma potassium is >7 mmol/L or the ECG has abnormalities associated with hyperkalaemia (widening of the QRS complex, loss of the P wave, peaking of the T wave or a sine wave pattern) and plasma potassium is > 6 mmol/L:
1 Give 10 mL of calcium chloride 10% IV over 5 min. This can be repeated every 5 min up to a total dose of 40 mL. Calcium chloride is more toxic to veins than calcium gluconate, but provides more calcium per ampoule (272 mg of calcium in 10 mL of calcium chloride 10%; 94 mg of calcium in 10 mL of calcium gluconate 10%).

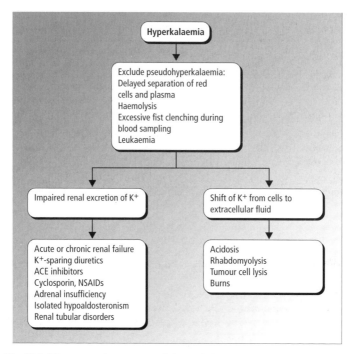

Fig. 42.3 Diagnosis of patients with hyperkalaemia.

2 Give 25 g of dextrose (50 mL of dextrose 50%) with 10 U of soluble insulin IV over 30 min. This will usually reduce plasma potassium for several hours. Check blood glucose after dextrose/insulin has been given to exclude rebound hypoglycaemia.

3 If hyperkalaemia is associated with a severe metabolic acidosis (arterial pH <7.2), give sodium bicarbonate 50 mmol (50 mL of 8.4% solution) IV over 30 min. This concentration of bicarbonate is irritant to veins and should preferably be given via a central line. Bicarbonate should not be given if alveolar ventilation is impaired (as shown by a raised $Pa\text{co}_2$).

4 Stop potassium supplements or any drugs (e.g. ACE inhibitors, potassium-retaining diuretics) which may be contributing to hyperkalaemia. Start calcium resonium (15 g 8-hly PO or 30 g by retention enema).

5 Recheck plasma potassium after 2 h. If hyperkalaemia is due to acute renal failure, renal replacement therapy may need to be started to prevent a recurrence: discuss this with a nephrologist.

Mild or moderate hyperkalaemia

• Stop potassium supplements or any drugs (e.g. ACE inhibitors, potassium-retaining diuretics) which may be contributing to hyperkalaemia, and reduce the dietary intake of potassium.

• Start calcium resonium (15 g 8-hly PO or 30 g daily by retention enema) in patients with hyperkalaemia complicating renal failure.

Hypokalaemia (Fig. 42.4)

Hypokalaemia may result in muscle weakness and arrhythmias. When plasma potassium falls below 2.5 mmol/L, muscle necrosis may occur; below 2 mmol/L, there may be ascending paralysis, resembling Guillain–Barré syndrome (p. 256). Arrhythmias may occur when plasma potassium is <3 mmol/L, especially in patients with underlying cardiac disorders or taking antiarrhythmic drugs.

Principles of management

• Treat the underlying disorder: hypokalaemia is most often due to diuretic therapy or gut loss of potassium, and replacement of salt and water may also be needed.

• In patients with arrhythmias, target plasma potassium is 4–4.5 mmol/L.

• Magnesium depletion commonly coexists with potassium depletion: check plasma magnesium (normal range 0.75–1.25 mmol/L) in patients with hypokalaemia, and correct hypomagnesaemia with IV or oral supplements.

Severe hypokalaemia or hypokalaemia associated with arrhythmias

• Attach an ECG monitor.

• Give potassium by IV infusion, initally 40 mmol over 4 h, and then recheck potassium. Give further potassium as needed, up to 200 mmol

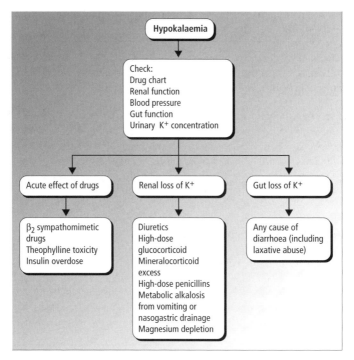

Fig. 42.4 Diagnosis of hypokalaemia.

over 24 h. The maximum rate of infusion should not exceed 20 mmol/h.
• Potassium given via a peripheral vein may cause pain at the infusion site and tissue necrosis if there is extravasation: administration via a central vein is preferable.

Mild or moderate hypokalaemia without arrhythmias
• Give oral potassium, e.g. Sando-K 2 tablets (12 mmol per tablet) 8-hly PO for 3–7 days, and increase the dietary intake of potassium.
• If hypokalaemia is due to the use of a loop diuretic, consider adding a potassium-retaining diuretic (e.g. amiloride or spironolactone) (avoid in patients with renal impairment).

Table 42.7 Classification of plasma calcium concentration

Plasma total calcium concentration (mmol/L)*	Clinical classification
>3.5	Severe hypercalcaemia
3.0–3.5	Moderate hypercalcaemia
2.6–3.0	Mild hypercalcaemia
2.2–2.6	Normal range
1.9–2.2	Mild hypocalcaemia
1.5–1.9	Moderate hypocalcaemia
<1.5	Severe hypocalcaemia

*Plasma total calcium concentration should be corrected for the plasma albumin concentration (which is a major determinant of the physiologically important ionized calcium fraction): add/subtract 0.2 mmol/L from the total calcium for each 10 g by which plasma albumin is below/above 40 g/L.

Calcium

Derangements of plasma calcium concentration (Table 42.7) result from disordered handling of calcium by the gut, kidneys or bone.
• Calcium exists in the extracellular fluid in three forms: the physiologically important ionized fraction (50%), the protein-bound fraction (40%) and a small fraction (10%) complexed to anions. Most laboratories measure total calcium, which should be corrected for the plasma albumin concentration (a major determinant of the ionized calcium fraction): add/subtract 0.2 mmol/L from the total calcium for each 10 g by which plasma albumin is below/above 40 g/L.

Hypercalcaemia

Causes of hypercalcaemia are given in Table 42.8, and investigation in Table 42.9.

Table 42.8 Causes of hypercalcaemia

Common
Malignancy involving bone (carcinoma of breast or bronchus, myeloma and
  lymphoma)
Primary hyperparathyroidism
Chronic renal failure with hyperparathyroidism and treatment with calcium and
  vitamin D metabolites

Uncommon
Sarcoidosis
Thyrotoxicosis
Other malignancies
Vitamin D therapy
Familial benign hypercalcaemia

Electrolyte disorders

Table 42.9 Investigation in hypercalcaemia

Full blood count
Creatinine, sodium and potassium
Uncuffed sample for calcium, phosphate, total protein, albumin, alkaline
  phosphatase
Chest X-ray
ECG

If the cause of hypercalcaemia is not known:
Serum and urine protein electrophoresis
Parathyroid hormone
C-reactive protein and ESR
Thyroid function tests

Table 42.10 Forced saline diuresis in severe hypercalcaemia complicated by reduced conscious level or cardiac arrhythmias

Put in a urinary catheter to monitor urine output
Put in a central venous line to monitor central venous pressure (CVP)
Give normal saline 1L 2-hly IV
Give frusemide 40 mg/h IV
If the CVP rises above +10 cm water, slow the infusion rate or give additional
  diuretic
Check plasma potassium and calcium 2-hly. Give IV potassium as required
When plasma calcium is <3.5 mmol/L, stop the forced saline diuresis and give
  normal saline without diuretic 1L 6- to 8-hly IV

• Hypercalcaemia may result in constipation, thirst, polyuria and confusional state.
• Severe hypercalcaemia (total calcium >3.5 mmol/L) is most often seen in patients who are known to have malignancies involving bone (carcinoma of the breast or bronchus, myeloma, lymphoma), but may sometimes be the presenting complaint. Much less commonly it is due to primary hyperparathyroidism.

Principles of management
• Correct hypovolaemia and increase the renal excretion of calcium.
• Inhibit accelerated bone resorption.
• Treat the underlying disorder.
• Avoid thiazides and immobilization, which contribute to hypercalcaemia.

Moderate or severe hypercalcaemia (total calcium >3 mmol/L)
1 The first-line treatment is rehydration. In patients with mild symptoms, oral rehydration (a fluid intake of at least 2–3 L/day) may be sufficient. Patients with more severe symptoms should receive normal saline IV. Options are:
  • normal saline 1 L 6–8-hly IV;

- forced saline diuresis (Table 42.10): this is potentially hazardous and should only be used when a rapid reduction in plasma calcium is essential (e.g. because the patient is comatose or has major cardiac arrhythmias);
  - dialysis may be needed in severe hypercalcaemia complicated by renal failure: seek expert advice from a nephrologist.

2 If plasma calcium remains >3 mmol/L despite rehydration, drug therapy to inhibit osteoclast-mediated bone resorption is indicated. The most commonly used agents are given in Table 42.11.

3 Specific treatment will be needed to prevent a recurrence of hypercalcaemia (e.g. chemotherapy for malignancies, surgery for primary hyperparathyroidism).

Electrolyte disorders

Table 42.11 Drug therapy in moderate or severe hypercalcaemia

Class of drug	Indication
Biphosphonate	First choice in hypercalcaemia due to non-haematological malignancy or primary hyperparathyroidism
Calcitonin	Failure to respond to biphosphonate
Glucocorticoid	Hypercalcaemia due to lymphoma, myeloma, vitamin D toxicity and sarcoidosis

Table 42.12 Causes of hypocalcaemia

Following parathyroidectomy
Idiopathic hypoparathyroidism
Acute pancreatitis
Hypomagnesaemia
Chronic renal failure
Malignancy (either involving bone, with increased osteoblastic activity, or in
    response to chemotherapy, with phosphate released from tumour cells forming
    complexes with plasma calcium)
Multiple citrated blood transfusions
Rhabdomyolysis
Septic shock
Pseudohypoparathyroidism

Hypocalcaemia

Causes of hypocalcaemia are given in Table 42.12.
• Acute severe hypocalcaemia (with tetany) is most commonly seen in patients with chronic renal failure after elective subtotal parathyroidectomy,
• Be aware that hyperventilation may also cause carpopedal spasm.

Acute severe hypocalcaemia with tetany
• Give 10 mL of calcium gluconate 10% IV over 5 min, followed by a continuous infusion of calcium gluconate. Add the contents of 10 10 mL ampoules of calcium gluconate to 900 mL of dextrose 5% (withdraw 100 mL from a 1 L bag), giving a concentration of roughly 1 mg elemental calcium per ml, and infuse at 50 mL/h until symptoms are relieved or corrected plasma calcium is >1.9 mmol/L.
• Seek expert advice on further management.

43 Acid–base disorders and arterial blood gases

When to check acid–base status and arterial blood gases

Disorders of acid–base status and arterial blood gases are common in acute illness. They may provide a clue to the diagnosis in syndromes such as hypotension or coma, and be a guide to the severity of specific disorders (e.g. pneumonia or diabetic ketoacidosis). Indications for checking acid–base status and arterial blood gases are given in Table 43.1

• All acutely ill patients should have oxygen saturation measured by non-invasive oximetry, and arterial blood gases should be checked if Sao_2 is < 90%. Central cyanosis is an unreliable sign of inadequate oxygen saturation.

Arterial blood sampling

1 Samples may be taken from the radial, brachial or femoral arteries. The radial artery of the non-dominant hand is the preferred site. If you use the brachial artery, the elbow should be fully extended over a pillow to prevent movement of the artery during sampling.

2 Put on gloves. Inject 1 mL of lignocaine 1% into the skin and around the artery using an orange (25 G) needle: pain leads to hyperventilation, which will acutely lower arterial Pco_2. Sampling should be done with a blue (23 G) needle and a heparinized 5 mL syringe (draw up 1 mL of heparin 1000 U/mL to heparinize the barrel, then expel the excess) or a commercially available preheparinized syringe (again having expelled the excess).

3 Locate the artery with your index and middle fingers to establish its course. Advance the needle, angled at about 45°, into the segment between your fingers. Sample 3 mL of blood. After removing the

Table 43.1 When to check acid–base status and arterial blood gases

Syndromes
Cardiac arrest
Severe hypotension
Acute severe chest pain
Acute breathlessness
Coma
Sepsis
Severe poisoning
Undiagnosed critical illness

Specific disorders
Pulmonary oedema
Pulmonary embolism
Pneumonia
Severe asthma ($Sao_2 < 92\%$)
Exacerbation of chronic obstructive
    pulmonary disease
Diabetic ketoacidosis
Renal failure
Liver failure

needle, put a folded gauze swab over the puncture site; you or an assistant should maintain pressure over the site for 10 min to achieve haemostasis.

4 Expel any bubbles from the syringe. Remove the needle directly into a disposal bin and cap the syringe. Invert the syringe several times to ensure good mixing of blood and heparin. Analyse the sample within 5 min or transport in a mixture of ice and water for analysis within 30 min. The inspired oxygen concentration should be stated to allow interpretation of arterial Po_2.

Interpreting the results: acid–base status
Ignore all the results apart from the directly measured variables: Po_2, Pco_2 and pH/hydrogen ion concentration. Conversion of pH units to hydrogen ion concentration is given in Table 43.2

Table 43.2 Acidity of arterial blood: conversion of pH units to hydrogen ion concentration (nmol/L)

	0	1	2	3	4	5	6	7	8	9
7.0	99	97	95	93	91	89	87	85	83	81
7.1	79	78	76	74	72	71	69	68	66	65
7.2	63	62	60	59	58	56	55	54	53	51
7.3	50	49	48	47	46	45	44	43	42	41
7.4	40	39	38	37	36	35	35	34	33	32
7.5	31	30	30	30	29	28	28	27	26	26
7.6	25	25	24	23	23	22	22	21	21	20

Acid–base disorders

• Use Tables 43.3 and 43.4 or Fig. 43.1 to determine the type and severity of acid–base disorder.
• Causes of specific acid–base disorders are given in Tables 43.5–43.8.

Management of acid–base disorders

• This is largely directed at the underlying causes.
• The use of bicarbonate in patients with metabolic acidosis remains controversial, but is generally indicated if the acidosis is severe (pH <7.2, hydrogen ion concentration >60 nmol/L) and is associated with hypotension. Give sodium bicarbonate 50 mmol (50 mL of 8.4% solution) IV over 30 min, and recheck arterial pH after a further 30 min. Repeat the dose if needed until arterial pH is >7.2.

Table 43.3 Classification of acid–base disorders according to arterial hydrogen ion concentration/pH and P_{CO_2}

Arterial P_{CO_2} (kPa)	Arterial hydrogen ion concentration (nmol/L) or pH		
	$[H^+] > 45$ pH < 7.35	35–45 7.35–7.45	<35 >7.45
<4.7	Metabolic acidosis with respiratory compensation or Metabolic acidosis + respiratory alkalosis, e.g. • Pulmonary oedema • Salicylate poisoning • Hepatorenal syndrome	Respiratory alkalosis with metabolic compensation	Respiratory alkalosis or Respiratory alkalosis + metabolic alkalosis, e.g. • Acute liver failure with vomiting, nasogastric drainage or severe hypokalaemia • Peritoneal dialysis for chronic renal failure
4.7–6.0	Metabolic acidosis	Normal acid–base status	Metabolic alkalosis
>6.0	Respiratory acidosis with partial metabolic compensation or Respiratory acidosis + metabolicacidosis, e.g. • Cardiopulmonary arrest • COPD complicated by circulatory failure or sepsis • Severe pulmonary oedema • Combined respiratory and renal failure • Severe tricyclic poisoning	Respiratory acidosis with metabolic compensation, e.g. • COPD with chronic CO_2 retention	Metabolic alkalosis + respiratory acidosis, e.g. • Diuretic therapy + COPD with chronic CO_2 retention

COPD, chronic obstructive pulmonary disease.

Table 43.4 Grading of severity of acid–base disorders

Arterial pH	Acid–base status	Arterial hydrogen ion concentration (nmol/L)
<7.2	Severe acidosis	>60
7.2–7.3	Moderate acidosis	50–60
7.3–7.35	Mild acidosis	45–50
7.35–7.45	Normal range	35–45
7.45–7.5	Mild alkalosis	30–35
7.5–7.6	Moderate alkalosis	20–30
>7.6	Severe alkalosis	<20

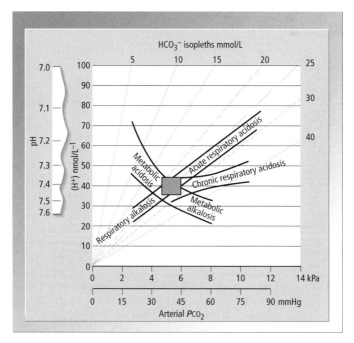

Fig. 43.1 Acid–base diagram relating arterial hydrogen ion concentration (nmol/L) or pH to Pa_{CO_2} within the body. The shaded rectangle is the normal range. The 95% confidence limits of hydrogen ion concentration/Pa_{CO_2} relationships in single disturbances of acid–base balance are shown. From Flenley DC. *Lancet* 1971; **1**: 961.

Table 43.5 Causes of respiratory acidosis (inadequate alveolar ventilation resulting in a raised arterial P_{CO_2})

Site of lesion	Causes
Brain	Stroke
	Mass lesion with brainstem compression
	Encephalitis
	Sedative drugs
	Status epilepticus
Spinal cord	Cord compression
	Transverse myelitis
	Poliomyelitis, rabies
Peripheral nerve	Guillain–Barré syndrome
	Critical illness polyneuropathy
	Toxins
	Acute intermittent porphyria
	Vasculitis, e.g. SLE
	Diphtheria
Neuromuscular junction	Myasthenia gravis
	Eaton–Lambert syndrome
	Botulism
	Toxins
Muscle	Hypokalaemia
	Hypophosphataemia
	Rhabdomyolysis
Thoracic cage and pleura	Crushed chest
	Morbid obesity
	Kyphoscoliosis
	Ankylosing spondylitis
Lungs and airways	Upper airways obstruction
	Severe acute asthma
	Chronic obstructive pulmonary disease
	Severe pneumonia
	Severe pulmonary oedema

Table 43.6 Causes of respiratory alkalosis

1 *Pulmonary disorders with hyperventilation*
  Acute asthma
  Pneumonia
  Pulmonary embolism
  Pulmonary oedema
2 *Primary hyperventilation*
  Anxiety and pain
  Central nervous system disorders, e.g. stroke, bacterial meningitis
3 *Liver failure*
4 *Sepsis syndrome*
5 *Salicylate poisoning*

Table 43.7 Causes of metabolic acidosis

1 *Lactic acidosis*
  Inadequate tissue perfusion due to hypotension, low cardiac output or sepsis
  Prolonged hypoxaemia
  Muscle contraction: status epilepticus
  Metformin
2 *Diabetic, alcoholic* and starvation ketoacidosis*
3 *Poisoning*
  Carbon monoxide
  Ethanol
  Ethylene glycol
  Methanol
  Paracetamol
  Salicylates
  Tricyclics
  Toluene (glue sniffing)
4 *Renal failure*
5 *Renal tubular acidosis*
6 *Loss of bicarbonate from the gut*
  Severe diarrhoea

* Alcoholic ketoacidosis: due to alcohol binge plus starvation; often associated with pancreatitis; hyperglycaemia may occur but is mild (<15 mmol/L); treat with IV dextrose infusion.

Table 43.8 Causes of metabolic alkalosis

1 *Loss of gastric acid*
  Prolonged vomiting
  Gastric aspiration
2 *Diuretic therapy*
3 *Severe and prolonged potassium deficiency*
4 *Mineralocorticoid and glucocorticoid excess*

Table 43.9 Estimation of the alveolar–arterial oxygen difference

Establish Fio_2, the fractional concentration of oxygen in inspired gas (0.21 in air)
Measure Pao_2 and $Paco_2$, the partial pressures of oxygen and carbon dioxide
(in kPa) in arterial blood
Estimate the partial pressure of oxygen in alveolar gas (PAo_2) from the simplified
  form of the alveolar gas equation:

  $$PAo_2 = [Pio_2 - (Paco_2/R)]$$

  where Pio_2 is the partial pressure of inspired oxygen (see box to derive Pio_2 from
  Fio_2) and R is the respiratory quotient (can be taken to be 1)

Fio_2	0.21	0.24	0.28	0.31	0.35	0.40	0.60	1.0
Pio_2	19.9	22.8	26.5	29.4	33.2	37.9	56.9	94.8

Subtract Pao_2 from PAo_2 to give the alveolar–arterial oxygen difference, which in
  normal subjects is less than 2.6 kPa.

Interpreting the results: arterial Po_2

The arterial Po_2 must be related to the inspired oxygen concentration. Table 43.9 shows how to estimate the alveolar–arterial oxygen difference, which is a measure of the efficiency of gas exchange by the lungs.

• In a patient breathing air, arterial hypoxaemia is defined as an arterial $Po_2 < 10.7\,kPa$, and respiratory failure as an arterial $Po_2 < 8\,kPa$.

• Respiratory failure is subdivided according to the arterial Pco_2. Type I respiratory failure is when $Paco_2$ is normal or low ($<6\,kPa$); type II respiratory failure is when $Paco_2$ is high ($>6\,kPa$).

Oxygen therapy

• Oxygen should be given to patients with hypoxaemia (oxygen saturation by oximetry $<90\%$), hypotension, low cardiac output, respiratory distress or cardiorespiratory arrest. Where possible, arterial blood gases should be measured before oxygen is started.

• Oxygen should be prescribed as carefully as any other drug, specifying the delivery device to be used and the oxygen flow rate. The characteristics of commonly used oxygen delivery devices are given in Table 43.10.

• Initial Fio_2 should be 40–60%, except for patients with type II respiratory failure ($Paco_2 > 6\,kPa$), who should start with 24% oxygen, and patients with cardiorespiratory arrest, who should receive 100% oxygen.

• Arterial blood gases should be checked within 2 h of starting oxygen, and Fio_2 adjusted accordingly. An adequate response is defined as a $Pao_2 > 8\,kPa$ or $Sao_2 > 90\%$.

• Hypoxaemic patients at risk of arrhythmias or respiratory failure should be monitored continuously by oximetry.

Acid–base disorders

Acid–base disorders

Table 43.10 Oxygen delivery devices

Device	Indication	Concentration of oxygen delivered	Advantages	Disadvantages
High-flow mask	Type II respiratory failure	24–60%, determined by the Venturi valve used and the flow rate of oxygen	• Delivers an accurate FiO_2 • Reduces the risk of CO_2 retention in type II respiratory failure	• New mask needed if FiO_2 has to be changed • Uncomfortable to wear for long periods
Low-flow mask	Type I respiratory failure	28–60%, depending on the oxygen flow rate, degree of leakage between the mask and face, and ventilatory minute volume.	• Simple and cheap • No need to change mask if FiO_2 has to be changed	• FiO_2 provided by a given oxygen flow rate is variable • At oxgen flow rates <5 L/min significant rebreathing may

occur, with risk of CO_2 retention in type II respiratory failure

Nasal cannulae	Patients with COPD or recovering from other causes of respiratory failure	Flow rate (L/min) Approx. O_2 conc. (%) 2 28 4 35 6 40 8 50 10 60 Depends on the oxygen flow rate and ventilatory minute volume; 2 L/min gives an FiO_2 of roughly 25–30%	• Prevent rebreathing and so reduce the risk of CO_2 retention in type II respiratory failure • Comfortable to wear for long periods • Nasal irritation with flow rates > 3 L/min

COPD, chronic obstructive pulmonary disease.

44 Acute adrenal insufficiency

Consider the diagnosis in any patient with unexplained hypotension who
• has been taking chronic corticosteroid therapy (prednisolone >7.5 mg daily or equivalent); or
• has clinical features suggestive of adrenal insufficiency (Table 44.1).
Causes of acute adrenal insufficiency are given in Table 44.2. Treatment requires correction of fluid depletion as well as steroid replacement therapy.

Priorities

1 If the patient is unconscious, initial resuscitation is as for any cause of coma (Chapter 6). Check blood glucose: if <3.5 mmol/L, give 50 mL of 50% dextrose IV via a large vein.
2 If systolic BP is <90 mmHg, give colloid 500 mL IV over 15–30 min.
3 If acute adrenal insufficiency is possible, take blood for measurement of cortisol and corticotrophin levels and other investigations (Table 44.3) and give hydrocortisone 100 mg IV, followed by a continuous infusion of 10 mg/h over the first 24 h.
4 Start antibiotic therapy for suspected sepsis (p. 103):
   • if a source of sepsis is evident;
   • if the white cell count is <3 or >20 × 10^9/L; or
   • if the temperature is <36 or >38°C.

Further management

1 Fluid replacement
• If systolic BP remains <90 mmHg after 500 mL colloid, put in a central line and infuse colloid to keep the central venous pressure 5–10 cm water (see p. 43).

Table 44.1 Clinical features of adrenal insufficiency

Common to primary and secondary adrenal insufficiency
Tiredness, weakness, anorexia, weight loss
Postural hypotension
Nausea, vomiting, diarrhoea
Hyponatraemia, hypoglycaemia, mild normocytic anaemia, lymphocytosis, eosinophilia

Primary adrenal insufficiency and associated disorders
Hyperpigmentation
Hyperkalaemia
Vitiligo
Autoimmune thyroid disease

Secondary adrenal insufficiency and associated disorders
Pale skin without marked anaemia
Amenorrhoea, decreased libido and potency
Scanty axillary and pubic hair
Small testicles
Secondary hypothyroidism
Headache, visual symptoms
Diabetes insipidus

Reference: Oelkers W. *New England Journal of Medicine* 1996; **335**: 1206–12.

Acute adrenal insufficiency

- If systolic BP is >90 mmHg, give normal saline 1 L every 6–8 h until the fluid deficit has been corrected, as judged by clinical improvement and the absence of postural hypotension.
- Hyperkalaemia is common in acute hypoadrenalism and potassium should not be added if plasma potassium is >5 mmol/L.

2 Steroid replacement
- Continue hydrocortisone 100 mg IV daily until vomiting has stopped.

Table 44.2 Causes of acute adrenal insufficiency

Adrenal causes

1 Rapid withdrawal of chronic corticosteroid therapy
2 Sepsis or surgical stress in patients with chronic adrenal dysfunction from
   Chronic corticosteroid therapy
   Autoimmune adrenalitis
   Other causes, e.g. tuberculosis, AIDS-related infections
3 Bilateral adrenal haemorrhage, necrosis or thrombosis
   Fulminant meningococcal sepsis (Waterhouse–Friderichsen syndrome)
   Coagulation disorders
   Heparin or warfarin therapy

Pituitary causes

Postpartum pituitary necrosis (Sheehan syndrome)
Necrosis or bleeding into a pituitary macroadenoma
Head trauma (often associated with diabetes insipidus)
Sepsis or surgical stress in patients with hypopituitarism

Table 44.3 Urgent investigation in suspected acute adrenal insufficiency

Creatinine, sodium and potassium, glucose*
Plasma cortisol and corticotrophin (10 mL blood in a heparinized tube, for later
   analysis)†
Full blood count
Blood culture
Urine microscopy and culture
Chest X-ray
ECG

* Typical biochemical findings in acute adrenal insufficiency, raised creatinine, low
sodium (120–130 mmol/L), raised potassium (5–7 mmol/L), low glucose.

† A plasma cortisol level of > 700 nmol/L in a critically ill patient effectively excludes
adrenal insufficiency.

Table 44.4 Commonly used corticosteroids

Steroid	Estimated potency	
	Glucocorticoid	Mineralocorticoid
Hydrocortisone (cortisol)	1	1
Prednisolone	4	0.25
Methylprednisolone	5	<0.01
Dexamethasone	30	<0.01

The normal glucocorticoid output of the adrenals is equivalent to 20–40 mg of hydrocortisone or 5–10 mg of prednisolone daily; with stress this may increase 10-fold.

Acute adrenal insufficiency

• Maintenance therapy is with hydrocortisone 30 mg PO daily, which is given in divided doses (20 mg in the morning and 10 mg in the evening) and fludrocortisone 50–300 µg PO daily.

3 Diagnosis

To confirm the diagnosis in equivocal cases (where the initial cortisol level is borderline), use the short tetracosactrin (Synacthen) test. Primary and secondary hypoadrenalism can be distinguished by measuring corticotrophin (high in primary and low in secondary hypoadrenalism).

• The test should be done when the patient has recovered, as hydrocortisone (but not fludrocortisone) must be stopped for 24 h before the test.

• Give 250 µg of tetracosactrin IV or IM before 10 a.m. Measure plasma cortisol before and 60 min after. With normal adrenal function, plasma cortisol is at least 550 nmol/L before or after administration of tetracosactrin. In patients with primary hypoadrenalism, tetracosactrin does not stimulate cortisol secretion, because the adrenal cortex is already maximally stimulated by endogenous corticotrophin. In severe secondary hypoadrenalism, plasma cortisol does not increase because of adrenocortical atrophy. However, in secondary hypoadrenalism which is mild or of recent onset, the test may be normal.

Problems

The patient on long-term corticosteroid therapy or receiving replacement therapy: when should the dose be increased?
- Mild infection: double the usual dose.
- Minor surgery*: 100 mg hydrocortisone IV 6-hly for 24 h starting with the premedication, then return to usual dose.
- Severe infection or major surgery: give hydrocortisone IV as for minor surgery but continue for 72 h or until taking oral fluids. After this, give the same dose orally (and restart fludrocortisone) and gradually taper over 2 weeks to the usual maintenance dose.

* Surgery not involving a body cavity or major limb bone.

45 Thyrotoxic crisis

• Consider the diagnosis in any patient with fever, abnormal mental state, sinus tachycardia or atrial fibrillation who also has signs of thyrotoxicosis.

• The mortality of untreated thyrotoxic crisis is high. If the diagnosis is suspected, antithyroid treatment must be started before biochemical confirmation.

Priorities

1 Make a clinical diagnosis

• The signs may not be prominent in the elderly, or may be masked by other illness. Check for goitre, thyroid bruit and ophthalmopathy.

• Investigations required urgently are given in Table 45.1.

• Identify the likely precipitant (Table 45.2).

2 Treat heart failure

This is usually associated with fast atrial fibrillation.

• Give oxygen, attach an ECG monitor and pulse oximeter and obtain an ECG.

• Cardioversion of atrial fibrillation is very unlikely to be successful until the patient is euthyroid: give digoxin to control the ventricular rate.

• There is relative digoxin resistance (increased renal excretion and reduced action on AV conduction) so high doses are needed:

  • loading dose 0.5 mg IV over 30 min; followed by

  • 0.25 mg IV over 30 min every 2 h until the heart rate is < 100/min or up to a total dose of 1.5 mg;

  • maintenance dose: 0.25–0.5 mg daily PO.

• Give a loop diuretic (frusemide or bumetanide) as required.

Table 45.1 Urgent investigation in suspected thyrotoxic crisis

Thyroid function (TSH, free T3 and free T4*) (for later analysis)
Creatinine, sodium and potassium
Full blood count
Blood glucose
Blood culture
Urine microscopy and culture
Chest X-ray
ECG
Arterial blood gases and pH

TSH, thyroid-stimulating hormone; T3, tri-iodothyronine; T4, thyroxine.

*If severely ill, increased production of reverse tri-iodothyronine may lead to near normal thyroxine levels.

Table 45.2 Precipitants of thyrotoxic crisis

Infection
Surgical stress
Trauma
Iodine: amiodarone; radiographic contrast media; radio-iodine
Pulmonary embolism
Myocardial infarction

3 Start beta-blockade

If there is no heart failure, give propranolol 40–160 mg 6-hly PO, aiming to reduce the heart rate to < 100/min. Diltiazem 60–120 mg 6-hly PO can be used if beta-blockade is contraindicated because of asthma.

Table 45.3 Antithyroid treatment in thyrotoxic crisis

Drug	Regimen
Carbimazole or Propylthiouracil	• 15–30 mg 6-hly by mouth or nasogastric tube, reducing to 10–20 mg 8-hly after 24 h • 150–300 mg 6-hly by mouth or nasogastric tube, reducing to 100–200 mg 8-hly after 24 h
Iodine	• Do not start within 4 h of carbimazole or propylthiouracil • Give 0.1–0.3 mL of aqueous iodine oral solution (Lugol's solution) 8-hly by mouth or nasogastric tube • Stop after 2 days if propylthiouracil is used or after 1 week with carbimazole

Thyrotoxic crisis

4 Start anticoagulation

• Give heparin by IV infusion or low-molecular-weight heparin SC (p. 404) to patients with atrial fibrillation or if pulmonary embolism is suspected (p. 183)

• Other patients should receive heparin 5000 units 8-hly SC as prophylaxis against venous thromboembolism.

5 Start antithyroid treatment (Table 45.3)

• Start either propylthiouracil or carbimazole (which act principally by inhibiting thyroxine synthesis).

• After 4 h, start iodine (which inhibits secretion of thyroxine). If iodine is started before antithyroid drugs, excess thyroxine may be produced, leading to an exacerbation of the crisis.

• Give dexamethasone 2 mg 6-hly PO to inhibit hormone release from the thyroid and reduce the peripheral conversion of thyroxine to tri-iodothyronine.

6 Other supportive management

• Treat severe agitation with chlorpromazine (50 mg 8-hly PO; or 25 mg 8-hly IM; or by rectal suppository 100 mg 6–8-hly).

- Treat sepsis (Chapter 10).
- Reduce fever by fanning, tepid sponging or paracetamol (avoid aspirin as it displaces thyroxine from thyroid-binding globulin).
- Give fluid replacement guided by measurement of CVP.

Problems

Failure to improve
- Check that precipitants have not been missed
- Exchange transfusion or peritoneal dialysis/haemodialysis may be considered in a patient who fails to improve within 24–48h. Seek expert advice from an endocrinologist.

46 Hypothermia (including myxoedema coma)

- Hypothermia is defined as a core temperature below 35°C.
- Coma occurs if the core temperature falls below 27°C.
- Measure rectal temperature with a low-reading thermometer in any patient admitted with a reduced level of consciousness who has been exposed to the cold.
- At high risk are the elderly (in whom hypothermia is often the consequence of acute illness) and those living rough (due to the combination of alcohol and cold exposure).

Priorities

1 **If unconscious**, start resuscitation as for coma from any cause (see Chapter 6).

2 **Give oxygen, attach an ECG monitor and put in a peripheral IV line.**

- Ventricular fibrillation may occur at core temperatures below 28–30°C. Precipitants include central vein cannulation, chest compression, endotracheal intubation and IV injection of adrenaline. DC countershock may not be effective until core temperature is >30°C. Continue cardiopulmonary resuscitation for longer than usual (as hypothermia protects the brain from ischaemic injury).
- Sinus bradycardia does not need treatment: temporary pacing is only indicated for complete heart block.

3 **Check blood glucose**. Treat hypoglycaemia. Raised blood glucose (10–20 mmol/L) is common (due to insulin resistance) and should not be treated with insulin because of the risk of hypoglycaemia on rewarming.

4 **Check for underlying illness** (e.g. pneumonia, stroke, myocardial infarction, fractured neck of femur).

- Investigations required urgently are given in Table 46.1.

Table 46.1 Urgent investigation of the patient with hypothermia

Blood glucose

Creatinine, sodium, potassium

Full blood count

Arterial pH and gases (corrected for temperature*)

Blood culture

Thyroid function (if age > 50 or suspected thyroid disease) (for later analysis)

Blood and urine for drug screen if no other cause for hypothermia is evident

ECG

Chest X-ray

X-ray pelvis and hips if history of a fall or clinical signs of fractured neck
  of femur

* For each 1°C decrease in body temperature below 37°C, arterial pH increases by 0.015, Pao_2 decreases by 4.4% and $Paco_2$ decreases by 7.2%.

NB: Blood levels of skeletal and cardiac muscle enzymes are raised in hypothermia, even in the absence of myocardial infarction.

- Consider poisoning with alcohol or psychotropic drugs if no other cause of hypothermia is evident (see Chapter 11).
- As pneumonia is a common cause and complication of hypothermia, give co-amoxiclav 1.2 g IV or cefotaxime 1 g IV once blood cultures have been taken. Further doses need not be given until the core temperature is >32°C.

5 **Fluid replacement**
- Most hypothermic patients are volume-depleted (due in part to cold-induced diuresis).
- If the chest X-ray does not show pulmonary oedema, start an IV infusion of normal saline 1 L over 4 h via a warming coil: further fluid therapy should be guided by the blood pressure, CVP and urine output.

6 **Active rewarming** (Table 46.2) may be indicated if core temperature is <30°C, or there is VF refractory to DC shock: take into consideration the age of the patient and concurrent illness.

Table 46.2 Methods of active rewarming

Peritoneal dialysis (p. 467)

Inhalation of warmed oxygen (via endotracheal tube: oxygen is warmed in a waterbath humidifier. Monitor the gas temperature at the mouth and maintain it around 44°C: this will require modification of most ventilators)

Oesophageal thermal probe

Cardiopulmonary bypass

Further management—passive rewarming

If the core temperature is 30–35°C the patient can be treated by passive external rewarming, aiming for a slow rise in core temperature around 0.5°C/h. Nurse in a side-room heated to 20–30°C on a ripple mattress with the blankets supported by a bed cage. Give warmed humidified oxygen by face mask. Monitor:

- rectal temperature (hourly, or preferably using a rectal probe allowing a continuous display);
- oxygen saturation by pulse oximeter (continuous display);
- ECG supraventricular arrhythmias (e.g. atrial fibrillation) are common and usually resolve as core temperature returns to normal;
- blood pressure (hourly): if systolic BP falls below 100 mmHg, reduce the rate of rewarming and give further IV fluid.
- CVP (hourly) NB: Do not put in a central line until core temperature is >30°C as it may precipitate VF;
- blood glucose (4-hourly);
- urine output by bladder catheter (hourly).

Treatment of myxoedema coma

The physical signs of hypothermia from whatever cause closely resemble those of myxoedema coma: however, if there is other evidence of hypothyroidism (Table 46.3), thyroid hormone and hydrocortisone should be given.

Hypothermia

Table 46.3 Features suggesting myxoedema in the patient with hypothermia

Preceding symptoms of hypothyroidism: weight gain with reduced appetite, dry skin
and hair loss
Previous radio-iodine treatment for thyroxicosis
Thyroidectomy scar
Hyponatraemia (plasma sodium <130 mmol/L)
Macrocytosis
Failure of core temperature to rise 0.5°C/h with external rewarming

NB: Slowly relaxing tendon reflexes are a non-specific feature of hypothermia.

Hypothermia

Table 46.4 Thyroid hormone replacement in myxoedema coma

Day 1–3	T3 10 µg 8-hly IV
Day 4–6	T3 20 µg 12-hly IV
Day 7–14	T3 20 µg 8-hly IV
Week 3–4	T4 50 µg once daily PO

1 Check for concurrent illness and continue antibiotic therapy and
passive external rewarming as above.
2 Take blood for thyroid hormones, TSH and cortisol before starting
treatment.
3 Start thyroid hormone replacement with tri-iodothyronine (T3)
(Table 46.4) or thyroxine (T4):
  • Tri-iodothyronine has a shorter half-life than thyroxine which is
  advantageous if haemodynamic problems develop and the dose has
  to be reduced.

- An alternative regimen is thyroxine 400–500 µg as a bolus IV or via a nasogastric tube. No further replacement therapy should be given for 1 week.

4 Give hydrocortisone 100 mg 12-hly IV in case there is panhypopituitarism (see p. 364).

Hypothermia

Infectious Diseases

47 Acute medical problems in the patient with HIV/AIDS

- Human immunodeficiency virus positive (HIV+) patients get common diseases as well as those that reflect their immune deficiency. The spectrum of HIV infection is summarized in Table 47.5.
- Establish who knows about the HIV diagnosis among the patient's relatives and friends and be sensitive to their needs. HIV+ patients have often made 'living wills'—find out if one exists.
- Take appropriate safety precautions when handling any body fluid and label all specimens as high risk (Table 47.1).
- Informed consent should be obtained before testing for HIV.
- The management of acute medical problems in the patient with HIV/AIDS is often complex, and you should seek expert advice early on.

HIV/AIDS

Breathlessness

Pulmonary infection (especially with *Pneumocystis carinii*) remains the commonest acute presentation of HIV+ patients. Other causes to consider are given in Table 47.2.

1 Attach a pulse oximeter and check arterial blood gases: the patient may be severely hypoxaemic with minimal lung signs. Give oxygen to maintain arterial oxygen saturation >90%. Investigations needed urgently are given in Table 47.3.

2 Your clinical assessment and the chest X-ray appearance may provide clues to the likely diagnosis (Table 47.2).

- Dual pathology is relatively frequent, and definitive diagnosis depends on microbiological findings.
- Initial treatment for suspected *Pneumocystis carinii* pneumonia (PCP) is given in Table 47.4.
- Seek expert advice from a chest physician on further manage-

Table 47.1 Care of the HIV+ patient: safety precautions

Cover all abrasions with a waterproof plaster

Wear latex gloves and plastic apron when handling urine, faeces, drain fluid or blood

Wear mask and visor or goggles for tracheobronchial suctioning

Wear a single-use, non-absorbent surgeon's gown for inserting central lines, intra-arterial lines or invasive procedures such as endoscopy

Seek immediate advice after any needlestick injury

ment. Examination of induced sputum and bronchoscopic alveolar lavage are often helpful in making a diagnosis.

Neurological problems

With improved PCP prophylaxis, HIV+ patients are presenting more frequently with neurological problems.

Confusion with or without headache

• Consider toxoplasmosis, cryptococcal meningitis (p. 252), cerebral lymphoma and progressive multifocal leucoencephalopathy. HIV encephalopathy is diagnosed by exclusion of other causes.

• Arrange urgent cranial CT or MRI.

• Perform an LP if the scan is normal. Send CSF for cell count; protein concentration; glucose (fluoride tube); Gram, Ziehl–Neelsen and India ink stains; and serological tests for *Cryptococcus* and *Toxoplasma gondii*.

• If no diagnosis can be made, give empirical treatment for toxoplasmosis with pyrimethamine and sulphadiazine, and repeat the scan after 2–3 weeks.

• Seek expert advice from an infectious diseases physician or neurologist.

Table 47.2 Diagnostic clues in the breathless HIV+ patient

Diagnosis	Clinical features	Chest X-ray features
Pneumocystis carinii pneumonia (PCP)	Dyspnoea, often of slow onset Dry cough Lungs clear, or sparse basal crackles Fever	Perihilar haze common Lobar consolidation rare Pleural effusion rare Apical shadowing if prophylaxis has been with nebulized pentamidine
Mycobacterium tuberculosis infection	Cough Haemoptysis Fever	Usually typical of tuberculosis: multiple areas of consolidation, often with cavitation, in one or both upper lobes
Mycobacterium avium intracellulare infection	Cough Dyspnoea Fever	Often normal
Bacterial pneumonia (p. 206)	Commoner in smokers Productive cough Focal signs Fever	Focal consolidation
Cytomegalovirus pneumonitis	Clinically indistinguishable from PCP (dual infection may occur)	Diffuse bilateral interstitial shadowing
Kaposi's sarcoma	No fever Dyspnoea More common in homosexual men and Africans than IV drug users May be associated with cutaneous Kaposi's sarcoma	Diffuse bilateral interstitial shadowing, more nodular than PCP May be unilateral and associated with hilar adenopathy Pleural effusion strongly suggestive

Table 47.3 Urgent investigation of the breathless HIV+ patient

Chest X-ray

Arterial blood gases

Full blood count

Blood culture (positive in most patients with *Mycobacterium avium-intracellulare* infection: use specific myobacterial culture bottles)

Creatinine, sodium and potassium

Sputum if available for Gram and Ziehl–Neelsen stain and culture

Other investigations to discuss with a chest physician

Examination of induced sputum

Fibreoptic bronchoscopy (for bronchoalveolar lavage or transbronchial biopsy)

Table 47.4 Initial treatment of suspected *Pneumocystis carinii* pneumonia

Antimicrobial therapy with co-trimoxazole or pentamidine

Co-trimoxazole

120 mg/kg in 2–4 divided doses by mouth or IV for 14 days

Causes haemolysis in glucose-6-phosphate dehydrogenase deficient patients (African/Mediterranean)

Pentamidine

4 mg/kg once daily IV

May cause renal impairment

Steroid therapy

Start immediately if moderate or severe PCP (breathless at rest; Pao_2 breathing air <8 kPa; extensive interstitial shadowing on chest X-ray)

Give prednisolone 1 mg/kg PO daily for 5 days

Table 47.5 Spectrum of HIV infection

Group 1 Acute infection (a mononucleosis-like syndrome associated with sero-conversion)

Group 2 Asymptomatic infection

Group 3 Persistent generalized lymphadenopathy

Group 4 Other disease

Constitutional disease (e.g. fever, weight loss, diarrhoea)*

Neurological disease (HIV encephalopathy, opportunistic infection, central nervous system lymphoma)

Secondary infectious diseases

- *Pneumocystis carinii pneumonia*
- Cytomegalovirus chorioretinitis, colitis, pneumonitis or adrenalitis
- *Candida albicans*: oral thrush*, oesophagitis
- *Mycobacterium avium-intracellulare:* localized or disseminated infection
- *Mycobacterium tuberculosis* infection*
- *Cryptococcus neoformans*: meningitis or disseminated infection
- *Toxoplasma gondii*: encephalitis or intracerebral mass lesions
- Herpes simplex virus: severe mucocutaneous lesions, oesophagitis
- *Cryptosporidium* diarrhoea
- *Isospora belli* diarrhoea

Secondary neoplasms

- Kaposi's sarcoma (cutaneous and visceral)
- Lymphoma (brain, bone marrow, gut)

Other conditions (thrombocytopenia, non-specific interstitial pneumonitis)*

AIDS is diagnosed in an HIV+ patient with group 4 disease, except those marked *.

HIV/AIDS

Focal upper motor neurone signs

- Consider toxoplasmosis or lymphoma.
- Arrange urgent cranial CT or MRI.
- Perform an LP if the scan is normal, and send CSF for investigation as above.

• If focal lesions (ring-enhancing, with surrounding oedema on CT), treat as toxoplasmosis.
• Seek expert advice from an infectious diseases physician or neurologist.

Impaired vision
• Suspect cytomegalovirus retinitis: fundoscopy shows characteristic infiltrates, similar in appearance to soft exudates.
• Seek an urgent ophthalmological opinion.
• Treatment is with ganciclovir (or cidofovir or foscarnet if ganciclovir is contraindicated; both are nephrotoxic). Ganciclovir causes severe marrow suppression when given with zidovudine, which should be temporarily stopped.

48 Septic arthritis

- Consider the diagnosis in any patient with fever and joint swelling (particularly if only one large joint is involved).
- Other causes of acute arthritis are given in Table 48.1.

Priorities

1 Your clinical assessment should address the following points:
- Does the patient have arthritis or periarticular inflammation (bursitis, tendinitis or cellulitis)? Painful limitation of movement of the joint suggests arthritis.
- Is the patient at risk of septic arthritis? Septic arthritis usually follows a bacteraemia (e.g. from pneumonia or urinary tract infection, or IV drug use) in a patient at risk because of rheumatoid arthritis, the presence of a prosthetic joint, or immunocompromise.
- Could this be a crystal arthritis (gout or pseudogout): is there a history of previous similar attacks of arthritis?
- Could this be a reactive arthritis: is there an associated rash, diarrhoea, urethritis or uveitis?
- Could this be gonococcal arthritis (Table 48.2)?

2 Aspirate the joint and send synovial fluid for cell count (in an EDTA tube; normal cell count is $<180/mm^3$, most mononuclear); Gram stain; culture; and microscopy under polarized light for crystals.
- If you are not familiar with joint aspiration, ask the help of a rheumatologist or orthopaedic surgeon.
- Both crystal and septic arthritis give rise to a purulent effusion, although the white cell count is usually higher in septic arthritis ($50\,000–200\,000/mm^3$).
- Bloodstaining of the effusion is common in pseudogout but rare in sepsis.

3 Other investigations needed are given in Table 48.3.

Table 48.1 Causes of acute arthritis

Usually mono- or oligoarthritis
Acute crystal arthritis: gout and pseudogout
Non-gonococcal septic arthritis (see Table 48.2)
Haemarthrosis (in haemophilia, or on warfarin)
Osteoarthritis
Trauma (causing internal derangement, haemarthrosis or fracture, or acute synovitis from penetrating injury)
Infective endocarditis (acute sterile synovitis or tenosynovitis)
HIV infection (acute sterile synovitis)

Usually polyarthritis
Gonococcal arthritis (see Table 48.2)
Reactive arthritis following gut or genitourinary infection
Rheumatic diseases, e.g. rheumatoid arthritis, systemic lupus erythematosus
Viral infections, e.g. rubella, hepatitis B and C, infectious mononucleosis

Further management

Organisms on Gram stain of synovial fluid, or high probability of septic arthritis

1 Start antibiotic therapy IV (Table 48.4).
  • Intra-articular administration is not needed.
  • The antibiotic regimen may need modification in the light of blood and synovial fluid culture results: discuss this with a microbiologist.
  • Antibiotic therapy for non-gonococcal septic arthritis usually needs to be given IV for 2–4 weeks.
2 If septic arthritis is confirmed, seek advice on further management from a rheumatologist or orthopaedic surgeon.
  • Aspirate the joint daily until an effusion no longer reaccumulates.
  • While the infection is resolving, the joint should be immobilized using a splint or cast.
  • Physiotherapy should be started early.
  • Give an NSAID for pain relief (e.g. indomethacin or diclofenac).
  •

Table 48.2 Comparison of gonococcal and non-gonococcal septic arthritis

	Gonococcal	Non-gonococcal
Organisms	*Neisseria gonorrhoeae*	*Staphylococcus aureus* (60%) Gram-negative rods (18%) Beta-haemolytic streptococci (15%) *Streptococcus pneumoniae* (3%)
Patient profile	Young, healthy, sexually active	Elderly, rheumatoid arthritis, prosthetic joint, IV drug use, immunocompromised
Initial presentation	Migratory polyarthralgia, tenosynovitis, dermatitis	Single hot, swollen, painful joint
Joints involved	Often polyarticular, esp. knee and wrist	Usually monoarticular, esp. knee
Other signs	Tenosynovitis, rash	Source of bacteraemia
Gram stain of synovial fluid	<25% positive	50–75% positive
Culture of synovial fluid	25% positive	85–95% positive
Blood culture	<10% positive	50% positive
Genitourinary culture (swab of urethra, cervix and anorectum)	80% positive	Not indicated
Response to antibiotics	Within a few days; outcome excellent	Takes weeks; joint drainage must be adequate; outcome often poor

References: Baker D G, Schumacher H R Jr. Acute monoarthritis. *New England Journal of Medicine* 1993; **329**: 1013–20. Goldenberg D L. Septic arthritis. *Lancet* 1998; **351**: 197–202.

Septic arthritis

Table 48.3 Investigation in suspected septic arthritis

Joint aspiration
X-ray joint to exclude osteomyelitis and for baseline
Chest X-ray to exclude pneumonia
Full blood count
C-reactive protein and ESR
Blood culture (x 2)
Urine microscopy and culture
Swab of urethra, cervix and anorectum if gonococcal infection is possible (see Table 48.2)

Table 48.4 Initial antibiotic therapy for suspected septic arthritis

Organisms on Gram stain	Initial antibiotic therapy (IV, high dose)
Gram-positive cocci	Flucloxacillin + benzylpenicillin (or vancomycin if penicillin allergic or suspected MRSA)
	Vancomycin
Gram-negative cocci	Ceftriaxone or cefotaxime
Gram-negative rods	Cefuroxime + gentamicin
None seen: gonococcal infection unlikely	Flucloxacillin + benzylpenicillin (or vancomycin if penicillin allergic or suspected MRSA) + gentamicin
None seen: gonococcal infection likely	Ceftriaxone or cefotaxime

Septic arthritis

• In patients with gonococcal arthritis, sexual partners should be traced.

No organisms on Gram stain of synovial fluid and low probability of septic arthritis

1 Consider the other causes of acute arthritis (Table 48.1).

• Pseudogout is the commonest cause of acute mono-or oligo-arthritis in the elderly.

2 Hold off antibiotic therapy (pending the results of blood and synovial fluid culture for definite exclusion of infection).

• Treat with an NSAID (e.g. indomethacin 50 mg 6-hly PO, covered with a proton-pump inhibitor in the elderly or patients with previous peptic ulceration).

• If gout is confirmed (also check plasma urate) and fails to respond to an NSAID, use colchicine. Allopurinol should not be started until the acute attack has completely resolved.

Septic arthritis

49 Fever on return from abroad

• Malaria is the most common single cause of fever after travel to the tropics, accounting for 30–40% of cases. Its clinical features are non-specific, and diagnosis requires examination of a blood film for parasites.

• Chemoprophylaxis against malaria does not ensure full protection and may prolong the incubation period.

• Exclude malaria or typhoid in any patient with a febrile illness presenting within 2 months of return from an endemic area (most of Africa, Asia, Central and South America).

• Consider other causes of febrile illness unrelated to travel, such as community-acquired pneumonia (p. 204) and urinary tract infection.

Priorities

1 Admit to a single room and nurse with standard isolation technique until the diagnosis is established.

2 Your clinical assessment should include these questions:

• Which countries travelled to and through? Travel in urban or rural areas or both?

• Immunizations before travel?

• Malaria prophylaxis taken as prescribed?

• Known or possible exposure to infection (including sexually transmitted diseases) (Table 49.1)?

• When did symptoms first appear (Table 49.2)?

• Treatments taken?

Physical signs which may be found in tropical infections are given in Table 49.3.

Clinical features of malaria and typhoid are summarized in Tables 49.4 and 49.5.

Table 49.1 Specific exposures and tropical infections

Exposure	Infection or disease
Raw or undercooked foods	Enteric infections, hepatitis, trichinosis
Drinking untreated water; milk, cheese	Salmonellosis, shigellosis, hepatitis, brucellosis
Freshwater swimming	Schistosomiasis, leptospirosis
Sexual contact	HIV, syphilis, hepatitis, gonococcaemia
Insect bites	Malaria, dengue fever (mosquitoes); typhus, Crimean–Congo haemorrhagic fever, borreliosis, tularaemia (ticks); Chagas' disease (triatomine bugs); African trypanosomiasis (tsetse flies)
Animal exposure or bites	Rabies, Q fever, tularaemia, borreliosis, viral haemorrhagic fevers, plague
Exposure to infected persons	Lassa, Marburg or Ebola viruses; hepatitis; typhoid; meningococcaemia

Reference: Humar A, Keystone J. Evaluating fever in travellers returning from tropical countries. *British Medical Journal* 1996; **312**: 953–6.

Fever

3 In patients who have travelled to rural west Africa within the previous 3 weeks, a viral haemorrhagic fever must be considered, particularly if pharyngitis is a prominent symptom: seek advice from an infectious diseases physician on management (before blood samples are taken).

4 Investigations needed urgently are given in Table 49.6.

Further management

This will depend on the clinical syndrome and likely pathogens:

1 Septic shock

• Antimicrobial therapy for patients who have travelled in endemic regions must cover falciparum malaria (Appendix) and typhoid (either

Table 49.2 Typical incubation periods for selected tropical infections

Short (<10 days)
Arboviral infections (including dengue fever)
Enteric bacterial infections
Typhus (louse-borne, flea-borne)
Plague
Paratyphoid
Haemorrhagic fevers

Medium (10–21 days)
Malaria
Typhoid fever
Scrub typhus, Q fever, spotted fever group
African trypanosomiasis
Brucellosis
Leptospirosis

Long (>21 days)
Viral hepatitis
Malaria
Tuberculosis
HIV
Schistosomiasis (Katayama fever)
Amoebic liver abscess
Visceral leishmaniasis
Filariasis

ciprofloxacin, cefotaxime or chloramphenicol IV; infections acquired in the Indian subcontinent, Middle East and South-East Asia may be multiple antibiotic-resistant and treatment should be modified in the light of sensitivity results).

• Patients with falciparum malaria must also receive antibiotics to cover Gram-negative infection (as mixed infections may occur).

• See Chapter 10 for general management of sepsis syndrome and septic shock.

Table 49.3 Possible signs in selected tropical infections

Sign	Infection or disease
Rash	Dengue fever, typhoid, typhus, syphilis, gonorrhoea, Ebola virus, brucellosis
Jaundice	Hepatitis, malaria, yellow fever, leptospirosis relapsing fever
Lymphadenopathy	Rickettsial infections, brucellosis, dengue fever, HIV, Lassa fever, visceral leishmaniasis
Hepatomegaly	Amoebiasis, malaria, typhoid, hepatitis, leptospirosis
Splenomegaly	Malaria, relapsing fever, trypanosomiasis, typhoid, brucellosis, kala-azar, typhus, dengue fever
Eschar (painless ulcer with black centre and erythematous margin)	Typhus, borreliosis, Crimean–Congo haemorrhagic fever
Haemorrhage	Lassa, Marburg or Ebola viruses; Crimean–Congo haemorrhagic fever; Rift Valley fever; dengue; yellow fever; meninococcaemia; epidemic louse-borne typhus; Rocky Mountain spotted fever

Reference: Humar A, Keystone J. Evaluating fever in travellers returning from tropical countries. *British Medical Journal* 1996; **312**: 953–6.

Fever

2 Chest X-ray shadowing

• Consider pulmonary tuberculosis and *Legionella* pneumonia in addition to the common causes of community-acquired pneumonia (Chapter 24).

3 Meningism

• Perform a lumbar puncture. If the CSF shows no organisms but a high lymphocyte count, consider tuberculous meningitis (p. 251), leptospirosis, or brucellosis.

• See Chapter 30 for the management of bacterial meningitis.

Table 49.4 Falciparum malaria: clinical features

Prodromal symptoms of malaise, headache, myalgia, anorexia and mild fever
Paroxysms of fever lasting 8–12 h
Dry cough, abdominal discomfort, diarrhoea and vomiting common
Moderate tender hepatosplenomegaly (without lymphadenopathy)
May be jaundiced

Cerebral malaria
Reduced conscious level
Focal or generalized fits common
Abnormal neurological signs may be present (including opisthotonos, extensor
    posturing of decorticate or decerebrate pattern, sustained posturing of limbs,
    conjugate deviation of the eyes, nystagmus, dysconjugate eye movements,
    bruxism, extensor plantar responses, generalized flaccidity)
Retinal haemorrhages common (papilloedema may be present but is unusual)
Abnormal patterns of breathing common (including irregular periods of apnoea and
    hyperventilation)

Reference: Molyneux M, Fox R. Diagnosis and treatment of malaria in Britain.
British Medical Journal 1993; **306**: 1175–80.

Fever

Table 49.5 Typhoid: clinical features

Insidious onset with malaise, anorexia and fever
Abdominal pain, distension and tenderness
Initial constipation followed later by diarrhoea
Headache
Dry cough
Liver and spleen often palpable after first week
Erythematous macular rash (rose spots) on upper abdomen and anterior chest may
    occur during second week

Table 49.6 Investigation of fever on return from abroad

Urgent:

Full blood count (neutropenia is seen in both malaria and typhoid; a low platelet count is common in falciparum malaria)

Blood film for malarial parasites if travel to or through an endemic area; the intensity of the parasitaemia is variable and, if the diagnosis is suspected but the film is negative, repeat blood films every 8 h for 2–3 days (rapid immunochromatographic detection of circulating parasite antigen with dipstick strip test now also available)

Creatinine, sodium and potassium

Blood glucose

Blood culture (positive in 70–90% of patients in the first week of typhoid)

Throat swab

Urine stick test, microscopy and culture

Stool microscopy and culture

Chest X-ray

Lumbar puncture if neck stiffness present

For later analysis:

Liver function tests

Serology as appropriate (e.g. for suspected viral hepatitis, *Legionella* pneumonia, typhoid, amoebic liver abscess, leptospirosis)

Fever

• If there are other features suggesting leptospirosis (haemorrhagic rash, conjunctivitis, renal failure, jaundice), give benzylpenicillin 600 mg 4-hly IV for 7 days. Alternative antibiotics are erythromycin or tetracycline.

4 Jaundice

• Always consider falciparum malaria.

• Others causes are hepatitis A and B (but with these infections patients are afebrile when jaundice appears), leptospirosis, cytomegalovirus and Epstein–Barr virus infection.

• Ask advice from a gastroenterologist.

Appendix: Treatment of malaria

Treatment of falciparum malaria

All patients with falciparum malaria should be admitted to hospital in view of potential complications until confirmed 0% parasitaemia.

Patient seriously ill or unable to take tablets
• Quinine should be given by IV infusion.
• Loading dose: 20 mg/kg (up to a maximum of 1.4 g) of quinine salt given over 4 h by IV infusion (omit if quinine, quinidine or mefloquine given within the previous 24 h), followed after 8–12 h by:
• Maintenance dose: 10 mg/kg (up to a maximum of 700 mg) of quinine salt given over 4 h by IV infusion 8- to 12-hly, until the patient can swallow tablets to complete the 7-day course. Reduce the maintenance dose to 5–7 mg/kg of quinine salt if IV treatment is needed for more than 48 h.
• The course of quinine should be followed by either a single dose of 3 tablets of Fansidar (each tablet contains pyrimethamine 25 mg and sulfadoxine 500 mg), **or** (if Fansidar-resistant) doxycycline 200 mg daily PO for 7 days when renal function has returned to normal.

Patient is not seriously ill (parasitemia <2%, fever <39°C, no complications) and can swallow tablets
• Quinine 600 mg of quinine salt 8-hly PO for 7 days, **followed by either** a single dose of 3 tablets of Fansidar, **or** (if Fansidar-resistant) doxycycline 200 mg daily PO for 7 days when renal function has returned to normal.
or
• Mefloquine 20–25 mg/kg (of mefloquine base) (up to a maximum of 1.5 g) as a single dose or preferably 2–3 divided doses 6–8 h apart PO. It is not necessary to give Fansidar or doxycycline after treatment with mefloquine. Mefloquine resistance has been reported in several countries.

Points in the management of severe falciparum malaria
1 **Obtain expert advice** (see below).
2 **Hypotension**
    • Give colloid (or blood if PCV <20%/haemoglobin <7g/dL) to

maintain CVP at +5 cm water (avoid higher levels because of the risk of pulmonary oedema).
- Start inotropic/vasopressor therapy if systolic BP remains <90 mmHg despite fluids (p. 480).
- Start antibiotic therapy for Gram-negative sepsis after taking blood cultures, with cefotaxime + gentamicin.

3 **Hypoglycaemia**
- Is a common complication: blood glucose should be checked 4-hly, or if conscious level deteriorates, or fits occur.
- If blood glucose is <3.5 mmol/L, give 50 mL of 50% dextrose IV and start an IV infusion of 10% dextrose (initially 1 L 12-hly) via a large peripheral or central vein.

4 **Fits**
- Recheck blood glucose.
- Manage along standard lines (p. 263).
- Exclude coexistent bacterial meningitis by CSF examination. (NB: Lumbar puncture should not be done within 1 h of a major seizure.)

5 **Pulmonary oedema**
- May occur from excessive IV fluid or ARDS (p. 168).

Treatment of benign malarias

P. vivax *and* ovale *malaria*
- Chloroquine 600 mg of chloroquine base PO, followed by a single dose of 300 mg after 6–8 h, followed by 300 mg daily for 2 days.
- Then give primaquine 15 mg daily PO for 14–21 days to eradicate the exoerythrocytic cycle. Check for glucose-6-phosphate dehydrogenase deficiency first as the drug can cause haemolysis in patients who are deficient in the enzyme: if G6PD-deficient, give 30 mg once weekly for 8 weeks.

P. malariae *malaria*
Chloroquine alone is sufficient, following the above regimen.

Infective species not known, or mixed infection

Initial treatment should be with quinine or mefloquine, as for falciparum malaria.

UK reference centres for advice on malaria treatment

London

Hospital for Tropical Diseases
4 St Pancras' Way
London NW1 OPE
Tel.: 020 7387 4411

Lister Unit
Northwick Park Hospital
Harrow, Middlesex
HA1 3UJ
Tel: 020 8869 2831 or 020 8869 2833 (office hours)
         020 88643232 and bleep duty registrar (out of hours)

Birmingham

Department of Infection and Tropical Medicine
Birmingham Hartlands Hospital
Birmingham B9 5SS
Tel: 0121 7666611 extensions 4382 or 4403 or 4535

Liverpool

School of Tropical Medicine
Pembroke Place
Liverpool L3 5QA
Tel.: 0151 7089393

Oxford

John Warin Ward
Churchill Hospital
Headington
Oxford OX3 7LJ
Tel.:   01865 741841

Glasgow

Scottish Centre for Infections and Environmental Health
Clifton House
Clifton Place
Glasgow G3 7LN
Tel.:   0141 3001130

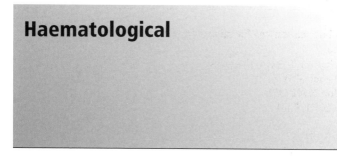

Haematological

50 Management of anticoagulation

See Tables 50.1–50.6.

Table 50.1 Indications for unfractionated heparin (UFH) or low-molecular-weight heparin (LMWH)

Prevention of deep vein thrombosis (UFH and LMWH)
Treatment of deep vein thrombosis or pulmonary embolism (UFH and LMWH)
Treatment of unstable angina (UFH and LMWH)
As adjunct to thrombolytic therapy with alteplase (UFH)
Treatment of acute peripheral arterial occlusion (UFH)
Acute atrial fibrillaiton (UFH)
Perioperatively, after withdrawal of warfarin (UFH)

Unfractionated heparin for treatment is best given by continuous IV infusion; the infusion rate is adjusted to maintain the activated partial thromboplastin time (APTT) at 1.5–2.5 x control (see Table 50.2)
Low-molecular-weight heparins are given by subcutaneous injection; monitoring of the APTT is not required

---

Table 50.2 Unfractionated heparin by infusion

Loading dose
5000–10 000 U (100 U/kg) IV over 5 min

Infusion
25 000 U made up in saline to 50 mL (500 U/mL)
Start the infusion at 1400 U/h (2.8 mL/h) using a syringe pump
Check the activated partial thromboplastin time (APTT) at 6 h
Adjust the dose as follows:

Activated partial thromboplastin (APTT) time (target 1.5–2.5 x control)	*Action*
>7.0	Stop infusion for 30–60 min and then reduce infusion rate by 500 U/h. Recheck APTT in 4 h
5.1–7.0	Reduce infusion rate by 500 U/h. Recheck APTT in 4 h
4.1–5.0	Reduce infusion rate by 300 U/h. Recheck APTT in 10 h
3.1–4.0	Reduce infusion rate by 100 U/h. Recheck APTT in 10 h
2.6–3.0	Reduce infusion rate by 50 U/h. Recheck APTT in 10 h
1.5–2.5	No change in infusion rate. Recheck APTT in 10 h
1.2–2.4	Increase infusion rate by 200 U/h. Recheck APTT in 10 h
<1.2	Increase infusion rate by 400 U/h. Recheck APTT in 4 h

After each change in infusion rate, wait 10 h before next APTT estimation unless
   APTT ratio is > 5 or <1.2, in which case check 4-hly
Check APTT daily
Heparin can cause an immune-mediated thrombocytopenia, which may be
   complicated by thrombosis: check the platelet count daily if given for longer than
   5 days and stop heparin immediately if this falls

Reference: *Drug and Therapeutics Bulletin* 1992; **30**: 77–80.

Table 50.3 Indications for warfarin anticoagulation

Indication	Target INR
Prevention of deep vein thrombosis	2–2.5
Treatment of deep vein thrombosis or pulmonary embolism	2–3
Treatment of recurrent deep vein thrombosis or pulmonary embolism	3–4.5
Atrial fibrillation: prevention of thromboembolism	2–3
Atrial flutter or fibrillation: in preparation for cardioversion	2–3
Rheumatic mitral stenosis (in sinus rhythm or atrial fibrillation)	2–3
Bioprosthetic heart valve*	2–3
Mechanical prosthetic heart valve†	2–4.5
Acute myocardial infarction: treatment of left ventricular mural thrombus	2–3

* Patients with bioprosthetic heart valves are often given warfarin for 3 months after surgery until endothelialization occurs, and aspirin thereafter; in patients with chronic atrial fibrillation, warfarin should be continued indefinitely.

† The target range depends on the exact type of mechanical prosthetic heart valve and its location (aortic or mitral) and whether previous emboli have occurred.

Anticoagulation

Table 50.4 Clinical conditions affecting the response to warfarin*

Increased anticoagulation
Impaired liver function
Congestive heart failure
Renal failure
Malabsorptive states
Hyperthyroidism

Decreased anticoagulation
Hypothyroidism
Transfusion of whole blood or fresh frozen plasma
Diet high in vitamin K (green vegetables)
Hereditary resistance to warfarin

* Drug interactions with warfarin are common and can be serious. When starting or stopping a treatment in a patient taking warfarin, check the list in the *British National Formulary* for an interaction.

Table 50.5 Starting warfarin

Day	International Normalized Ratio (INR), best checked 09.00–10.00 h	Dose of wafarin (mg) to be given that evening (17.00–18.00 h)
1	1.4 or above	Establish cause of coagulation disorder. Do not start warfarin before discussion with a haematologist
	<1.4	10
2	<1.8	10
	1.8	1
	>1.8	0.5
3	<2.0	10
	2.0–2.1	5
	2.2–2.3	4.5
	2.4–2.5	4
	2.6–2.7	3.5
	2.8–2.9	3
	3.0–3.1	2.5
	3.2–3.3	2
	3.4	1.5
	3.5	1
	3.6–4.0	0.5
	>4.0	Give none.
4	<1.4	Ask advice from a haematologist
	1.4	8
	1.5	7.5
	1.6–1.7	7
	1.8	6.5
	1.9	6
	2.0–2.1	5.5
	2.2–2.3	5
	2.4–2.6	4.5
	2.7–3.0	4
	3.1–3.5	3.5
	3.6–4.0	3
	4.1–4.5	Miss 1 day, then give 2 mg
	>4.5	Miss 2 days, then give 1 mg

Reference: Fennerty A *et al*. Anticoagulants in venous thromboembolism. *British Medical Journal* 1988; **297**: 1285–8.

Anticoagulation

Table 50.6 Management of over-anticoagulation or bleeding in a patient taking warfarin

International Normalized Ratio	Clinical condition	Action*
>1.5	Major bleeding† or rapid reversal for surgery needed	Stop warfarin Give vitamin K 5 mg IV + fresh frozen plasma 1 L (15 mL/kg) IV
>8	No bleeding or minor bleeding	Stop warfarin; restart when INR is <5 If there is minor bleeding, give vitamin K 0.5 mg IV + fresh frozen plasma 1L IV If the patient is at increased risk of bleeding, give vitamin K 0.5 mg IV Repeat the dose of vitamin K if INR remains >5 after 24 h
6–8	No bleeding or minor bleeding	Stop warfarin; restart when INR is <5
<6 but >0.5 units above target value	No bleeding	Reduce dose or stop warfarin; restart when INR is <5

* Full reversal of anticoagulation in a patient with a mechanical prosthetic heart valve carries a risk of valve thrombosis: discuss management with a haematologist.

† If there is unexpected bleeding at therapeutic INR, a structural lesion (e.g. carcinoma of bladder or large bowel) must be excluded.

Anticoagulation

51 Sickle cell crisis

• The most common manifestation of sickle cell disease in adults is a vaso-occlusive crisis with infarction of bone marrow.

• Suspect a vaso-occlusive crisis in any black, Arabic, Indian or Mediterranean patient with acute pain in the spine, abdomen, chest or joints. Most patients with sickle cell disease will know their diagnosis.

• Pain can be severe and requires adequate doses of analgesic, which vary between individuals. Ask patients which analgesic they usually have for crises, and at what dose.

Priorities

1 Make a working diagnosis from
• the sickle solubility test and blood film;
• the presence of a likely precipitant (infection, dehydration, strenuous exercise, exposure to cold and psychological stress);
• the exclusion of other causes where possible.

2 Relieve pain
• Discuss the patient's previous requirement for analgesics and how much has been taken in the past 24 h.

• If the pain is severe, give **morphine** 5–25 mg IM at 2–4-hly intervals or by continuous SC or IV infusion: give a loading dose of 10 mg SC (5 mg if < 50 kg), followed by an infusion of 150 µg/kg/h; or **diamorphine** 5–25 mg SC at 2–4-hly intervals; or **pethidine** 50–150 mg IM at 2–4-hly intervals if morphine or diamorphine are not tolerated.

• A non-steroidal anti-inflammatory agent can be used for mild pain and should be given to all patients with bone or joint crisis unless contraindicated (renal failure, peptic ulceration).

3 Give humidified oxygen

Give humidified oxygen at 4–6 L/min if oxygen saturation is <92%. Keep the patient warm.

4 Has the crisis been precipitated by infection?

Assess the patient for evidence of infection. Investigations required urgently are given in Table 51.1.

• Fever usually <37.5°C may occur without infection (reflecting tissue necrosis). Suspect infection if the temperature is >37.5°C.

• Adults with sickle cell disease are effectively splenectomized and thus at particular risk of infection with capsulate bacteria: pneumococcus, meningococcus and *H. influenzae* type B.

Table 51.1 Urgent investigation of suspected vaso-occlusive crisis of sickle cell disease

---

Steady-state haemoglobin and haemoglobin electrophoresis (from clinic card if diagnosis established)

Full blood count, reticulocyte count and film*

Sickle solubility test† (Hb electrophoresis as soon as practicable)

Blood culture (x2)

Urine microscopy and culture

Chest X-ray

Creatinine, sodium and potassium

Blood group and antibody screen

Oxygen saturation by pulse oximetry

Arterial blood gases (if oxygen saturation < 90%, chest X-ray shadowing or respiratory symptoms)

---

* Blood film in sickle cell disease (homozygous SS): normochromic normocytic anaemia; raised reticulocyte count; in adults, Howell–Jolly bodies (reflecting hyposplenism), usually sickle cells. Numerous target cells indicate Hb SC.

† Sickle solubility test indicates the presence of HbS, and is therefore positive in both homozygotes (SS) and heterozygotes (AS—sickle cell trait) and also double heterozygotes (S beta Thal, SC).

• Suspect salmonella gastroenteritis if there is diarrhoea and vomiting
• Antibiotic therapy should be started after taking blood for culture. If there is no clinical focus of infection, give coamoxiclav.

5 Is there chest involvement?

This carries a relatively high mortality and is shown by pleuritic chest pain with X-ray shadowing. It is impossible to distinguish vaso-occlusive infarction from pneumonia with certainty and you should assume that both are present.

• Give oxygen 28–60% by mask and monitor oxygen saturation by pulse oximetry, aiming to maintain $Sao_2 > 90\%$. Recheck arterial gases after 4 h or if deterioration occurs.

• Discuss with a haematologist. Ventilation and exchange transfusion are needed if Pao_2 cannot be maintained above 9 kPa (70 mmHg) with 60% oxygen by mask.

• Start antibiotic therapy (see p. 211).

6 Is there neurological involvement?

This is an indication for exchange transfusion (Table 51.2). Seek advice from a haematologist.

7 Is there priapism?

• Priapism presents with groin pain and painful penile erection. If not adequately treated, it may result in permanent erectile failure.
• Give etilefrine 100 mg PO.

Table 51.2 Indications for exchange transfusion in complications of sickle cell disease

Neurological involvement: stroke, transient ischaemic attack or fits
Lung involvement ($Pao_2 < 9$ kPa with Fio_2 60%)
Rapidly falling haemoglobin
Priapism

• Contact a urologist to give intracavernous infusion of etilefrine 6–10 mg (repeated after 1 h if no response).
• If there is no response after 24 h of etilefrine therapy, consider exchange transfusion. The results are variable.
• Continue etilefrine 50 mg nocte for the prevention of recurrent priapism.

Further management

1 Titration of analgesia
• Increments in morphine or diamorphine of 2–5 mg every 2 h can be given titrated against the emergence of breakthrough pain.
• Pethidine increments should not exceed 10 mg and the maximum dose must be 150 mg in 2 h. Pethidine metabolites may cause major seizures.
• Monitor conscious level, respiratory rate and oxygen saturation by pulse oximetry.
• Give an oral laxative, antiemetic and antipruritic.

2 Fluid intake
• Ensure a fluid intake of $3 L/m^2$ body surface area/day (see p. 436) for calculation of BSA from height and weight).
• Unless symptoms are very mild, start with an IV infusion of dextrose saline.

3 Monitor haemoglobin
• Check the full blood count daily: discuss management with a haematologist if the haemoglobin is falling or reticulocytes are absent (which may indicate an aplastic or sequestration crisis).
• Do not transfuse without discussion with a haematologist.

4 Reducing analgesia
• Reduce doses in the same steps required when titrating upwards.
• Introduce oral analgesics as soon as possible, at least 48 h before discharge and typically when the parenteral doses fall to the following thresholds: morphine or diamorphine 5 mg, pethidine 75 mg. Analgesic conversions are given in Table 51.3.

Table 51.3 Approximate analgesic conversions

Analgesic	Conversion (mg/mg) to morphine tablets (Sevredol)
Morphine or diamorphine SC	1 : 2
Pethidine IM	2 : 1

Problems

Vaso-occlusive crisis or acute abdomen?

• There is no clear distinction and the patient should be assessed jointly with the surgical team (Chapter 36).

• It is usually reasonable to delay surgery longer than usual and to proceed if deterioration occurs despite treatment directed at vaso-occlusive crisis.

Sickle crises causing increased anaemia

These are much less common than vaso-occlusive crises:

• Sequestration crisis (in the sinuses of the enlarged spleen in children).

• Aplastic crisis (reduced marrow erythropoiesis, e.g. after parvovirus infection).

• Increased haemolysis crisis (following infections).

The clue is the rapid fall in haemoglobin. These crises must be recognized early because transfusion can be life-saving. Seek advice from a haematologist.

52 Anaphylaxis and anaphylactic shock

Suspect anaphylaxis if, after an IV or IM injection, insect sting or exposure to a potential allergen, the patient develops:

- skin and mucosal urticaria, erythema and angio-oedema;
- wheeze and breathlessness;
- tachycardia and hypotension.

  Causes of anaphylactic reaction are given in Table 52.1.

Priorities

Severe anaphylactic reaction (anaphylactic shock)

1 Give oxygen 60–100%, put in an IV cannula, check the BP and attach an ECG monitor. Lay the patient flat and raise the foot of the bed.

- **If there is respiratory distress, call an anaesthetist**. This may be due to upper airways obstruction from oedema of the larynx or epiglottis, and may require endotracheal intubation or emergency tracheotomy.

- **If cardiac arrest appears imminent,** give adrenaline 0.5 mg (5 mL of 1 in 10 000 solution) by slow IV injection over 5 min, stopping if the patient's condition improves.

- For other patients, give **adrenaline 0.5–1 mg (0.5–1 mL of 1 in 1000 solution) IM.**

- Start an IV infusion of colloid IV, 500 mL over 15 min

- If there is bronchospasm, give nebulized salbutamol. IV aminophylline (p. 195) can be added if needed.

2 Give chlorpheniramine 10–20 mg IV over 1 min and hydrocortisone 300 mg IV.

3 If systolic BP remains <100 mmHg:

- Arrange transfer to the ITU.
- Give adrenaline 0.5–1 mg (0.5–1 mL of 1 in 1000 solution) IM every 10 min.

Table 52.1 Causes of anaphylactic and anaphylactoid reaction*

Drugs
Antibiotics, most commonly beta-lactam class
Radiographic contrast media
Parenteral iron
Streptokinase
Neuromuscular blocking agents
Thiopentone
Vitamin K

Blood products

Allergen extracts

Bee and wasp stings

* Anaphylactic and anaphylactoid reactions to drugs are clinically indistinguishable. Anaphylactoid reactions are due to direct triggering of the release of mediators by the drug itself and may therefore occur after the first dose.

• Continue IV colloid infusion, giving a further 500 mL over 30 min. When the patient's condition is stable, put in a CVP line to guide fluid management.

• If multiple doses of adrenaline are needed, consider starting an infusion (which must be given via a central line) (p. 480).

• If the patient has been taking a non-cardioselective beta-blocker and is resistant to adrenaline, give glucagon (50 µg/kg by IV bolus followed by an infusion of 1–5 mg/h) or salbutamol by IV infusion (p. 195).

Further management

1 Admit to hospital for 24 h as relapses can occur.
2 Give hydrocortisone 300 mg 6-hly IV for 2–4 doses and chlorpheniramine 8 mg 8-hly PO for 24–48 h.

3 Inform the patient of the drug responsible for the reaction.
  • A bracelet engraved with this information may be obtained from Medic-Alert Foundation International; telephone enquiries 0800 581420).
  • Patients at high risk of anaphylaxis should carry adrenaline for self-injection in the event of further exposure to allergen. Consult the *British National Formulary* for a suitable device.

4 If anaphylaxis was due to a drug, report the reaction to the Committee on Safety of Medicines (see the *Adverse reactions to drugs* section of the *British National Formulary*).

5 Specific allergen immunotherapy (desensitization) is indicated in the case of severe anaphylactic reaction to bee or wasp stings: seek advice from a clinical immunologist.

Minor anaphylactic reaction

Give chlorpheniramine 10 mg IV (repeated only if symptoms recur).

Section 3
Procedures

53 Central vein cannulation

Central vein cannulation has many potential complications (Table 53.1): give careful consideration to the need for the procedure and the choice of vein.

Indications

1 Measurement of central venous pressure (CVP):
  - transfusion of large volumes of fluid required;
  - fluid challenge in patients with oliguria or hypotension;
  - to exclude hypovolaemia when the clinical evidence is equivocal.
2 Insertion of a pulmonary artery (Swan–Ganz) catheter or temporary pacing wire.
3 Administration of some drugs (e.g. dopamine) and IV feeding solutions.
4 No suitable peripheral veins for IV infusion.

Technique

Choosing the approach
- See Table 53.2. The right internal jugular and right subclavian are the two most commonly used veins. The right internal jugular vein is preferable to the left as it is contralateral to the thoracic duct and the circulation of the dominant cerebral hemisphere.
- **Cannulation of the internal jugular vein** is generally associated with fewer complications than with the subclavian vein, and **is the preferred approach in patients with bleeding tendency** (platelet count $< 100 \times 10^{12}/L$ or prothrombin time $> 1.5 \times$ control (because of the risk of uncontrollable bleeding from inadvertent puncture of the subclavian

419

Table 53.1 Complications of central vein cannulation

During placement
Arterial puncture or laceration
Pneumothorax (via internal jugular or subclavian vein) or tension pneumothorax
Haemothorax
Cardiac tamponade (can be caused by central venous line introduced by any route, if its tip lies below the pericardial reflection and it perforates the vessel wall; least likely via internal jugular vein)
Injury to adjacent nerves
Air embolism

After placement
Infection: local infection and/or bacteraemia
Venous thrombosis

Table 53.2 Choice of route for central vein cannulation

Vein	Comment
Internal jugular	Use in preference to the subclavian vein if there is bleeding tendency or respiratory compromise
Subclavian	Overall complication rate higher than via internal jugular vein
Femoral	Safe route if rapid access required. Use for placing pacing wire if access via internal jugular or subclavian veins is not possible. Can be used (with caution) after thrombolytic therapy if access via antecubital fossa vein not possible. Drawbacks are increased risk of infection and venous thrombosis
Antecubital fossa vein	Use if thrombolytic therapy has been given. Often difficult to place pacing wire via this route

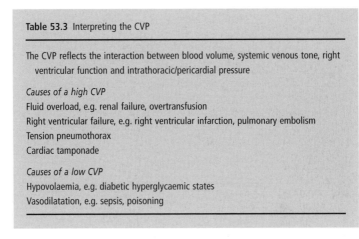

Table 53.3 Interpreting the CVP

The CVP reflects the interaction between blood volume, systemic venous tone, right ventricular function and intrathoracic/pericardial pressure

Causes of a high CVP
Fluid overload, e.g. renal failure, overtransfusion
Right ventricular failure, e.g. right ventricular infarction, pulmonary embolism
Tension pneumothorax
Cardiac tamponade

Causes of a low CVP
Hypovolaemia, e.g. diabetic hyperglycaemic states
Vasodilatation, e.g. sepsis, poisoning

Central vein cannulation

artery) **or respiratory disease** (because of the greater risk of pneumothorax with subclavian access).

• The femoral vein is a safe route if rapid access is required (e.g. for placement of temporary pacing wire in a haemodynamically unstable patient). Its drawbacks are an increased risk of infection and venous thrombosis.

• An antecubital fossa vein can be used to place a central line for infusions, but manipulation of a pacing wire or pulmonary artery catheter via this route can be very difficult.

• Consider using **ultrasound** to locate the internal jugular or subclavian veins before venepuncture if previous access has been difficult or the patient is at risk of complications (e.g. bleeding disorder).

Venepuncture
Internal jugular vein puncture—high approach reducing the risk of pneumothorax (Fig. 53.2)

1 Remove the pillow and position the patient with head-down tilt of the bed if possible (to fill out the vein and reduce the risk of air embolism in hypovolaemic patients).

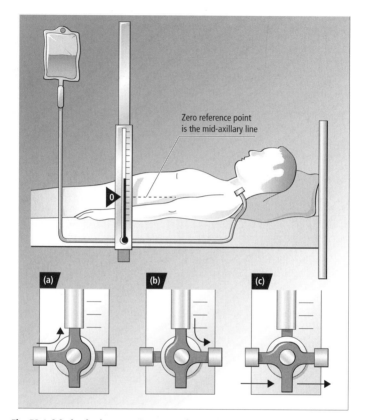

Fig. 53.1 Method of measuring central venous pressure: CVP line with position of three-way tap for: a, priming the manometer; b, measuring CVP; c, fluid infusion. Redrawn from Davidson TI. *Fluid Balance*. Oxford: Blackwell Scientific Publications 1987; 38.

2 Turn the patient's head to the left. Locate the right carotid artery. The internal jugular vein is superficial, lateral and parallel to the artery.
3 Prepare and drape the skin.
4 Infiltrate the skin and subcutaneous tissues over the anterior edge

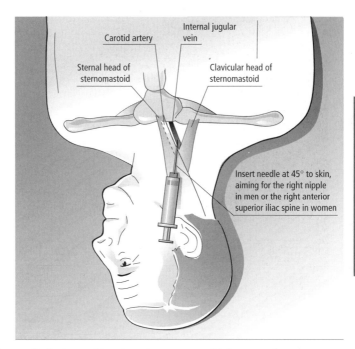

Fig. 53.2 Right internal jugular vein puncture—high approach.

of the sternocleidomastoid muscle at the level of the thyroid cartilage with 5 mL of lignocaine 1%.

5 Nick the skin over the vein with a small scalpel blade.

6 Identify the line of the carotid artery with your left hand. Insert the needle just lateral to this at an angle of 45° to the skin, aiming for the right nipple in men or the right anterior superior iliac spine in women (Fig. 53.2). Advance slowly whilst aspirating for blood. The vein lies superficially so do not advance more than a few centimetres.

7 If you do not hit the vein, slowly withdraw the needle to just under the skin, aspirating for blood as you do so (as you may have inadvertently transfixed the vein). Advance again, aiming slightly more medially.

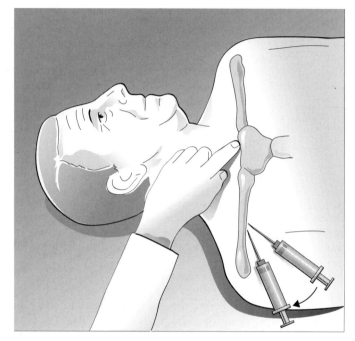

Fig. 53.3 Right subclavian vein puncture—infraclavicular approach.

Right subclavian vein puncture: infraclavicular approach (Fig. 53.3)

1 Remove the pillow and position the patient with head-down tilt of the bed if possible (to fill out the vein and reduce the risk of air embolism in hypovolaemic patients).

2 Define the suprasternal notch, the sternoclavicular joint and the acromioclavicular joint.

3 Prepare and drape the skin.

4 Infiltrate the skin and subcutaneous tissues with 5–10 mL of lignocaine 1%, starting from a point one finger's breadth below the junction of the medial one-third and lateral two-thirds of the clavicle. Infiltrate up to and just below the clavicle.

5 Nick the skin with a small scalpel blade.

6 Advance the needle along the same track until it touches the clavicle. Move the tip stepwise down the clavicle until it is lying just below it. Then swing the needle round so that it it now pointing just above the suprasternal notch. Slowly advance the needle whilst aspirating for blood. Make a conscious effort to keep the track of the needle parallel to the bed (to avoid puncturing the subclavian artery or pleura).

7 If the vein is not found, withdraw slowly whilst aspirating. Flush the needle to make sure it is not blocked. Try again, aiming slightly more cranially.

Right femoral vein puncture (Fig. 53.4)

1 Place the patient in a supine position. The leg should be slightly abducted and externally rotated. Identify the femoral artery below the inguinal ligament: the femoral vein lies medially.

2 If time allows, shave the groin. Prepare and drape the skin.

3 Infiltrate the skin and subcutaneous tissues with 5–10 mL of lignocaine 1%.

4 Nick the skin with a small scalpel blade.

5 Place two fingers of your left hand on the femoral artery to define its position. Holding the syringe in your right hand, place the tip of the needle at the entry site on the skin. Move the syringe slightly laterally, and advance the needle at an angle of around 30° to the skin whilst aspirating for blood. The vein is usually reached 2–4 cm from the skin surface.

6 If the vein is not found, withdraw slowly whilst aspirating. Flush the needle to make sure it is not blocked. Try again, aiming slightly to the left or right of your initial pass.

Placement of the cannula using a guidewire-through-needle technique (Seldinger technique)

1 Once you have punctured the vein, check that you can aspirate blood easily.

2 Remove the syringe, capping the needle with your finger to prevent entry of air.

3 Pass the flexible end of the guidewire down the needle. If there is any resistance to the passage of the wire, withdraw it and check you are still in the vein by aspirating blood. Change the angle of the needle or rotate the bevel. If there is still resistance, but you are

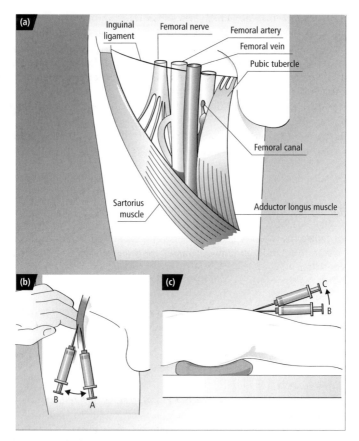

Fig. 53.4 Right femoral vein puncture: (a) anatomy of the femoral vein; (b) and (c) technique. From Rosen M *et al. Handbook of Percutaneous Central Venous Catheterization.* 2nd edn. London: WB Saunders, 1993.

confident the needle is in the vein, try a new wire with a flexible J shaped end.

4 When half the length of the wire is in the vein, remove the needle. Place the cannula and dilator over the wire and advance it into position.

- A cannula inserted via the subclavian vein sometimes passes into the internal jugular vein rather than the SVC. This can be checked for by aspirating 5 mL of blood and then injecting it swiftly whilst a colleague listens with the diaphragm of a stethoscope over the ipsilateral internal jugular vein. A bruit signifies misplacement.

5 Attach the infusion set.

6 Fix the cannula to the skin with a suture or a transparent adhesive dressing.

7 If the cannula has been placed via the internal jugular or subclavian veins, a chest X-ray should be taken to confirm correct positioning and absence of pneumothorax.

Troubleshooting

Arterial puncture
If you inadvertently puncture the artery, apply pressure for 5 min and then reattempt venepuncture.

Pneumothorax
- If the patient is being mechanically ventilated, this may become a tension pneumothorax and you must insert a chest drain even if it is small (see p. 455).
- For management of pneumothorax in patients who are not ventilated, see p. 217.

Misplacement of a cannula inserted via the subclavian vein in the internal jugular vein
The cannula must be repositioned. Infusion of hypertonic solutions into the internal jugular vein may cause venous thrombosis.

Frequent ventricular extrasystoles or ventricular tachycardia
May indicate that the tip of the cannula is lying against the tricuspid valve. Withdraw the cannula a few centimetres.

Line infection
Staphylococcus aureus and *epidermidis* are the most common pathogens, but infection with Gram-negative rods and fungi may occur in immunocompromised patients.

Obviously infected line

Diagnosed if there is tenderness, erythema and purulent discharge at the skin exit site.

• The cannula must be removed and the tip sent for culture.

• If the patient is febrile, take blood cultures and start antibiotic therapy. Initial treatment should be with IV gentamicin plus flu-cloxacillin (or vancomycin if penicillin allergic or suspected MRSA). If cultures show *Staph. aureus* sepsis with bacteraemia, IV antistaphylo-coccal therapy should be given for 2 weeks. For *Staph. epidermidis* and Gram-negative sepsis, give IV therapy until the patient has been afebrile for 24–48 h. For *Pseudomonas* sepsis, give IV therapy for 7 –10 days.

Possibly infected line

Diagnosed if there is fever or other systemic signs of sepsis, but no signs at the skin exit site.

• Take blood cultures from both a peripheral vein and via the cannula.

• The decision to remove the cannula before culture results are back depends on the likelihood of it being infected, how long the cannula has been in and if there is another source of infection possible.

• If both blood cultures grow the same organism, the cannula must be removed and antibiotic therapy given as above.

54 Pulmonary artery catheterization

• Remember that pulmonary artery catheterization is diagnostic and not therapeutic: make sure that the patient is adequately resuscitated and receives appropriate treatment while the catheter is being placed.
• Data derived from pulmonary artery catheterization may be misleading because of errors in measurement and artefact, and you should not let it replace clinical assessment.

Indications

1 **Pulmonary oedema:**
   • to titrate further therapy if the patient is not improving with initial management (p. 167);
   • to differentiate acute respiratory distress syndrome (ARDS) from cardiogenic pulmonary oedema (p. 168).
2 **Hypotension** despite a central venous pressure of 10 cm water or more (i.e. not due to hypovolaemia):
   • to titrate further therapy with fluids and inotropic–vasopressor agents (p. 41).
3 **Suspected ventricular septal rupture after myocardial infarction** (p. 147) only if echocardiography is not available.

Technique

Preparation
1 Set up the equipment (Fig. 54.1).
2 The pressure transducer must be zeroed and calibrated. The reference point for zero is usually taken at the fourth intercostal space in the mid-axillary line, with the patient supine.

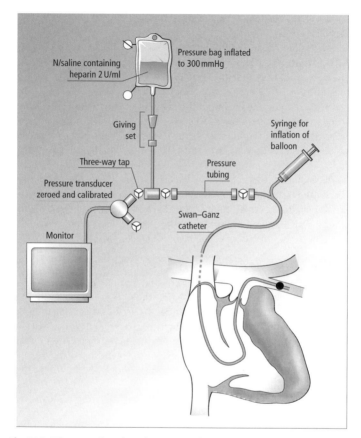

Fig. 54.1 Diagram showing the set-up of equipment for pulmonary artery catheterization. When the balloon is inflated, flow around the tip of the catheter ceases. The measured pressure is transmitted back from the pulmonary veins (as these are valveless) and gives an estimate of left atrial and left ventricular end-diastolic pressures.

3 Connect the patient to an ECG monitor and put in a peripheral venous cannula.

4 Prepare the skin and apply drapes as for temporary cardiac pacing.

5 Check that the catheter can pass down the cannula, and check the balloon by inflating it with air (usually 1.5 mL). Leave the syringe attached.

6 Attach the manometer line to the channel of the distal (pulmonary artery) lumen and flush the dead space. If the catheter also has a proximal (right atrial) lumen, flush this channel with heparinized saline and leave the syringe attached.

Cannulating a central vein

See Chapter 53. The internal jugular vein is the preferred route of access, as the risk of pneumothorax and arterial puncture is lower than with subclavian vein access. It is more difficult to manipulate the catheter into the pulmonary artery with femoral vein access.

Placement of the catheter

1 Insert the catheter for about 10 cm and inflate the balloon fully. Advance it guided by X-ray screening, or the pressure waveform (Fig. 54.2) and the distance inserted (Table 54.1).

• Do not advance more than 10–15 cm unless the waveform changes because of the risk of knotting.

• Always deflate the balloon before withdrawing the catheter to prevent it tearing the tricuspid or pulmonary valves.

Table 54.1 Expected distance (cm) from point of insertion via right internal jugular vein in the adult

Location	Distance (cm)
Right atrium	10–15
Right ventricle	25–35
Pulmonary artery	35–40
Wedge position	40–50

Catheterization

Catheterization

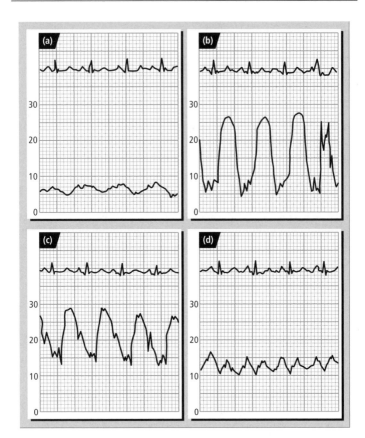

Fig. 54.2 Diagram showing the typical pressure waveforms (mmHg) on insertion of a pulmonary artery catheter: (a) right atrium; (b) right ventricle; (c) pulmonary artery; (d) wedge position.

• Ventricular extrasystoles and non-sustained ventricular tachycardia are common during manipulation of the catheter through the right heart and do not need treatment.
• Passage across the tricuspid valve can sometimes be helped by the patient taking a deep inspiration.

2 When the waveform changes from pulmonary artery to wedge, deflate the balloon. The trace should promptly change back to pulmonary artery.

Measuring the wedge pressure
• Move the catheter to find a position where the wedge pressure is reliably obtained with the balloon fully or near-fully inflated. The volume needed should be noted. If this is less than 1.3 mL, the catheter tip is too peripheral: withdraw it a little.
• Criteria of a satisfactory wedge position are given in Table 54.2.
• The wedge pressure fluctuates with respiration and should be measured at end-expiration when pleural pressure is around zero. Large swings in pleural pressure occur in patients with severe airways obstruction, which can make interpretation of the wedge pressure trace difficult or impossible.
• Avoid keeping the balloon inflated in the wedge position for more than 15 s (to minimize the risk of pulmonary artery rupture).

Catheterization

Table 54.2 Criteria of a satisfactory wedge position

1 The mean wedge pressure:
   is lower than or equal to the PA diastolic pressure
   is lower than the mean PA pressure

2 The waveform is characteristic of the left atrial waveform
   (see Fig. 54.2)

3 The wedge waveform promptly:
   disappears on deflation of the balloon
   reappears on reinflation

4 The balloon has to be inflated to its maximum volume (or close to this) to obtain
   the wedge pressure

5 Blood aspirated from the wedge position has an oxygen saturation of > 95%

Aftercare
• Obtain a chest X-ray to check the position of the catheter.
• The catheter should be fast-flushed hourly to prevent thrombus formation at the tip.
• Remove the catheter within 72 h to reduce the risk of infection. If needed, a new catheter can be put in, preferably at a different site.
• If infection related to the catheter is suspected: see p. 427.

| Troubleshooting |

The catheter will not enter the pulmonary artery
• This can be a problem in patients with low cardiac output, tricuspid regurgitation or a dilated right heart.
• If you cannot advance the catheter despite screening, use a guidewire to stiffen it. Disconnect the catheter from the manometer line and pass the guidewire down the distal channel.

Damping of the pressure trace
This may be due to kinking of the catheter or manometer line; air bubbles in the system; or thrombus partially occluding the lumen of the catheter: several fast flushes should clear this.

Problems with measuring the wedge pressure
No change in waveform when you inflate the balloon
• If there is no resistance to inflation, suspect balloon rupture.
• If there is normal resistance, the catheter has slipped back. If the catheter outside the skin has not been kept sterile with a sheath, a new catheter should be inserted.

Ramp increase in pressure when you inflate the balloon
• This indicates that the balloon has inflated eccentrically with occlusion of the tip ('over-wedging'). The ramp increase in pressure reflects the continuous flush infusion.
• Deflate the balloon and reinflate it until a satisfactory trace is obtained.

Catheterization

Tachypnoeic patient
• End-expiration is brief in a patient with rapid respiration and, as the monitor averages values obtained over several seconds, the digital display of the wedge pressure is misleading.
• The solution is to print out the pressure trace, marking end-expiration (most chart recorders will have an event marker), and measure the pressure from this.

Spontaneous wedging
• This indicates that the catheter is positioned too peripherally. Some migration peripherally commonly occurs after insertion as the catheter warms and becomes more flexible.

Catheterization

Table 54.3 Pressure measurements: normal values

Site*	Pressure (mmHg)
Central vein or right atrium	Mean 0–8
Right ventricle	Systolic 15–30
	Diastolic 0–8
Pulmonary artery (PA)	Systolic 15–30
	Diastolic 3–12†
	Mean 9–16
PA wedge pressure‡	Mean 1–10

* The reference point for zero is taken at the fourth intercostal space in the mid-axillary line (the level of the tricuspid valve), with the patient lying flat.

† Pressures in the low-resistance pulmonary circulation normally equilibrate at end-diastole, and so the pulmonary artery diastolic pressure can substitute for the wedge pressure, providing: (a) the heart rate is less than 120/min; (b) pulmonary hypertension is not present (PA systolic < 30 mmHg, PA mean < 20 mmHg).

‡ PA wedge pressure is measured at end-expiration, when pleural pressure is around zero and the intravascular pressure is closest to the physiologically relevant transmural pressure.

Catheterization

Table 54.4 Derived variables

Variable	Formula	Normal range	Units
Body surface area	$\sqrt{\text{Height (inches)} \times \text{Weight (lb)}/3131}$; or $\sqrt{\text{Height (cm)} \times \text{Weight (kg)}/3600}$	—	m^2
Cardiac index	$CI = CO/BSA$	2.5–4.2	$L/min/m^2$
Systemic vascular resistance	$[(MAP - RAP)/CO \times 80]$	770–1500	$dyne.s/cm^5$
Pulmonary vascular resistance	$[(MPAP - MPAWP)/CO \times 80]$	25–125	$dyne.s/cm^5$
Arterial oxygen transport (Do_2)	$[0.134 \times CO \times Hba \times Sao_2]$	950–1300	ml/min
Systemic oxygen consumption (Vo_2)	$[0.134 \times CO \times (Hba \times Sao_2 - Hbv \times Svo_2)]$	180–320	ml/min
Alveolar–arterial oxygen gradient $(A - aDo_2)$ (see p. 360)	$Fio_2 \times 94.8 - (Pao_2 + Paco_2)$	<3	kPa

BSA, Body surface area; CI, cardiac index; CO, cardiac output (L/min); Fio_2, fractional concentration of oxygen in inspired gas; Hba, haemoglobin concentration of arterial blood (g/dL); Hbv, haemoglobin concentration of venous blood (g/dL); MAP, mean systemic arterial pressure; MPAWP, mean pulmonary artery wedge pressure; MRAP, mean right atrial pressure; Sao_2, oxygen saturation of systemic arterial blood (%); Svo_2, oxygen saturation of mixed venous blood (%).

References: Barry WH, Grossman W. Range of normal resting hemodynamic values. In: Braunwald E, ed. *Heart Disease: A Textbook of Cardiovascular Medicine*, 2nd edn. Philadelphia: WB Saunders, 1984. Mosteller RD. Simplified calculation of body surface area. *New England Journal of Medicine* 1987; **317**: 1098.

• Pull the catheter back until you find a position at which the balloon has to be fully or near-fully inflated to give a wedge pressure.

Special considerations

Suspected ventricular septal rupture
• Prepare four heparinized 2 mL syringes ready for sampling, with blind hubs and ice if the samples will have to be transported to the laboratory.
• Take samples in the right atrium, right ventricle and pulmonary artery and from a systemic artery.
• A step-up in oxygen saturation of > 10% between right atrium and right ventricle indicates a left to right shunt at ventricular level.
• The size of the shunt is given by the ratio of pulmonary to systemic flow ($Q_P : Q_S$), calculated as follows:

$Q_P : Q_S = (Art - RA)/(Art - PA)$, where Art is systemic arterial oxygen saturation (So_2), RA is right atrial So_2, and PA is pulmonary arterial So_2.

Left bundle branch block
• Complete heart block is a rare and usually transient complication because the catheter may induce additional right bundle block as it passes through the right heart.
• Put in the catheter under screening, with a temporary pacing wire to hand in case this is needed.

Catheterization

55 Temporary cardiac pacing

Indications

These are given in Table 55.1.

Technique

Preparation
1 Check the screening equipment and make sure a defibrillator and other resuscitation equipment are to hand.
2 Connect an ECG monitor and put in a peripheral venous cannula. Make sure the ECG leads are off the chest (so they are not confused with the pacing wire when screening).
3 Put on mask, gown and gloves. Prepare the skin and apply drapes to a wide area. If it is likely that permanent pacing will be needed, use the right side in right-handed patients.
4 Check that the wire will pass down the cannula. Temporary pacing wires are usually 5 or 6 French and require a cannula one size larger.

Cannulation of a central vein
See Chapter 53.
• The wire is usually easier to manipulate via the right internal jugular vein, but may be fixed more comfortably via the right subclavian vein.
• The femoral vein can be used if access via the internal jugular or subclavian veins is not possible.

Placement of the wire (Figs 55.1 & 55.2)
1 Advance the wire into the right atrium and direct it towards the apex of the right ventricle (just medial to the lateral border of the cardiac silhouette): it may cross the tricuspid valve easily.

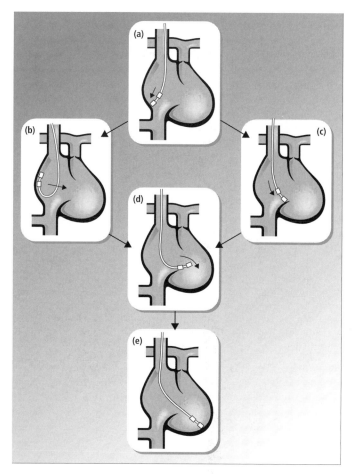

Fig. 55.1 Placement of a ventricular pacing wire from the superior vena cava (via internal jugular or subclavian veins). (a) Catheter advanced to the low right atrium. (b) Further advancement produces a loop or bend in the distal catheter, which is then rotated medially. (c) Alternatively, catheter in low right atrium deflects off tricuspid annulus directly into the right ventricle. (d) Superior orientation of the catheter tip in the ventricle requires clockwise torque during advancement to avoid the interventricular septum. (e) Final catheter position in the right apex. Catheter position in (b) is suitable for atrial pacing.

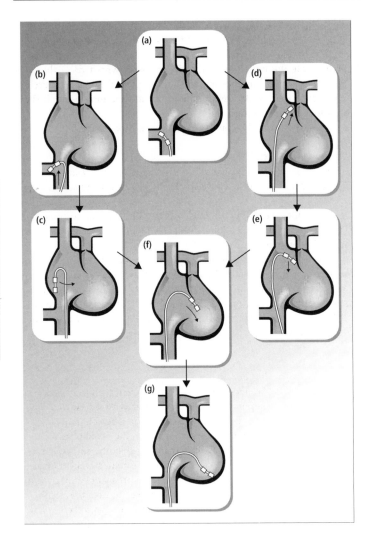

2 If you have difficulty, form a loop of wire in the right atrium. With slight rotation and advancement of the wire, the loop should prolapse across the tricuspid valve.

3 Manipulate the wire so that the tip curves downwards at the apex of the right ventricle and lies in a gentle S shape within the right atrium and ventricle (Fig. 55.3). Displacement of the wire may occur if there is too much or not enough slack.

4 Attach the wire to the connecting leads and pacing box.

Checking the threshold

1 Set the box to 'demand' mode with a pacing rate faster than the intrinsic heart rate. Set the output at 3 V. This should result in paced rhythm.

2 If it does not, you need to find a better position. Before moving from a position that may have taken a long while to achieve, make sure the problem is not due to loose connections: check these are all secure.

3 Progressively reduce the output until there is failure to capture: the heart rate drops abruptly and pacing spikes are seen but not followed by paced beats. A threshold of <1 V is ideal. A threshold a little above this is acceptable if it is stable and if the procedure has been difficult or if there is a large infarct or other factors expected to cause a high threshold (Table 55.2).

Temporary cardiac pacing

Fig. 55.2 (*Opposite.*) Placement of a ventricular pacing wire from the inferior vena cava (via femoral vein). (a) Catheter is advanced to the hepatic vein. (b) Catheter tip engages proximal hepatic vein and is advanced further. (c) A loop or bend is formed in the distal catheter, which is then rotated medially. (d) Alternatively, the catheter is advanced to the high medial right atrium. (e) With advancement, a bend is formed in the catheter, which is then quickly withdrawn or 'snapped' back to the level of the tricuspid orifice. (f) After crossing the tricuspid valve, the catheter is advanced with counterclockwise torque to avoid the interventricular septum. (g) Final catheter position in the right ventricular apex. Catheter positions in (c) and (d) can be used for atrial pacing. Figures 55.1 and 55.2 reproduced with permission from *Cardiac Pacing*. Ed. Ellenbogen KA. Boston: Blackwell Scientific Publications 1992; 178–9.

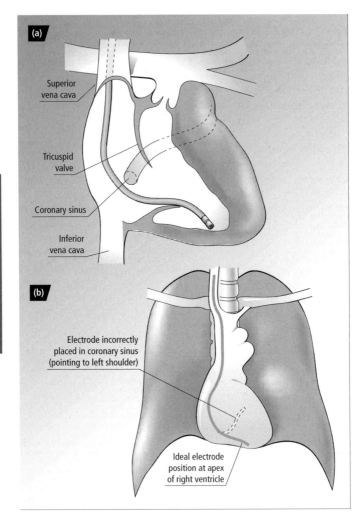

(a)

Superior
vena cava

Tricuspid
valve

Coronary sinus

Inferior
vena cava

(b)

Electrode incorrectly
placed in coronary sinus
(pointing to left shoulder)

Ideal electrode
position at apex
of right ventricle

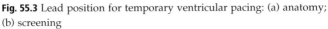

Fig. 55.3 Lead position for temporary ventricular pacing: (a) anatomy;
(b) screening

Table 55.1 Indications for temporary cardiac pacing

In acute myocardial infarction
Asystole
Complete heart block
Right bundle branch block with new left anterior hemiblock or left posterior hemiblock*
New left bundle branch block
Mobitz type II second degree AV block
Mobitz type I (Wenckebach) second degree AV block with hypotension not responsive to atropine
Sinus bradycardia with hypotension or recurrent sinus pauses not responsive to atropine
Atrial or ventricular overdrive pacing for incessant ventricular tachycardia

Unrelated to myocardial infarction
Sinus or junctional bradycardia associated with haemodynamic compromise and unresponsive to atropine
Second-degree AV block or sinus arrest if associated with syncope or near-syncope
Complete heart block associated with syncope or near-syncope, or ventricular rate < 40/min
Atrial or ventricular overdrive pacing for incessant ventricular tachycardia

Preoperative
Sinus node disease/second-degree Mobitz type I (Wenckebach) AV block/bundle branch block (including bifascicular block) only if history of syncope or pre-syncope
Second-degree Mobitz type II AV block
Complete heart block

*Left anterior hemiblock gives left axis deviation (S wave > R in lead II); left posterior hemiblock gives right axis deviation (S wave > R in lead I).

Temporary cardiac pacing

Table 55.2 Causes of failure to capture and/or sense

Wire malpositioned or displaced
Ventricular perforation
Myocardial fibrosis (from previous infarction or cardiomyopathy)
Drugs (Class I anti-arrhythmics)
Lead contacts not secure

4 Check the stability of the wire. Set the box at a rate faster than the intrinsic heart rate, with an output of 1 V. Ask the patient to cough forcefully, sniff and breathe deeply. Watch the monitor for loss of capture.

Placement of a flotation pacing wire without screening
1 Hold the electrode above the chest wall in the approximate shape in which it is expected to lie. Note the proximal marker which is level with the hub of the central cannula.
2 Check that the balloon inflates and deflates easily.
3 Insert the pacing wire with the balloon deflated. As soon as it is judged to be beyond the tip of the sheath, inflate the balloon. Insert to the previously noted marker then deflate the balloon.
4 Attach the pacing leads and box.
5 Check threshold as above.

Final points
1 Set the output at more than three times the threshold or 3 V, whichever is higher. Set the mode to 'demand'. If the patient is now in sinus rhythm at a rate >50/min, set a back-up rate of 50/min. If there is AV block or bradycardia, set at 70–80/min (90–100/min if there is cardiogenic shock).
2 Remove the insertion sheath to reduce the risk of lead displacement. Take care not to displace the lead as you do this. If there is any doubt about the stability of the position, leave the sheath in since this will make subsequent repositioning easier.

3 Suture the wire to the skin close to the point of insertion and cover it with a dressing. The rest of the wire should be looped and fixed to the skin with adhesive tape.

4 Obtain a chest X-ray to confirm a satisfactory position of the wire and exclude a pneumothorax.

Aftercare

1 Check the pacing threshold daily. The threshold usually rises to 2–3 × its initial value over the first few days after insertion.

2 If infection related to the wire is suspected: see p. 427).

Troubleshooting

Tachyarrhythmias

• Ventricular extrasystoles and non-sustained ventricular tachycardia are common as the wire crosses the tricuspid valve and do not require treatment.

• If non-sustained VT recurs, check that the position of the wire is still satisfactory and that excess slack has not formed in the area of the tricuspid valve.

Failure to capture and/or sense (Table 55.2)

• The threshold normally increases by a factor of about 2–3 after insertion because of endocardial oedema.

• The most common reason for failure to capture and/or sense is wire displacement.

• Check that the wire tip is pointing downwards at the apex of the right ventricle.

• A position in an epicardial vein looks similar to the correct one, but the wire may be seen more easily and tends to curve round at the apex.

• A wire misplaced in the coronary sinus points towards the left shoulder (Fig. 55.2).

• If a threshold <1 V cannot be found after trying alternative sites, accept a high threshold in a stable position.

Temporary cardiac pacing

Perforation

1 Suspect perforation with:
- failure to capture and/or sense;
- pericardial chest pain;
- diaphragmatic pacing at low output (3 V or less).

2 Are there signs of cardiac tamponade (p. 175)? If so, arrange urgent echocardiography and pericardial drainage.

3 Reposition or replace the wire.

56 Pericardial aspiration

Aspiration should only be attempted if the pericardial effusion is large (echo separation > 2 cm), to minimize the risk of complications (Table 56.1).

Indications

1 **Cardiac tamponade** (p. 175). Echocardiography must be done first to confirm the presence of a pericardial effusion unless there is cardiac arrest from presumed tamponade.
2 **Pericardial effusion due to suspected bacterial pericarditis** (p. 172).

Special equipment

1 Long needle (15 cm, 18 G) or long 'cannula over needle' intravenous cannula (e.g. Wallace).
2 Guidewire (80 cm or more, 0.035' diameter, with J end).
3 Dilator (5–7 French).
4 Pigtail catheter (60 cm long, 5–7 French diameter, multiple side-holes).
5 Drainage bag and connector.

Technique

Preparation
1 Arrange either X-ray or echocardiographic screening
2 Lay the patient semirecumbent in the screening room and propped up so the effusion pools anteriorly and inferiorly.

Table 56.1 Complications of pericardial aspiration

Vasovagal reaction
Penetration of a cardiac chamber (usually right ventricle) (may result in acute tamponade)
Laceration of a coronary artery (may result in acute tamponade)
Arrhythmia
Pneumothorax
Perforation of stomach or colon

- Connect an ECG monitor. Ensure you have venous access.
- Take blood for group and save.
- Ensure that resuscitation equipment including a defibrillator is to hand.
- Give sedation with midazolam (2 mg (elderly 1 mg) IV over 30 s, followed after 2 min by increments of 0.5–1 mg if sedation not adequate; usual range 2.5–7.5 mg).

3 Put on gown, mask and gloves. Prepare the skin from mid-chest to mid-abdomen and put on drapes.
4 Anaesthetize the skin and subcutaneous tissue overlying the angle between the xiphisternum and the left costal margin with a 25 G (orange) needle, and then use a 21 G (green) needle to infiltrate local anaesthetic along a track running from this point cranially (Fig. 56.1).
5 Make a small skin incision.

Insertion of the catheter

1 Attach the long needle or 'cannula over needle' to a 10-mL syringe containing lignocaine and advance it slowly along the anaesthetized track aiming for the suprasternal notch. Angle it at about 30° so that it passes just under the costal margin. Every centimetre or so, inject some lignocaine and aspirate.
2 As soon as fluid is aspirated, remove the syringe and introduce about 20 cm of the guidewire (if you are using a 'cannula over needle', the needle will have to be withdrawn first). See *Troubleshooting* if there is doubt as to whether the fluid is pericardial effusion or blood.

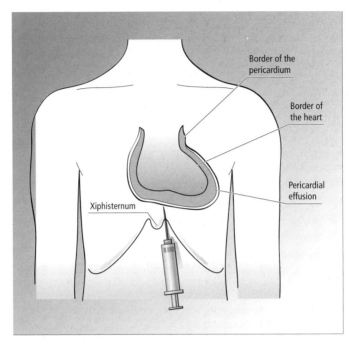

Fig. 56.1 Pericardial aspiration.

3 Check the position of the guidewire by screening. It should loop freely within the cardiac shadow.

4 Dilate the track.

5 Introduce the pigtail catheter over the guidewire. Keep the guidewire taut and, whilst screening, push the catheter through the pericardium and about 20 cm into the pericardial cavity. If a pigtail catheter is not available, fluid can be aspirated through the sheath of a large Seldinger-type central venous cannula.

6 Take specimens for microscopy, culture and cytology. Then aspirate to dryness and/or connect to drainage bag.

7 Insert a skin suture and loop it over the catheter several times, tying it each time. Attach the connector and drainage bag via a three-way tap. Fix securely with adhesive tape.

Pericardial aspiration

| Troubleshooting |

You cannot enter the effusion
• Check that the diagnosis is correct and that the effusion does not look solid or loculated.
• Consider the apical or left parasternal routes, but check first with echocardiography that there is sufficient fluid (>2cm separation or fluid) and no lung along the proposed needle track.

The pigtail catheter will not pass over the guidewire into the pericardial space
• Check that the guidewire is correctly positioned within the cardiac shadow.
• Check that the guidewire is held taut and not looped.
• Use a larger dilator.

You aspirate heavily bloodstained fluid
• The possibilities are: haemorrhagic effusion (common in malignancy or Dressler syndrome); venous puncture; right heart puncture; or laceration of a coronary artery with haemopericardium.
• Keep hold of the needle, but remove the syringe and empty into a clean pot. Blood will clot, but even heavily bloodstained effusion will not.
• Remove 5 mL more fluid and reinject whilst imaging using echocardiography. The cavity containing the needle tip will be marked by microbubbles.
• If you are still in doubt, compare the haematocrit of the fluid with that of a venous sample (both sent in EDTA tubes), or connect to a pressure monitor: right ventricular penetration is shown by a characteristic waveform (Fig. 54.2, p. 432).

Pericardial aspiration

57 DC cardioversion

Indications

Conversion of ventricular and supraventricular tachyarrhythmias.

Technique

Ventricular fibrillation or pulseless ventricular tachycardia:
Give immediate unsynchronized shock starting at 200 J (p. 4).

Other tachyarrhythmias
Preparation

1 Record a 12-lead ECG and check the arrhythmia. If you are not sure that cardioversion is indicated, discuss the case with a cardiologist.

• Fast atrial fibrillation in a patient with mitral valve disease or impaired myocardial function is unlikely to respond and is better treated by control of the ventricular rate (p. 27).

• Tachyarrhythmias caused by digoxin toxicity (p. 123) should be treated conservatively (nodal or atrial tachycardia) or initially with lignocaine (VT).

2 Preparation of the patient before DC cardioversion is summarized in Table 57.1. Put in a peripheral venous cannula, and check that resuscitation equipment and drugs are to hand.

3 Contact an anaesthetist. A brief general anaesthetic is preferable to sedation with a benzodiazepine.

4 Change the leads from the bedside to the defibrillator monitor. Adjust the leads until the R waves are significantly higher than the T waves and check that the synchronizing marker falls consistently on the QRS complex and not the T wave.

Table 57.1 Checklist before elective DC cardioversion of atrial flutter or fibrillation

Nil by mouth
For at least 4 h before the procedure

Anticoagulation
Anticoagulation is not mandatory for atrial fibrillation or flutter reliably known to be
of less than 2 days' duration in the absence of structural heart disease, but it is
advisable to give aspirin 300 mg daily PO, and low-molecular-weight heparin
before and for 24 h after cardioversion
If the patient has been in atrial fibrillation or flutter for more than 2 days, ensure
that warfarin anticoagulation has been given for at least 3 weeks, with INR
consistently > 2.0. Check that the current INR is >2.0

Plasma potassium
Check that this is > 3.5 mmol/L

Plasma digoxin
Check that there are no features to suggest toxicity (nausea, xanthopsia, slow AF,
frequent ventricular extrasystoles) and that, if the dose is high
(> 0.25 mg/day), renal function is normal

Thyroid function
In patients with atrial fibrillation, check that thyroid function is normal:
cardioversion of atrial fibrillation due to thyrotoxicosis (which may be otherwise
occult) is unlikely to be successful

Suspected brady–tachy syndrome
Consider inserting a temporary pacing wire because asystole or severe bradycardia
may complicate DC cardioversion

Transoesophageal echocardiography*
Atrial fibrillation or flutter of < 2 days' duration associated with structural disease
of the heart in an unanticoagulated patient
Embolic event after previous cardioversion
Atrial thrombus shown on previous echocardiography

*NB: Thrombus forms after cardioversion so transoesophageal echocardiography is
not a substitute for anticoagulation in elective routine cases.

Table 57.2 Initial charge for DC cardioversion

	Initial charge	Mode
Ventricular fibrillation or pulseless ventricular tacycardia	200 J	Unsynchronized
Ventricular tachycardia	200 J	Synchronized
Atrial fibrillation	200 J	Synchronized
Atrial flutter	100 J	Synchronized
Other supraventricular arrhythmias	50–100 J	Synchronized
Digoxin toxicity possible	25 J	Synchronized

In synchronized mode, the machine will not discharge until it senses an R wave, to ensure that the shock is delivered during and not after the QRS complex.

Countershock

1 Place gel pads on the sternum and over the cardiac apex. Gel pads should be changed every 3 shocks, and strong pressure should be applied to the chest wall with the paddles to prevent the shock from arcing and to reduce transthoracic impedance.

2 Initial charges are given in Table 57.2.

• If digoxin toxicity is possible, use a low initial charge (25 J) and consider giving lignocaine 100 mg before the shock.

3 Make sure the procedure is done safely.

• The first shock should be charged either on the patient's chest or in the machine, and not in the air.

• The paddles should then be kept on the chest for subsequent shocks as required.

• If the defibrillator is charged but then not needed, it should be discharged with the paddles back in the machine.

• The operator should call to all staff that the defibrillator is being charged and again before delivering the shock, and should look to make sure that no one is in contact directly or indirectly with the patient before the shock is delivered.

DC cardioversion

4 If the first shock fails to convert the arrhythmia, double the charge or use the maximum charge (360 J).

Aftercare

1 Record a 12-lead ECG.

2 Consider prophylactic antiarrhythmic therapy to maintain sinus rhythm (see Chapter 2).

3 Continue warfarin anticoagulation for at least 3 weeks after successful cardioversion of atrial flutter or fibrillation of more than 48 h duration, as atrial mechanical activity may not recover for several days after reversion to sinus rhythm. If there is mitral stenosis, or a history of embolic stroke or transient ischaemic attack, anticoagulation should be permanent.

4 Apply hydrocortisone cream to avoid painful dermatitis.

DC cardioversion

58 Insertion of a chest drain

Drainage of a pneumothorax (see p. 217) or large pleural effusion causing dyspnoea.

Technique

Preparation

1 Check the position of the pneumothorax or effusion by examination and inspection of the chest X-ray. Make sure you have not misdiagnosed an emphysematous bulla (p. 217).

2 Assemble the underwater seal (Fig. 58.1) and check that the connections fit.

3 Choose an appropriate drain, e.g. 16–20 French for low-viscosity effusions, 20–24 French for pneumothorax, 28 French for haemopneumothorax.

4 Position the patient lying flat or semirecumbent with the hand resting behind the neck. Put in a venous cannula (in the event of a vasovagal reaction requiring therapy).

5 Identify the fifth interspace in the mid-axillary line (level with the nipple in a man and the root of the breast in a woman): this is the safest site of insertion. Mark the site with a ballpoint pen.

6 Put on a mask and sterile gloves. Prepare and drape the skin.

Insertion of the tube

1 Draw up 20 mL of lignocaine 1%. Infiltrate the skin with 2–3 mL using a 25G (orange) needle, then change to a 21 G (green) needle to infiltrate subcutaneous tissues. Advance the needle into the thorax until air (or effusion fluid) is aspirated, then withdraw slightly and

Insertion of a chest drain

455

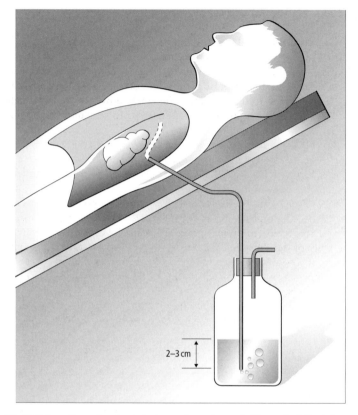

Fig. 58.1 Insertion of a chest drain: underwater seal. The end of the tube is 2–3 cm below the level of the water in the bottle. If intrapleural pressure rises above 2–3 cm water, air will bubble out. If intrapleural pressure becomes negative, water rises up the tube only to fall again when intrapleural pressure falls towards atmospheric. The system operates as a simple one-way valve. When the pneumothorax has resolved, the water level will generally be slightly negative throughout the respiratory cycle and reflect the normal fluctuation in intrapleural pressure, and when the patient coughs air will no longer bubble out. Redrawn from Brewis RAL. *Lecture Notes on Respiratory Disease*, 3rd edn. Oxford: Blackwell Scientific Publications, 1985; 290.

Insertion of a chest drain

infiltrate about 5 mL around the pleura, leaving a further 2–3 mL in the needle track as you withdraw.

• If you cannot freely obtain air or fluid, do not proceed further at this site, and ask advice from a senior colleague.

2 Make a 1–1.5 cm incision with a scalpel in line with and just above the edge of the lower rib of the intercostal space. Using a Spencer Wells or similar forceps, enlarge the track down to and through the pleura, wide enough for your little finger to pass into the pleural cavity.

3 Place two interrupted 3/0 silk sutures across the incision. These should be left loose so the tube can pass, and will be tied when the tube is removed. Place a 1/0 silk suture above the incision, which will be used to anchor the tube.

4 Take the tube off the trocar (which should not enter the thoracic cavity) and, holding the tip of the tube with the forceps, pass it into the pleural cavity. To drain a pneumothorax, direct the tube towards the apex of the thoracic cavity, until about 25 cm of drain is within the chest. The side-holes on the tube must be well within the chest or subcutaneous emphysema will result. To drain an effusion, direct the tube posterobasally.

5 Attach the underwater seal bottle.

6 Anchor the tube with the 1/0 silk suture wrapped and tied several times around the drain.

7 Place a pad of gauze between the skin and the tube, and tape the tube to the side of the chest.

Aftercare (see Fig. 58.2)

Note: The chest drain should not be clamped except if the underwater seal bottle is being changed or has to be elevated above the patient.

1 Obtain a chest X-ray after insertion of the drain to check the position of the tube and the size of the pneumothorax. If the lung has not re-expanded, apply 2.5 kPa suction to the outlet from the underwater seal bottle using a high-volume, low-pressure pump (e.g. Vernon Thompson pump).

2 Repeat the chest X-ray the following morning. If the lung is fully re-expanded, and the underwater seal bottle has stopped bubbling:

• stop suction;
• wait 24 h and then repeat the chest X-ray;
• if the lung remains fully re-expanded, and there is no bubbling in

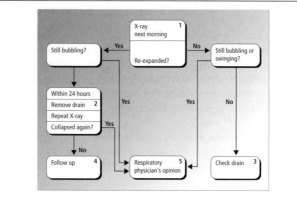

Explanatory notes

1   Chest X-ray If the underwater seal is *always* kept below the level of the chest, clamping is unnecessary and potentially dangerous. As far as possible, an X-ray film should be taken in the department, rather than on the ward with a portable machine; an expiration film is unnecessary.

2   Removal of chest drain Bubbling should have stopped for at least 24 hours. Since some patients find tube removal unpleasant, consider premedication. After removing the suture that holds the drain in place, withdraw the tube while the patient holds his or her breath in full inspiration. Use the two remaining sutures to seal the wound.

3   Check chest drain If the lung has not reinflated but there is no bubbling in the underwater bottle, then the tube is blocked or kinked—this can be corrected; or else the tube has become displaced—a replacement must be inserted through a clean incision.

4   Follow up Arrange for a chest clinic appointment in 7–10 days. The patient must be given a discharge letter and told to attend again immediately in the event of noticeable deterioration. Air travel should be avoided until changes seen on radiographs have resolved.

5   Respiratory physician's opinion Should advice from a specialist be required, transfer of continuing care is advisable. Important considerations in management are:
• assessing why re-expansion has not been achieved (for example, air leaking around the drain site, tube displaced or blocked, large persistent leak);
• the use of suction to re-expand the lung (this can be lengthy, requires appropriate equipment and pressure settings, influences how and where confirmatory radiographs are taken, and involves care from experienced nursing staff);
• whether early thoracic surgery would be appropriate (for example, failure of conservative measures, need to prevent recurrence);
• consideration of chemical pleurodesis in certain cases;
• management of surgical emphysema.

Fig. 58.2 Management of an intercostal drain. From Miller AC, Harvey JE. *British Medical Journal* 1993; **307**: 114–6.

Insertion of a chest drain

the underwater seal bottle when the patient coughs, remove the drain.

3 Consider premedication with morphine/cyclizine before removal of the drain. Take down the dressing. Cut and remove the suture which has anchored the drain. Ask the patient to hold his or her breath in full inspiration while the drain is withdrawn from the chest. An assistant should hold a gauze swab over the incision while you tie the two interrupted 3/0 silk sutures (to be removed after 5 days). Cover the incision with an adhesive dressing.

4 The patient can be discharged. Arrange follow-up in the chest clinic in 7–10 days, with a repeat chest X-ray taken prior to the appointment.

Troubleshooting

Pain
• Pain around the chest incision may occur. NSAIDs are usually effective, but initially opiates may be necessary.
• If the pain is distant from the incision, you should check the position of the cannula tip. If it is curled against the interior of the thoracic cavity, withdraw it slightly. There should be about 25 cm of intrathoracic tube in an adult of normal size

Fluid level does not swing with breathing
• **Tube kinked**: this usually occurs because of angulation over the ribs and may be corrected by releasing the dressing. Occasionally it is necessary to withdraw the drain slightly.
• **Tube blocked**: if the tube is too small, which is the most common fault, it can easily become blocked by secretions. It should be replaced by a larger one.
• **Wrong position**: if the drainage holes are wholly or partially extrapleural, which can be diagnosed from the chest film, the tube needs to be removed and another inserted.

Surgical emphysema
• A little localized subcutaneous air is usual.
• Increasing surgical emphysema may indicate malposition of the tube with a drainage hole in a subcutaneous position; if so, a new tube must be inserted.

Pneumothorax does not resolve

• If the tube is well positioned, of adequate size (the largest that can be comfortably inserted) and not blocked, this indicates a persisting bronchopleural fistula.

• Seek expert advice from a chest physician or thoracic surgeon. Some will resolve with increased suction.

59 Lumbar puncture

Indications

1 Suspected meningitis (p. 247) If you suspect bacterial meningitis, take blood cultures and start antibiotic therapy immediately (p. 248), before performing lumbar puncture.
2 Suspected subarachnoid haemorrhage (p. 243).
3 Suspected Guillain–Barré syndrome (p. 256).

Contraindications

1 Reduced level of consciousness.
2 Focal neurological signs (long tract or posterior fossa).
3 Papilloedema.
4 Generalized tonic–clonic seizure in the preceding hour.
5 Anticoagulation.
   Lumbar puncture may be performed in patients with contra-indications, but not before you have obtained expert advice from a neurologist or neurosurgeon.

Special equipment

1 Spinal needle. The disposable ones are usually sharper. Choose a 20 or 22 G needle.
2 Manometer and three-way tap.
3 Three plain sterile bottles (numbered) and a fluoride bottle for glucose (to be sent with a blood glucose sample, taken before LP).

Technique

Positioning the patient (Fig. 59.1)

1 Move the patient to the edge of the bed on their left side if you are right handed.

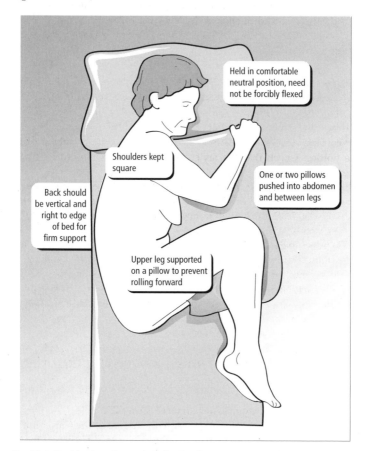

Fig. 59.1 Positioning the patient for lumbar puncture. Redrawn from Patten J. *Neurological Differential Diagnosis*. London: Harold Starke, 1977; 262.

2 The thoracolumbar spine should be maximally flexed. It does not matter if the neck is not flexed. Place a pillow between the knees to prevent torsion of the spine.

Choose the interspace to be used

1 Define the plane of the iliac crests which runs through L3–4. The spinal cord in the adult ends at the level of L1–2.

2 Choose either the L3–4 or L4–5 spaces. Mark the space using your thumbnail.

Lumbar puncture

1 Put on gloves and prepare the skin. It helps to place a drape on top of the patient so that you can recheck the position of the iliac crest if necessary.

2 Draw up lignocaine, assemble the manometer and undo the tops of the bottles. Check that the stylet of the needle moves freely. Place everything within easy reach.

3 Stretch the skin over the chosen space with the finger and thumb of your left hand, placed on the spinous processes of the adjacent vertebrae (Fig. 59.2). Put 0.5 mL of lignocaine in the skin and subcutaneous tissues with a 21 G (orange) needle.

4 Place the spinal needle on the mark, bevel uppermost, and advance it towards the umbilicus, taking care to keep it parallel to the ground.

5 The interspinous ligament gives some resistance, and you should notice increased resistance as you go through the tough ligamentum flavum. There is usually an obvious 'give' when the needle is through this. The dura is now only 1–2 mm away. Advance in small steps, withdrawing the stylet after each step.

6 Cerebrospinal fluid (CSF) should flow freely once you enter the dura. If the flow is poor, rotate the needle in case a nerve root is lying against it.

Measuring the opening pressure and collecting CSF

1 Connect the manometer and measure the height of the CSF column (the 'opening pressure'). The patient should uncurl slightly and try to relax at this stage.

2 Cap the top of the manometer with your finger, disconnect it from the needle and put the CSF in the glucose tube.

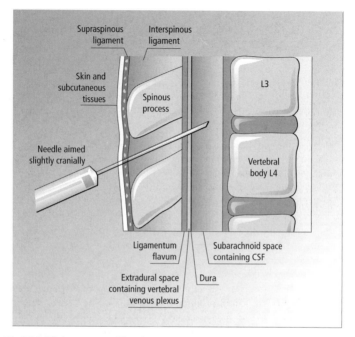

Fig. 59.2 The anatomy of lumbar puncture.

3 Collect three samples (about 2 mL each) in the plain sterile bottles.
4 Remove the needle and place a small dressing over the puncture site.

Interpreting CSF results

Normal values are given in Table 59.1, and CSF formulae in meningitis in Table 59.2.

Problems

You hit bone

1 Withdraw the needle. Recheck the patient's position and the bony landmarks. Try again, taking particular care to keep the needle parallel to the ground.

Table 59.1 Cerebrospinal fluid: normal values and correction for traumatic tap

Opening pressure	7–18 cm CSF
Cell count	0–5/mm³, all lymphocytes
Protein concentration	0.15–0.45 g/L (15–45 mg/dL)
Glucose concentration	2.8–4.2 mmol/L
CSF: blood glucose ratio	>50%

Correction of cell count and protein concentration in traumatic tap: for every 1000 RBC/mm³, subtract 1 WBC/mm³ and 0.015 g/L (15 mg/dL) protein

References: Normal reference values. *New England Journal of Medicine* 1986; 314: 39–49. Gottlieb AJ *et al*. *The Whole Internist Catalogue*. Philadelphia: W B Saunders, 1980: 127–8.

Table 59.2 CSF formulae in meningitis

	Pyogenic	Viral	Tuberculous	Cryptococcal
Cell count/mm³	>1000	<500	<500	<150
Predominant cell type	Polymorphs	Lymphocytes	Lymphocytes	Lymphocytes
Protein conc. (g/L)	>1.5	0.5–1.0	1.0–5.0	0.5–1.0
CSF: blood glucose	<50%	>50%	<50%	<50%

The values given are typical, but many exceptions occur.

Antibiotic therapy substantially changes the CSF formula in pyogenic bacterial meningitis, leading to a fall in cell count, increased proportion of lymphocytes and fall in protein level. However, the low CSF glucose level usually persists.

Lumbar puncture

2 If this fails, modify the angle of the needle in the sagittal plane.

3 If you are still unsuccessful, try another space, or consider trying with the patient sitting flexed forward.

Heavily bloodstained fluid

1 The possibilities are subarachnoid haemorrhage, traumatic tap or puncture of the venous plexus. If the fluid appears to be venous blood (slow ooze) try again in another space, after flushing the needle.

2 Subarachnoid haemorrhage results in uniformly bloodstained CSF (as shown by the red cell count in successive samples). Xanthochromia of the supernatant is always found from 12 h to 2 weeks after the bleed; centrifuge the CSF and examine the supernatant by spectrophotometry if available. Otherwise compare against a white background with a 'control' bottle filled with water.

Deteriorating conscious level after lumbar puncture

1 Give mannitol 20% 100–200 mL (0.5 g/kg) IV over 10 min. Check plasma osmolality: further mannitol may be given until plasma osmolality is 320 mosmol/kg.

2 Arrange transfer to the ITU in case intubation and ventilation are needed. If intubated, hyperventilate to an arterial P_{CO_2} of 4.0 kPa (30 mmHg).

3 Seek advice on further management from a neurologist or neurosurgeon.

Lumbar puncture

60 Peritoneal dialysis

Indications

Indications

- **Acute renal failure**, when other methods of renal replacement therapy are not possible or are contraindicated.
- **Elimination of some poisons** (e.g. lithium), when haemodialysis is not possible.
- **Core rewarming in hypothermia** (p. 374).

Contraindications

- Recent abdominal surgery.
- Hypercatabolic state.

Technique

Preparation
1 Prepare a 1L bag of dialysis fluid warmed to 37°C.
2 Lay the patient flat. Put in a peripheral IV cannula.
3 Confirm that the bladder is empty by ultrasound, or, if this is not available, by catheterization.
4 Shave the lower abdomen.
5 Put on gown, gloves and mask and prepare and drape the skin.

Inserting the catheter
1 The usual site for insertion is 2.5 cm below the umbilicus in the midline. If there is an operation scar here, use a more lateral site (avoid the area of the inferior epigastric artery, whose surface marking is a line joining the femoral artery with the umbilicus).

2 Infiltrate with 10–15 mL of lignocaine 1% down to and around the peritoneum.

3 Aspirate for gas (indicating perforation of bowel) and, if found, choose another site.

4 Insert an IV cannula into the peritoneal cavity and run in the prepared dialysis fluid using a standard IV giving set. Withdraw the cannula. (This step is optional but makes inserting the PD catheter easier.)

5 Incise the skin vertically with a narrow scalpel blade (e.g. no. 11) and insert the PD catheter over the obturator through the abdominal wall with a twisting action.

6 As soon as the tip is through the peritoneum (signalled by loss of resistance), rotate the catheter so that the black spot (which marks the direction of the curve) is facing inferolaterally. Withdraw the obdurator 2 cm. Advance the catheter, aiming downwards and laterally towards the pelvis, until two-thirds has been inserted. Then withdraw the obturator completely as you advance the catheter until only 2 cm is protruding.

7 Attach the right-angled end of the connecting set to the catheter, which should be held with a deep purse-string suture (3/0 silk).

8 Place gauze swabs around the catheter. Use a split gallipot to support it and the connecting piece if kinking could occur.

Peritoneal dialysis for acute renal failure

Choice of fluid

• PD fluid is available in 1 or 2 L bags. The osmolality of the fluid (which influences the shift of water from plasma to PD fluid) varies according to the dextrose concentration.

• Start with 1 L bags of 1.36% dextrose unless the patient is fluid-overloaded, in which case use dextrose of a higher concentration (2.27% or 3.86%).

Exchanges

1 Weigh the bags before and after use to calculate their fluid capacity (allow 1 mL/g) as they may not contain exactly 1 L.

2 Warm the fluid to 37°C. Add heparin (500 units/L) to reduce fibrin deposition on the catheter.

3 The exchange time consists of inflow time, dwell time and outflow time. Start with hourly exchanges, roughly 20 min each for inflow, dwell and outflow. If inflow and outflow take longer, omit the dwell time.

4 The exchange time can be increased after the first day if the patient's biochemistry and fluid status are satisfactory.

Monitoring

• See Table 60.1.

• Check plasma potassium 4 h after starting dialysis and then at least twice daily. If plasma potassium falls below 3.5 mmol/L, potassium should be added to the PD fluid to give a concentration of 4 mmol/L.

Table 60.1 Monitoring the patient during peritoneal dialysis

Hourly
Inflow volume estimated by weight
Volume of effluent
Volume of other fluid in or out

4-hly
Temperature
Pulse and blood pressure
Check plasma potassium 4 h after starting dialysis and then at least twice daily

8–12-hly
Blood glucose (some patients develop hyperglycaemia, particularly when
  hyperosmolar PD fluid is used)
Plasma biochemistry

Daily
Weight after drainage of PD fluid

Peritoneal dialysis

Peritoneal dialysis for core rewarming in hypothermia

Choice of fluid
• Use 1- or 2-L bags, potassium free.
• Warm the dialysate by running it through a blood-warming coil immersed in water heated to 54°C: this will give a dialysate temperature around 44°C when it enters the peritoneal cavity.

Exchanges
Run in rapidly and drain out immediately. Core temperature is usually restored to normal after 6–8 exchanges.

Monitoring
Check plasma potassium hourly. If this falls below 3.5 mmol/L, potassium should be added to the PD fluid to give a concentration of 4 mmol/L.

Table 60.2 Initial antibotic therapy for peritonitis complicating peritoneal dialysis

Vancomycin + gentamicin or *Ceftazidime*

Vancomycin
Loading dose: 500 mg intraperitoneally (IP)
Maintenance dose: 25 mg/L IP

Gentamicin
Loading dose: 1.7 mg/kg IP
Maintenance dose: 4 mg/L IP
Check a random blood level after 4 days and reduce the dose if this is 4 mg/L
   or more

Ceftazidime
500 mg/L IP

Peritoneal dialysis

Troubleshooting

Fluid accumulation or poor drainage
• Accumulation of 500–1000 mL is usual.
• Check that the catheter is not kinked as it leaves the abdomen. Syringe the catheter with saline.
• If fluid accumulation is progressive (often due to plugging of the end of the catheter by omentum), the catheter will have to be resited. The position of the catheter can be checked by ultrasound. Resiting is best done with a second catheter, leaving the first in place to prevent leakage of fluid down the track.

Peritonitis
• Shown by abdominal pain, fever and cloudy effluent.
• Aspirate 30 mL of effluent through the wall or port of the bag (sterilize the site with an alcohol swab).
• Divide 10 mL between aerobic and anaerobic blood culture bottles. Send 20 mL for cell count and centrifugation with Gram staining and culture of the sediment.
• Initial antibiotic therapy is given in Table 60.2.
• Antibiotic treatment should be continued for at least 5 days after clearing of the effluent (usually for a total of 7–10 days).

61 Insertion of a Sengstaken– Blakemore tube

Indication

Failure to control variceal bleeding despite pharmacological therapy (p. 276).

• A Sengstaken–Blakemore tube should only be used to control life-threatening variceal bleeding. If you have not had experience with its placement and use, it is better to manage the patient conservatively because of the risks of inhalation, mucosal ulceration and incorrect positioning.

• Balloon tamponade is not a definitive procedure. Plan ahead for variceal injection/banding or oesophageal transection.

Special equipment

1 Sengstaken–Blakemore tube (Fig. 61.1). If this has only three lumens, tape a standard medium-bore nasogastric tube with the perforations just above the oesophageal balloon to allow aspiration of the oesophagus. The lumens of the tube are not always labelled; if not, label them now with tape. If there is time, store the tube in the freezer section of a refrigerator to reduce its flexibility, which makes insertion easier.

2 Sphygmomanometer (for inflation of the oesophageal balloon).

3 Contrast medium (e.g. Gastrografin) 10 mL and 300 mL water or 5% dextrose (for inflation of the gastric balloon).

4 Bladder syringe for aspirating the oesophageal drainage tube.

Technique

Preparation of the patient

1 The patient should be intubated by an anaesthetist before insertion of the tube (to prevent misplacement of the tube in the trachea or inhalation of blood) if the conscious level is depressed (grade 2 or more (p. 297)).

2 Sedation with midazolam 2 mg (elderly 1 mg) IV over 30 s, followed after 2 min by increments of 0.5–1 mg if sedation not adequate; usual range 2.5–7.5 (mg) should be used only if the patient is particularly agitated and an anaesthetist is available in case intubation becomes necessary.

Insertion of the tube

1 Put on apron and gloves.

2 Anaesthetize the throat with lignocaine spray.

3 Lubricate the end of the tube with KY jelly and pass it through the gap between your index and middle fingers placed in the back of the oropharynx. This reduces the chance of the tube curling. Ask the patient to breathe quietly through his/her mouth throughout the procedure. You are unlikely to need a chock for the teeth.

4 If at any stage of the procedure the patient becomes dyspnoeic withdraw the tube immediately and start again after endotracheal intubation.

5 Assistants should suck blood from the mouth and from all lumens while you insert the tube.

6 Steadily advance the tube until it is inserted to the hilt.

7 Inflate the gastric balloon with the contrast mixture (310 mL). Insert a bung or clamp the tube. If there is resistance to inflation, deflate the balloon and check the position of the tube with X-ray screening.

8 Pull the tube back gently until resistance is felt.

9 Firm traction on the gastric balloon is usually sufficient to stop the bleeding since this occurs at the filling point of the varices in the lower few centimetres of the oesophagus. If not, inflate the oesophageal balloon:

- Connect the lumen of the oesophageal balloon to a sphygmomanometer via a 3-way tap (Fig. 61.2).
- Inflate to 40 mmHg and clamp the tube.

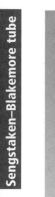

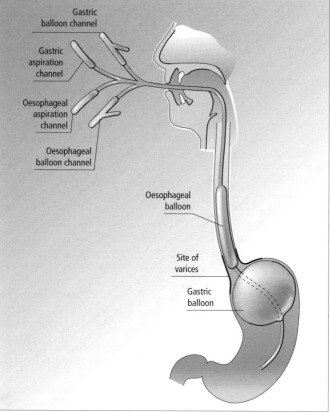

Fig. 61.1 Four-lumen Sengstaken–Blakemore tube in place to compress bleeding varices. Redrawn from Thompson R. *Lecture Notes on the Liver*. Oxford: Blackwell Scientific Publications, 1985; 37.

• The oesophageal balloon tends to deflate easily so the pressure must be checked every 2 h or so.

10 Place a sponge pad (as used to support endotrachaeal tubes in ventilated patients) over the side of the patient's mouth to prevent the tube rubbing.

11 Strap the tube to the cheek. Fixation with weights over the end of

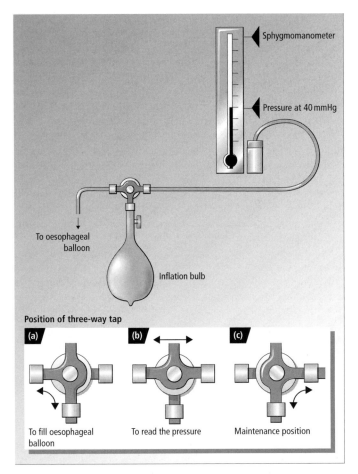

Sphygmomanometer

Pressure at 40 mmHg

To oesophageal
balloon

Inflation bulb

Position of three-way tap

(a)

To fill oesophageal
balloon

(b)

To read the pressure

(c)

Maintenance position

Fig. 61.2 Method of filling the oesophageal balloon and measuring its
pressure.

the bed is less effective, and may lead to displacement, especially in
agitated patients.

12 Mark the tube in relation to the teeth so that movement can be
detected more easily.

Aftercare

1 It is not necessary to deflate the oesophageal balloon every hour as sometimes recommended.

2 Aspirate the oesophageal channel every 30 min or more frequently if needed to prevent accumulation of secretions and to reduce the risk of inhalation.

3 Continue terlipressin infusion and other supportive therapy (p. 276).

4 Obtain a chest X-ray to check the position of the tube.

5 If facilities for variceal injection/banding are available, the tube should be removed in the endoscopy suite immediately before this, which can be done as soon as the patient is haemodynamically stable (and usually within 12 h).

6 If endoscopic therapy is not possible, discuss the case with the regional liver unit and arrange transfer if appropriate. Alternatively, start planning for oesophageal transection within 24 h if bleeding recurs when the balloon is deflated.

7 Do not leave the tube in for longer than 24 h because of the risk of mucosal ulceration.

8 Changing the side of the attachment to the cheek every 2 h reduces the risk of skin ulceration, but should be done carefully because of the risk of displacement.

Mistakes to avoid

1 Endotracheal placement of the tube. You should have a low threshold for intubation and ventilation.

2 Using air instead of contrast, which allows easy deflation of the balloon with consequent displacement of the tube.

3 Poor anchoring, or displacement when moving the patient.

4 Failure to plan ahead. Ask advice from a gastroenterologist regarding a definitive procedure (variceal injection or banding, oesophageal transection, shunt or embolization).

Appendices

62 Drug infusions

See Tables 62.1–62.7.

Table 62.1 Guide to drug infusions

Drug	Indication	Page reference
Acetylcysteine	Paracetamol poisoning	122
Alteplase	Thrombolysis	142
Aminophylline	Bronchospasm	195
Amiodarone	Treatment of VT/VF/AF	727
Doxapram	Respiratory failure	200
Heparin	Anticoagulation	404
Insulin	Diabetes	322
Isoprenaline	Bradycardia	11
Labetalol	Severe hypertension	162
Naloxone	Opiate antagonism	107
Nitroprusside	Severe hypertension	162
Salbutamol	Bronchospasm	195
Streptokinase	Thrombolysis	142

VF, ventricular fibrillation; VT, ventricular tachycardia; AF, atrial fibrillation.

Table 62.2 Guide to inotropic-vasopressor therapy

Cause of hypotension	Choice of therapy*	Dosage (μ/kg/min)
Left ventricular failure	Dobutamine if systolic BP is > 90 mmHg	5–40
Right ventricular infarction	Dopamine if systolic BP is 80–90 mmHg	5–40
Pulmonary embolism	Noradrenaline if systolic BP is < 80 mmHg	0.05–5
Cardiac tamponade, while awaiting pericardiocentesis	Noradrenaline	0.05–5
Septic shock	Noradrenaline	0.05–5
	Dobutamine should be added if cardiac output is low	5–40
Anaphylactic shock	Adrenaline	5–40

*All agents (with the exception of dobutamine) must be administered via a central vein, as tissue necrosis due to alpha-1 adrenergic vasoconstriction may occur if there is extravasation from a peripheral vein.

Table 62.3 Adrenaline and noradrenaline infusions: 2 mg in 50 ml (40 μg/ml)

Infusion volumes (ml/h)

Dose (μg/kg/min)	Weight (kg) 30	35	40	45	50	55	60	65	70	75	80	85	90	95	100	105	110	115	120
0.01	0.45	0.53	0.6	0.68	0.75	0.83	0.9	0.98	1.05	1.13	1.2	1.28	1.35	1.43	1.5	1.58	1.65	1.73	1.8
0.02	0.9	1.05	1.2	1.35	1.5	1.65	1.8	1.95	2.1	2.25	2.4	2.55	2.7	2.85	3	3.15	3.3	3.45	3.6
0.03	1.35	1.57	1.8	2.02	2.25	2.48	2.7	2.92	3.15	3.38	3.6	3.82	4.05	4.28	4.5	4.72	4.95	5.17	5.4
0.04	1.8	2.1	2.4	2.7	3	3.3	3.6	3.9	4.2	4.5	4.8	5.1	5.4	5.7	6	6.3	6.6	6.9	7.2
0.05	2.25	2.63	3	3.38	3.75	4.13	4.5	4.88	5.25	5.63	6	6.38	6.75	7.13	7.5	7.88	8.25	8.63	9
0.06	2.7	3.15	3.6	4.05	4.5	4.95	5.4	5.85	6.3	6.75	7.2	7.65	8.1	8.55	9	9.45	9.9	10.4	10.8
0.07	3.15	3.68	4.2	4.73	5.25	5.78	6.3	6.83	7.35	7.88	8.4	8.93	9.45	9.98	10.5	11	11.6	12.1	12.6
0.08	3.6	4.2	4.8	5.4	6	6.6	7.2	7.8	8.4	9	9.6	10.2	10.8	11.4	12	12.6	13.2	13.8	14.4
0.09	4.05	4.72	5.4	6.08	6.75	7.42	8.1	8.78	9.45	10.1	10.8	11.5	12.2	12.8	13.5	14.2	14.9	15.5	16.2
0.1	4.5	5.25	6	6.75	7.5	8.2	9	9.75	10.5	11.3	12	12.8	13.5	14.3	15	15.8	16.5	17.3	18
0.2	9	10.5	12	13.5	15	16.5	18	19.5	21	22.5	24	25.5	27	28.5	30	31.5	33	34.5	36
0.3	13.5	15.8	18	20.3	22.5	24.8	27	29.3	31.5	33.8	36	38.3	40.5	42.8	45	47.3	49.5	51.8	54
0.4	18	21	24	27	30	33	36	39	42	45	48	51	54	57	60	63	66	69	72
0.5	22.5	26.3	30	33.8	37.5	41.3	45	48.8	52.5	56.3	60	63.8	67.5	71.3	75	78.8	82.5	86.3	90
0.6	27	31.5	36	40.5	45	49.5	54	58.5	63	67.5	72	76.5	81	85.5	90	94.5	99	104	108
0.7	31.5	36.8	42	47.3	52.5	57.8	63	68.3	73.5	78.8	84	89.3	94.5	99.8	105	110	116	121	126
0.8	36	42	48	54	60	66	72	78	84	90	96	102	108	114	120	126	132	138	144
0.9	40.5	47.3	54	60.8	67.5	74.3	81	87.8	94.5	101	108	115	122	128	135	142	149	155	162
1	45	52.5	60	67.5	75	82.5	90	97.5	105	113	120	128	135	143	150	158	165	173	180

Table 62.4 Adrenaline and noradrenaline infusions: 4 mg in 50 ml (80 µg/ml)

Infusion volumes (ml/h)

Dose (µg/kg/min)	Weight (kg) 30	35	40	45	50	55	60	65	70	75	80	85	90	95	100	105	110	115	120
0.01	0.23	0.26	0.3	0.34	0.38	0.41	0.45	0.49	0.53	0.56	0.6	0.64	0.68	0.71	0.75	0.79	0.83	0.86	0.9
0.02	0.45	0.53	0.6	0.68	0.75	0.83	0.9	0.98	1.05	1.13	1.2	1.28	1.35	1.43	1.5	1.58	1.65	1.73	1.8
0.03	0.68	0.79	0.9	1.01	1.13	1.24	1.35	1.46	1.57	1.69	1.8	1.91	2.02	2.14	2.25	2.36	2.48	2.59	2.7
0.04	0.9	1.05	1.2	1.35	1.5	1.65	1.8	1.95	2.1	2.25	2.4	2.55	2.7	2.85	3	3.15	3.3	3.45	3.6
0.05	1.13	1.31	1.5	1.69	1.88	2.06	2.25	2.44	2.63	2.81	3	3.19	3.38	3.56	3.75	3.94	4.13	4.31	4.5
0.06	1.37	1.57	1.8	2.02	2.25	2.48	2.7	2.92	3.15	3.38	3.6	3.82	4.05	4.28	4.5	4.72	4.95	5.17	5.4
0.07	1.58	1.84	2.1	2.36	2.63	2.89	3.15	3.41	3.68	3.94	4.2	4.46	4.73	4.99	5.25	5.51	5.78	6.04	6.3
0.08	1.8	2.1	2.4	2.7	3	3.3	3.6	3.9	4.2	4.5	4.8	5.1	5.4	5.7	6	6.3	6.6	6.9	7.2
0.09	2.02	2.36	2.7	3.04	3.38	3.71	4.05	4.39	4.72	5.06	5.4	5.74	6.08	6.41	6.75	7.09	7.42	7.76	8.1
0.1	2.25	2.63	3	3.38	3.75	4.13	4.5	4.88	5.25	5.63	6	6.38	6.75	7.13	7.5	7.88	8.25	8.63	9
0.2	4.5	5.25	6	6.75	7.5	8.25	9	9.75	10.5	11.3	12	12.8	13.5	14.3	15	15.8	16.5	17.3	18
0.3	6.75	7.88	9	10.1	11.3	12.4	13.5	14.6	15.8	16.9	18	19.1	20.3	21.4	22.5	23.6	24.8	25.9	27
0.4	9	10.5	12	13.5	15	16.5	18	19.5	21	22.5	24	25.5	27	28.5	30	31.5	33	34.5	36
0.5	11.3	13.1	15	16.9	18.8	20.6	22.5	24.4	26.3	28.1	30	31.9	33.8	35.6	37.5	39.4	41.3	43.1	45
0.6	13.5	15.8	18	20.3	22.5	24.8	27	29.3	31.5	33.8	36	38.3	40.5	42.8	45	47.3	49.5	51.8	54
0.7	15.8	18.4	21	23.6	26.3	28.9	31.5	34.1	36.8	39.4	42	44.6	47.3	49.9	52.5	55.1	57.8	60.4	63
0.8	18	21	24	27	30	33	36	39	42	45	48	51	54	57	60	63	66	69	72
0.9	20.3	23.6	27	30.4	33.8	37.1	40.5	43.9	47.3	50.6	54	57.4	60.8	64.1	67.5	70.9	74.3	77.6	81
1	22.5	26.3	30	33.8	37.5	41.3	45	48.8	52.5	56.3	60	63.8	67.5	71.3	75	78.8	82.5	86.3	90
2	45	52.5	60	67.5	75	82.5	90	97.5	105	113	120	128	135	143	150	158	165	173	180
3	67.5	78.8	90	101	113	124	135	146	158	169	180	191	203	214	225	236	248	259	270
4	90	105	120	135	150	165	180	195	210	225	240	255	270	285	300	315	330	345	360

Table 62.5 Adrenaline and noradrenaline infusions: 8 mg in 50 ml (160 µg/ml)

Infusion volumes (ml/h)

Dose (µg/kg/min)	Weight (kg) 30	35	40	45	50	55	60	65	70	75	80	85	90	95	100	105	110	115	120
0.1	1.13	1.31	1.5	1.69	1.88	2.06	2.25	2.44	2.63	2.81	3	3.19	3.38	3.56	3.75	3.94	4.13	4.31	4.5
0.2	2.25	2.63	3	3.38	3.75	4.13	4.5	4.88	5.25	5.63	6	6.38	6.75	7.13	7.5	7.88	8.25	8.63	9
0.3	3.38	3.94	4.5	5.06	5.63	6.19	6.75	7.31	7.88	8.44	9	9.56	10.1	10.7	11.3	11.8	12.4	12.9	13.5
0.4	4.5	5.25	6	6.75	7.5	8.25	9	9.75	10.5	11.3	12	12.8	13.5	14.3	15	15.8	16.5	17.3	18
0.5	5.63	6.56	7.5	8.44	9.38	10.3	11.3	12.2	13.1	14.1	15	15.9	16.9	17.8	18.8	19.7	20.6	21.6	22.5
0.6.	6.75	7.88	9	10.1	11.3	12.4	13.5	14.6	15.8	16.9	18	19.1	20.3	21.4	22.5	23.6	24.8	25.9	27
0.7	7.88	9.19	10.5	11.8	13.1	14.4	15.8	17.1	18.4	19.7	21	22.3	23.6	24.9	26.3	27.6	28.9	30.2	31.5
0.8	9	10.5	12	13.5	15	16.5	18	19.5	21	22.5	24	25.5	27	28.5	30	31.5	33	34.5	36
0.9	10.1	11.8	13.5	15.2	16.9	18.6	20.3	21.9	23.6	25.3	27	28.7	30.4	32.1	33.8	35.4	37.1	38.8	40.5
1	11.3	13.1	15	16.9	18.8	20.6	22.5	24.4	26.3	28.1	30	31.9	33.8	35.6	37.5	39.4	41.3	43.1	45
2	22.5	26.3	30	33.8	37.5	41.3	45	48.8	52.5	56.3	60	63.8	67.5	71.3	75	78.8	82.5	86.3	90
3	33.8	39.4	45	50.6	56.3	61.9	67.5	73.1	78.8	84.4	90	95.6	101	107	113	118	124	129	135
4	45	52.5	60	67.5	75	82.5	90	97.5	105	113	120	128	135	143	150	158	165	173	180
5	56.3	65.6	75	84.4	93.8	103	113	122	131	141	150	159	169	178	188	197	206	216	225
6	67.5	78.8	90	101	113	124	135	146	158	169	180	191	203	214	225	236	248	259	270
7	78.8	91.9	105	118	131	144	158	171	184	197	210	223	236	249	263	276	289	302	315
8	90	105	120	135	150	165	180	195	210	225	240	255	270	285	300	315	330	345	360
9	101	118	135	152	169	186	203	219	236	253	270	287	304	321	338	354	371	388	405
10	113	131	150	169	188	206	225	244	263	281	300	319	338	356	375	394	413	431	405

Table 62.6 Dopamine and dobutamine infusions: 250 mg in 50 ml (50 mg/ml)

Infusion volumes (ml/h)

Dose (µg/kg/min)	Weight (kg)																		
	30	35	40	45	50	55	60	65	70	75	80	85	90	95	100	105	110	115	120
1	0.36	0.42	0.48	0.54	0.6	0.66	0.72	0.78	0.84	0.9	0.96	1.02	1.08	1.14	1.2	1.26	1.32	1.38	1.44
2	0.72	0.84	0.96	1.08	1.2	1.32	1.44	1.56	1.68	1.8	1.92	2.04	2.16	2.28	2.4	2.52	2.64	2.76	2.88
3	1.08	1.26	1.44	1.62	1.8	1.98	2.16	2.34	2.52	2.7	2.88	3.06	3.24	3.42	3.6	3.78	3.96	4.14	4.32
4	1.44	1.68	1.92	2.16	2.4	2.64	2.88	3.12	3.36	3.6	3.84	4.08	4.32	4.56	4.8	5.04	5.28	5.52	5.76
5	1.8	2.1	2.4	2.7	3	3.3	3.6	3.9	4.2	4.5	4.8	5.1	5.4	5.7	6	6.3	6.6	6.9	7.2
6	2.16	2.52	2.88	3.24	3.6	3.96	4.32	4.68	5.04	5.4	5.76	6.12	6.48	6.84	7.2	7.56	7.92	8.28	8.64
7	2.52	2.94	3.36	3.78	4.2	4.62	5.04	5.46	5.88	6.3	6.72	7.14	7.56	7.98	8.4	8.82	9.24	9.66	10.1
8	2.88	3.36	3.84	4.32	4.8	5.28	5.76	6.24	6.72	7.2	7.68	8.16	8.64	9.12	9.6	10.1	10.6	11	11.5
9	3.24	3.78	4.32	4.86	5.4	5.94	6.48	7.02	7.56	8.1	8.64	9.18	9.72	10.3	10.8	11.3	11.9	12.4	13
10	3.6	4.2	4.8	5.4	6	6.6	7.2	7.8	8.4	9	9.6	10.2	10.8	11.4	12	12.6	13.2	13.8	14.4
20	7.2	8.4	9.6	10.8	12	13.2	14.4	15.6	16.8	18	19.2	20.4	21.6	22.8	24	25.2	26.4	27.6	28.8
30	10.8	12.6	14.4	16.2	18	19.8	21.6	23.4	25.2	27	28.8	30.6	32.4	34.2	36	37.8	39.6	41.4	43.2
40	14.4	16.8	19.2	21.6	24	26.4	28.8	31.2	33.6	36	38.4	40.8	43.2	45.6	48	50.4	52.8	55.2	57.6
50	18	21	24	27	30	33	36	39	42	45	48	51	54	57	60	63	66	69	72
60	21.6	25.2	28.8	32.4	36	39.6	43.2	46.8	50.4	54	57.6	61.2	64.8	68.4	72	75.6	79.2	82.8	86.4
70	25.2	29.4	33.6	37.8	42	46.2	50.4	54.6	58.8	63	67.2	71.4	75.6	79.8	84	88.2	92.4	96.6	101
80	28.8	33.6	38.4	43.2	48	52.8	57.6	62.4	67.2	72	76.8	81.6	86.4	91.2	96	101	106	110	115
90	32.4	37.8	43.2	48.6	54	59.4	64.8	70.2	75.6	81	86.4	91.8	97.2	103	108	113	119	124	130
100	36	42	48	54	60	66	72	78	84	90	96	102	108	114	120	126	132	138	144

Table 62.7 Dopamine and dobutamine infusions: 500 mg in 50 ml (10 mg/ml)

Infusion volumes (ml/h)

Dose (µg/kg/min)	Weight (kg) 30	35	40	45	50	55	60	65	70	75	80	85	90	95	100	105	110	115	120
1	0.18	0.21	0.24	0.27	0.3	0.33	0.36	0.39	0.42	0.45	0.48	0.51	0.54	0.57	0.6	0.63	0.66	0.69	0.72
2	0.36	0.42	0.48	0.54	0.6	0.66	0.72	0.78	0.84	0.9	0.96	1.02	1.08	1.14	1.2	1.26	1.32	1.38	1.44
3	0.54	0.63	0.72	0.81	0.9	0.99	1.08	1.17	1.26	1.35	1.44	1.53	1.62	1.71	1.8	1.89	1.98	2.07	2.16
4	0.72	0.84	0.96	1.08	1.2	1.32	1.44	1.56	1.68	1.8	1.92	2.04	2.16	2.28	2.4	2.52	2.64	2.76	2.88
5	0.9	1.05	1.2	1.35	1.5	1.65	1.8	1.95	2.1	2.25	2.4	2.55	2.7	2.85	3	3.15	3.3	3.45	3.6
6	1.08	1.26	1.44	1.62	1.8	1.98	2.16	2.34	2.52	2.7	2.88	3.06	3.24	3.42	3.6	3.78	3.96	4.14	4.32
7	1.26	1.47	1.68	1.89	2.1	2.31	2.52	2.73	2.94	3.15	3.36	3.57	3.78	3.99	4.2	4.41	4.62	4.83	5.04
8	1.44	1.68	1.92	2.16	2.4	2.64	2.88	3.12	3.36	3.6	3.84	4.08	4.32	4.56	4.8	5.04	5.28	5.52	5.76
9	1.62	1.89	2.16	2.43	2.7	2.97	3.24	3.51	3.78	4.05	4.32	4.59	4.86	5.13	5.4	5.67	5.94	6.21	6.48
10	1.8	2.1	2.4	2.7	3	3.3	3.6	3.9	4.2	4.5	4.8	5.1	5.4	5.7	6	6.3	6.6	6.9	7.2
20	3.6	4.2	4.8	5.4	6	6.6	7.2	7.8	8.4	9	9.6	10.2	10.8	11.4	12	12.6	13.2	13.8	14.4
30	5.4	6.3	7.2	8.1	9	9.9	10.8	11.7	12.6	13.5	14.4	15.3	16.2	17.1	18	18.9	19.8	20.7	21.6
40	7.2	8.4	9.6	10.8	12	13.2	14.4	15.6	16.8	18	19.2	20.4	21.6	22.8	24	25.2	26.4	27.6	28.8
50	9	10.5	12	13.5	15	16.5	18	19.5	21	22.5	24	25.5	27	28.5	30	31.5	33	34.5	36
60	10.8	12.6	14.4	16.2	18	19.8	21.6	23.4	25.2	27	28.8	30.6	32.4	34.2	36	37.8	39.6	41.4	43.2
70	12.6	14.7	16.8	18.9	21	23.1	25.2	27.3	29.4	31.5	33.6	35.7	37.8	39.9	42	44.1	46.2	48.3	50.4
80	14.4	16.8	19.2	21.6	24	26.4	28.8	31.2	33.6	36	38.4	40.8	43.2	45.6	48	50.4	52.8	55.2	57.6
90	16.2	18.9	21.6	24.3	27	29.7	32.4	35.1	37.8	40.5	43.2	45.9	48.6	51.3	54	56.7	59.4	62.1	64.8
100	18	21	24	27	30	33	36	39	42	45	48	51	54	57	60	63	66	69	72

63 Respiratory function tests

See Tables 63.1–63.8.

Table 63.1 Choosing respiratory function tests

Condition	Tests
Asthma	Serial measurements of peak flow
Chronic obstructive pulmonary disease	Serial measurements of peak flow
	Spirometry before and after bronchodilator therapy
	Arterial blood gases
Interstitial lung disease	Spirometry
	Static lung volumes
	Carbon monoxide transfer factor
	Arterial blood gases
Extrathoracic airways obstruction	Flow/volume loop
Preoperative assessment	Spirometry
	Exercise test (6-min walk)

Table 63.2 Peak expiratory flow rate in males (L/min)

Height (ft/inches)	Age (years) 20–25	30	35	40	45	50	55	60	65	70
5'3"	572	560	548	536	524	512	500	488	476	464
5'6"	597	584	572	559	547	534	522	509	496	484
5'9"	625	612	599	586	573	560	547	533	520	507
6'0"	654	640	626	613	599	585	572	558	544	530
6'3"	679	665	650	636	622	608	593	579	565	551

Standard deviation 60 L/min.

Table 63.3 Peak expiratory flow rate in females (L/min)

Height (ft/inches)	Age (years) 20–25	30	35	40	45	50	55	60	65	70
4'9"	377	366	356	345	335	324	314	303	293	282
5'0"	403	392	382	371	361	350	340	329	319	308
5'3"	433	422	412	401	391	380	370	359	349	338
5'6"	459	448	438	427	417	406	396	385	375	364
5'9"	489	478	468	457	447	436	426	415	405	394

Standard deviation 60L/min.

Respiratory function tests

Table 63.4 Forced expiratory volume in 1 s (FEV₁) in males (L)

Height (ft/inches)	Age (years) 20–25	30	35	40	45	50	55	60	65	70
5'3"	3.61	3.45	3.30	3.14	2.99	2.83	2.68	2.52	2.37	2.21
5'6"	3.86	3.71	3.55	3.40	3.24	3.09	2.93	2.78	2.62	2.47
5'9"	4.15	4.00	3.84	3.69	3.53	3.38	3.22	3.06	2.91	2.75
6'0"	4.44	4.28	4.13	3.97	3.82	3.66	3.51	3.35	3.20	3.04
6'3"	4.69	4.54	4.38	4.23	4.07	3.92	3.76	3.61	3.45	3.30

Standard deviation 0.5 L.

Table 63.5 Forced expiratory volume in 1s (FEV₁) in females (L)

Height (ft/inches)	Age (years) 20–25	30	35	40	45	50	55	60	65	70
4'9"	2.60	2.45	2.30	2.15	2.00	1.85	1.70	1.55	1.40	1.25
5'0"	2.83	2.68	2.53	2.38	2.23	2.08	1.93	1.78	1.63	1.48
5'3"	3.09	2.94	2.79	2.64	2.49	2.34	2.19	2.04	1.89	1.74
5'6"	3.36	3.21	3.06	2.91	2.76	2.61	2.46	2.31	2.16	2.01
5'9"	3.59	3.44	3.29	3.14	2.99	2.84	2.69	2.54	2.39	2.24

Standard deviation 0.4 L.

Table 63.6 Forced vital capacity (FVC) in males (L)

Height (ft/inches)	Age (years) 20–25	30	35	40	45	50	55	60	65	70
5'3"	4.17	4.06	3.95	3.84	3.73	3.62	3.51	3.40	3.29	3.18
5'6"	4.53	4.42	4.31	4.20	4.09	3.98	3.87	3.76	3.65	3.54
5'9"	4.95	4.84	4.73	4.62	4.51	4.40	4.29	4.18	4.07	3.96
6'0"	5.37	5.26	5.15	5.04	4.93	4.82	4.71	4.60	4.49	4.38
6'3"	5.73	5.62	5.51	5.40	5.29	5.18	5.07	4.96	4.85	4.74

Standard deviation 0.6 L.

Table 63.7 Forced vital capacity (FVC) in females (L)

Height (ft/inches)	Age (years) 20–25	30	35	40	45	50	55	60	65	70
4'9"	3.13	2.98	2.83	2.68	2.53	2.38	2.23	2.08	1.93	1.78
5'0"	3.45	3.30	3.15	3.00	2.85	2.70	2.55	2.40	2.25	2.10
5'3"	3.83	3.68	3.53	3.38	3.23	3.08	2.93	2.78	2.63	2.48
5'6"	4.20	4.05	3.90	3.75	3.60	3.45	3.30	3.15	3.00	2.85
5'9"	4.53	4.38	4.23	4.08	3.93	3.78	3.63	3.48	3.33	3.18

Standard deviation 0.4 L.

Respiratory function tests

Table 63.8 FEV$_1$ as a percentage of forced vital capacity (%)

	Age (years) 20–25	30	35	40	45	50	55	60	65	70
Males*	82.5	80.6	78.7	76.9	75.0	73.1	71.3	69.4	67.5	65.7
Females†	81.0	79.9	78.8	77.7	76.6	75.5	74.3	73.2	72.1	71.0

* Standard deviation 7%.

† Standard deviation 6%.

Notes on Tables 63.2–63.8

• The mean ± 1 standard deviation includes 68% of healthy subjects; the mean ± 2 standard deviations includes 95% of healthy subjects.

• FEV$_1$ and FVC: the values shown are for people of European descent; for races with smaller thoraces (e.g. from the Indian subcontinent and Polynesia), subtract 0.4 L from the values given for FEV$_1$ and 0.7 L for FVC in males and 0.6 L in females.

Reference: Cotes JE. *Lung Function*, 4th edn. Oxford: Blackwell Scientific Publications, 1978.

64 Peripheral nervous system

See Tables 64.1 and 64.2, and Figure 64.1.

Table 64.1 Muscle groups: root and peripheral nerve supply

Movement	Muscle group	Main roots	Peripheral nerve
Shoulder abduction	Deltoid	C5	Axillary
Shoulder adduction	Latissimus dorsi	C7	Brachial plexus
	Pectoralis major	C5–7	Brachial plexus
Elbow flexion	Biceps	C5–C6	Musculocutaneous
	Brachioradialis	C6	Radial
Elbow extension	Triceps	C7	Radial
Wrist flexion	Flexor muscles of forearm	C7–C8	Median/ulnar
Wrist extension	Extensor muscles of forearm	C7	Radial
Finger flexion	Flexor muscles of forearm	C7–C8	Median/ulnar
Finger extension	Extensor muscles of forearm	C7	Radial
Finger abduction	Interossei	T1	Ulnar
	Abductor digiti minimi	T1	Ulnar
Thumb abduction	Abductor pollicis brevis	T1	Median
Hip flexion	Iliopsoas	L1–2	Femoral

Continued p. 492

Table 64.1 Continued

Movement	Muscle group	Main roots	Peripheral nerve
Hip extension	Gluteus maximus	L5–S1	Inferior gluteal
Hip abduction	Gluteus medius and minimus	L4–5	Superior gluteal
	Tensor fasciae latae	L4–5	Superior gluteal
Hip adduction	Adductors	L2–3	Obturator
Knee flexion	Hamstrings	S1	Sciatic
Knee extension	Quadriceps	L3–4	Femoral
Ankle dorsiflexion	Tibialis anterior	L4	Sciatic (peroneal)
Ankle plantarflexion	Gastrocnemius	S1–2	Sciatic (tibial)
Ankle eversion	Peroneus longus	L5–S1	Sciatic (peroneal)
Ankle inversion	Tibialis anterior	L4	Sciatic (peroneal)
	Tibialis posterior	L4–5	Sciatic (tibial)
Great-toe dorsiflexion	Extensor hallucis longus	L5	Sciatic (peroneal)

Reference: Medical Research Council Memorandum No. 45. *Aids to the Examination of the Peripheral Nervous System*. London: Her Majesty's Stationery Office, 1976.

Table 64.2 Tendon reflexes: root and peripheral nerve supply

Tendon reflex	Muscle	Main roots	Peripheral nerve
Biceps	Biceps	C5–6	Musculocutaneous
Supinator	Brachioradialis	C6	Radial
Triceps	Triceps	C7	Radial
Finger	Long finger flexors	C7–8	Median/ulnar
Knee	Quadriceps	L3–4	Femoral
Ankle	Gastrocnemius	S1–2	Sciatic (tibial)

Reference: Medical Research Council Memorandum No. 45. *Aids to the Examination of the Peripheral Nervous System*. London: Her Majesty's Stationery Office, 1976.

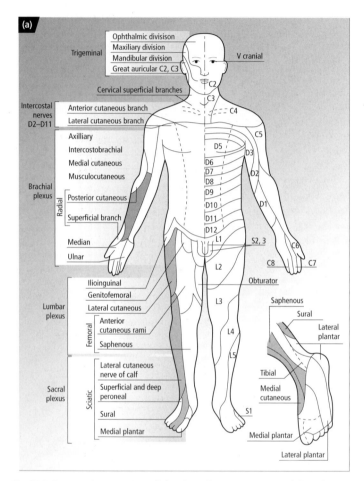

Fig. 64.1 Sensory innervation of the skin. Cutaneous areas of distribution of spinal segments and sensory fibres of the peripheral nerves: (a) anterior and (b) posterior views. From *Brain's Diseases of the Nervous System*, 10th edn. Oxford: Oxford University Press, 1993.

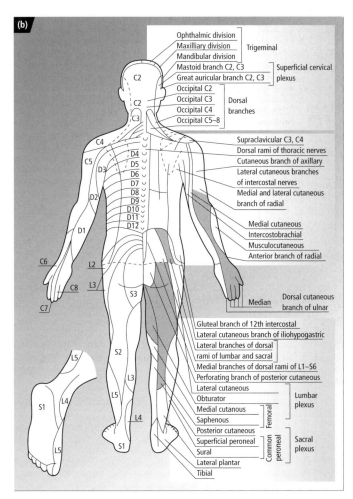

Fig. 64.1 *Continued*

Further reading

Many guidelines are now published on the Internet. Sites worth visiting include:

Agency for Healthcare Research and Quality (US), www.ahcpr.gov/clinic/cpgsix.htm
Database of Critically Appraised Guidelines (Institute of Health Sciences & University of Oxford), www.ihs.ox.ac.uk
National Guideline Clearinghouse (US), www.guideline.gov/index.asp

Section 1: Common Presentations

1 Cardiac arrest
Advanced Life Support Working Group of the European Resuscitation Council. The 1998 European Resuscitation Council guidelines for adult advanced life support. *British Medical Journal* 1998; **316,** 1863–1869.
Ballew, K.A. (1997) Recent advances: Cardiopulmonary resuscitation. *British Medical Journal* **314**, 1462–1465.

2 Cardiac dysrhythmias
Agency for Healthcare Research and Quality. Management of new onset atrial fibrillation: summary. www.ahrq.gov/clinic/atrial-sum.htm.
Cannom, D.S. & Prystowsky, E.N. (1999) Management of ventricular arrhythmias: detection, drugs and devices. *Journal of the American Medical Association* **281**, 172–179.
Ganz, L.I. & Friedman, P.L. (1995) Medical progress: Supraventricular tachycardia. *New England Journal of Medicine:* 162–173.
Mangrum, J.M. & DiMarco, J.P. (2000) Primary care: The evaluation

and management of bradycardia. *New England Journal of Medicine* **342**, 703–709.

Prystowsky, E.N., Benson, D.W. Jr, Fuster, V. *et al*. (1996) Management of patients with atrial fibrillation. *Circulation* **93**, 1262–1277.

Roden, D.M. (2000) Antiarrhythmic drugs: from mechanisms to clinical practice. *Heart* **84**, 339–346.

3 Hypotension

Hasdal, D., Topol, E.J., Califf, R.M., Berger, P.B. & Holmes, D.R. Jr (2000) Cardiogenic shock complicating acute coronary syndromes. *Lancet* **356**, 749–756.

Stainsby, D., MacLennan, S. & Hamilton, P.J. (2000) Management of massive blood loss: a template guide. *British Journal of Anaesthesia* **85**, 487–491.

4 Acute chest pain

Brauer, R.B., Liebermann-Meffert, D., Stein, H.J., Bartels, H. & Siewert, J.R. (1997) Boerhaave's syndrome: analysis of the literature and report of 18 new cases. *Diseases of the Esophagus* **10**, 64–68.

Fruergaard, P., Launbjerg, J., Hesse, B. *et al*. (1996) The diagnoses of patients admitted with acute chest pain but without myocardial infarction. *European Heart Journal* **17**, 1028–1034.

Lee, T.H. & Goldman, L. (2000) Primary care: Evaluation of the patient with acute chest pain. *New England Journal of Medicine* **342**, 1187–1195.

5 Acute breathlessness

Manning, H.L. & Schwartzstein, R.M. (1995) Mechanisms of disease: Pathophysiology of dyspnoea *New England Journal of Medicine* **333**, 1547–1553.

6 The unconscious patient

Plum, F. & Posner, J.B. (1980) The diagnosis of stupor and coma (3rd edn). Philadelphia. FA Davis.

7 Transient loss of consciousness

Linzer, M., Yang, E.H., Estes, N.A.M. III *et al*. (1997) Diagnosing syncope. Part 1: Value of history, physical examination, and electrocardiography. Part 2: Unexplained syncope. *Annals of Internal Medicine* **126**, 989–996; **127**, 76–86.

8 Acute confusional state

Hall, W. & Zador, D. (1997) The alcohol withdrawal syndrome. *Lancet* **349**, 1897–1900.

Young, L. & George, J. Guidelines for the Diagnosis and Management of Delirium in the Elderly *British Geriatrics Society* web site. www.bgs.org.uk

9 Headache

Ferrari, M.D. (1998) Migraine. *Lancet* **351**, 1043–1051.

Swannell, A.J. (1997) Polymyalgia rheumatica and temporal arteritis: diagnosis and management. *British Medical Journal* **314**, 1329–1332.

10 Sepsis syndrome

CME: Septicaemia. *Journal of the Royal College of Physicians of London* (2000) **34**, 418–444, 522–40.

Levi, M. & ten Cate, H. (1999) Current concepts: Disseminated intravascular coagulation. *New England Journal of Medicine* **341**, 586–592.

Pizzo, P.A. (1999) Current concepts: Fever in immunocompromised patients. *New England Journal of Medicine* **341**, 893–900.

11 Poisoning

Hirschfeld, R.M.A. & Russell, J.M. (1997) Current concepts: Assessment and treatment of suicidal patients. *New England Journal of Medicine* **337**, 910–915.

Jones, A.L. & Volans, G. (1999) Management of self poisoning. *British Medical Journal* **319**, 1414–1417.

National Poisons Information Service web site (TOXBASE). www.spib.axl.co.uk

Proudfoot, A.T. & Vale, J.A. , (1995) Paracetamol (acetaminophen) poisoning. *Lancet* **346**, 547–552.

Walker, E. & Hay, A. (1999) Carbon monoxide poisoning. *British Medical Journal* **319**, 1082–1083.

12 The critically ill patient

Goldhill, D.R., Worthington, L., Mulcahy, A., Tarling, M. & Sumner, A. (1999) The patient-at-risk team: identifying and managing seriously ill ward patients. *Anaesthesia* **54**, 853–860.

Section 2: Specific Problems

Cardiovascular

13 Acute myocardial infarction

Ryan, T.J., Anderson, J.L., Antman, E.M. *et al.* (1996) ACC/AHA guidelines for the management of patients with acute myocardial infarction: a report of the American College of Cardiology/American Heart Association task force on practice guidelines (committee on management of acute myocardial infarction). *Journal of the American College of Cardiology* **28**, 1328–1428. 1999 Update: *Journal of the American College of Cardiology* 1999; **34**: 890–911.

14 Unstable angina

Braunwald, E., Antman, E.M., Beasley, J.W. *et al.* (2000) ACC/AHA guidelines for the management of patients with unstable angina and non-ST-segment elevation mycardial infarction: executive summary and recommendations. *Circulation* **102**, 1193–1209.

Maynard, S.J., Scott, G.O., Riddell, J.W. & Adgey, A.A.J. (2000) Management of acute coronary syndromes. *British Medical Journal* **321**, 220–223.

Theroux, P. & Fuster, V. (1998) Acute coronary syndromes: unstable angina and non-Q-wave myocardial infarction. *Circulation* **97**, 1195–1206.

Yeghiazarians, Y., Braunstein, J.B., Askari, A. & Stone, P.H. (2000) Medical progress: Unstable angina. *New England Journal of Medicine* **342**, 101–114.

15 Aortic dissection

Hagan, P.G., Nienaber, C.A., Isselbacher, E.M. *et al.* (2000) The International Registry of Acute Aortic Dissection (IRAD): new insights into an old disease. *Journal of the American Medical Association* **283**, 897–903.

Pretre, R. & Von Segesser, L.K. (1997) Aortic dissection. *Lancet* **349**, 1461–1464.

16 Severe hypertension

Vaughan, C.J. & Delanty, N. (2000) Hypertensive emergencies. *Lancet* **356**, 411–417.

17 Pulmonary oedema

Ware, L.B. & Matthay, M.A. (2000) Medical progress: the acute respiratory distress syndrome. *New England Journal of Medicine* **342**, 1334–1349.

18 Pericarditis

Maisch, B. (1994) Pericardial diseases, with a focus on etiology, pathogenesis, pathophysiology, new diagnostic imaging methods and treatment. *Current Opinion in Cardiology* **9**, 379–388.

Vaitkus, P.T., Herrmann, H.C. & LeWinter, M.M. (1994) Treatment of malignant pericardial effusion. *Journal of the American Medical Association* **272**, 59–64.

19 Cardiac tamponade

Tsang, T.S.M., Oh, J.K. & Seward, J.B. (1999) Diagnosis and management of cardiac tamponade in the era of echocardiography. *Clinical Cardiology* **22**, 446–452.

20 Deep vein thrombosis

Kearon, C., Math, J.M., Newman, T.E. & Ginsberg, J.S. (1998) Noninvasive diagnosis of deep vein thrombosis. *Annals of Internal Medicine* **128**, 663–677.

Lensing, A.W.A., Prandoni, P., Prins, M.H. & Buller, H.R. (1999) Deep-vein thrombosis. *Lancet* **353**, 479–485.

21 Pulmonary embolism

British Thoracic Society, Standards of Care Committee (1997) Suspected acute pulmonary embolism: a practical approach. *Thorax* **52** (Suppl. 4), S1–S24.

Goldhaber, S.Z. (1998) Medical progress: Pulmonary embolism. *New England Journal of Medicine* **339**, 93–104.

Wells, P.S., Ginsberg, J.S., Anderson, D.R. *et al.* (1998) Use of a clinical model for safe management of patients with suspected pulmonary embolism. *Annals of Internal Medicine* **129**, 997–1005.

Respiratory

22 Acute asthma

Lipworth, B.J. (1997) Treatment of acute asthma. *Lancet* **350** (Suppl. II:): 18–23.

The British guidelines on asthma management. 1995 review and position statement. *Thorax* 1997; **52** (Suppl. I): S1–S21.

23 Acute exacerbation of chronic obstructive pulmonary disease
Barnes, P.J. (2000) Medical progress: Chronic obstructive pulmonary disease. *New England Journal of Medicine* **343**, 269–280.
British Thoracic Society guidelines (1997) Management of acute exacerbations of COPD. *Thorax* **52** (Suppl. 5), S16–S21.
Madison, J.M. & Irwin, R.S. (1998) Chronic obstructive pulmonary disease. *Lancet* **352**, 467–473.

24 Pneumonia
Bartlett, J.G., Breimann, R.F., Mandell, L.A., File, T.M. Jr & Community-acquired pneumonia in adults: guidelines for management. *Clinical Infectious Diseases* **1998** (26), 811–838.
Brown, P.D. & Lerner, S.A. (1998) Community-acquired pneumonia. *Lancet* **352**, 1295–1302.
Stout, J.E. & Yu, V.L. (1997) Current concepts: Legionellosis. *New England Journal of Medicine* **337**, 682–687.

25 Pneumothorax
Peek, G.J., Morcos, S. & Cooper, G. (2000) Regular review: the pleural cavity. *British Medical Journal* **320**, 1318–1321.
Sahn, S.A. & Heffner, J.E. (2000) Spontaneous pneumothorax. *New England Journal of Medicine* **342**, 868–874.

26 Haemoptysis
Sternbach, G. & Varon, J. (1995) Massive haemoptysis. *Intensive Care World* **12**, 74–78.

Neurological

27 Stroke
Gubitz, G. & Sandercock, P. (2000) Acute ischaemic stroke. *British Medical Journal* **320**, 692–696.
Intercollegiate Working Party for Stroke. National clinical guidelines for stroke. Royal College of Physicians, London: (2000) www.rcplondon.ac.uk

28 Transient ischaemic attack

Albers, G.W., Hart, R.G., Lutsep, H.L., Newell, D.W. & Sacco, R.L. (1999) Suppl. to the guidelines for the management of transient ischemic attacks. *Stroke* **30**, 2502–2511.

29 Subarachnoid haemorrhage

Edlow, J.A. & Caplan, L.R. (2000) Primary care: Avoiding pitfalls in the diagnosis of subarachnoid hemorrhage. *New England Journal of Medicine* 2000, 29–36.

30 Bacterial meningitis

Begg, N., Cartwright, K.A.V., Cohen, J. *et al.* (1999) Consensus statement on diagnosis, investigation, treatment and prevention of acute bacterial meningitis in immunocompetent adults. *Journal of Infection* **39**, 1–15.

Quagliarello, V.J. & Scheld, W.M. (1997) Drug therapy: Treatment of bacterial meningitis. *New England Journal of Medicine* **336**, 708–716.

31 Spinal cord compression

Husband, D.J. (1998) Malignant spinal cord compression: prospective study of delays in referral and treatment. *British Medical Journal* **317**, 18–21.

32 Guillain–Barré syndrome

Hahn, A.F. (1998) Guillain–Barré syndrome. *Lancet* **352**, 635–641.

33 Epilepsy

Delanty, N., Vaughan, C.J. & French, J.A. (1998) Medical causes of seizures. *Lancet* **352**, 383–390.

Greenberg, M.K., Barsan, W.G. & Starkman, S. (1996) Neuroimaging in the emergency patient presenting with seizure. *Neurology* **47**, 26–32.

Lowenstein, D.H. & Alldredge, B.K. (1998) Current concepts: Status epilepticus. *New England Journal of Medicine* **338**, 970.

Gastrointestinal/Liver/Renal

34 Acute upper gastrointestinal haemorrhage

Early management of bleeding oesophageal varices. *Drug and Therapeutics Bulletin* 2000, **38**, 37–40.

Joint Working Group guidelines for good practice in and audit of the management of upper gastrointestinal haemorrhage. *Journal of Royal College of Physicians of London* 1992, **26**, 281–289.

Rockall, T.A., Logan, R.F.A., Devlin, H.B. & Northfield, T.C. (1995) Incidence of and mortality from acute upper gastrointestinal haemorrhage in the United Kingdom. *British Medical Journal* **311**, 222–226.

35 Acute diarrhoea

Gorbach, S.L. (1997) Treating diarrhoea. *British Medical Journal* **314**, 1776.

Kelly, C.P., Pothoulakis, C. & LaMont, J.T. (1994) Current concepts: *Clostridium difficile* colitis. *New England Journal of Medicine* **330**, 257–262.

Tabaqchali, S. & Jumaa, P. (1995) Diagnosis and management of *Clostridium difficile* infection. *British Medical Journal* **310**, 1375–1380.

36 Acute abdominal pain

Baron, T.H. & Morgan, D.E. (1999) Current concepts: Acute necrotizing pancreatitis. *New England Journal of Medicine* **340**, 1412–1417.

37 Acute liver failure

Caraceni, P. & Van Thiel, D.H. (1995) Acute liver failure. *Lancet* **345**, 163–169.

Mas, A. & Rodes, J. (1997) Fulminant hepatic failure. *Lancet* **349**, 1081–1085.

Riordan, S.M. & Williams, R. (1997) Current concepts: Treatment of hepatic encephalopathy. *New England Journal of Medicine* **337**, 473–479.

38 Acute renal failure

Brady, H.R. & Singer, G.G. (1995) Acute renal failure. *Lancet* **346**, 1533–1540.

Couser, W.G. (1999) Glomerulonephritis. *Lancet* **353**, 1509–1515.

Klahr, S. & Miller, S.B. (1998) Current concepts: Acute oliguria. *New England Journal of Medicine* **338**, 671–675.

Thadhani, R., Pascual, M. & Bonventre, J.V. (1996) Medical progress: Acute renal failure. *New England Journal of Medicine* **334**, 1448–1460.

Endocrine/Metabolic

39–41 Diabetes

Joshi, N., Caputo, G.M., Weitekamp, M.R. & Karchmer, A.W. (1999) Primary care: Infections in patients with diabetes mellitus. *New England Journal of Medicine* **341**, 1906–1912.

Lebovitz, H.E. (1995) Diabetic ketoacidosis. *Lancet* **345**, 767–772.

Service, F.J. (1995) Medical progress: Hypoglycaemic disorders. *New England Journal of Medicine* **332**, 1144–1152.

42 Electrolyte disorders (sodium, potassium and calcium)

Adrogue, H.J. & Madias, N.E. (2000) Primary care: Hypernatraemia. *New England Journal of Medicine* **342**, 1493–1499.

Adrogue, H.J. & Madias, N.E. (2000) Primary care: Hyponatraemia. *New England Journal of Medicine* **342**, 1581–1589.

Bushinsky, D.A. & Monk, R.D. (1998) Calcium. *Lancet* **352**, 306–311.

Gennari, F.J. (1998) Current concepts: Hypokalaemia. *New England Journal of Medicine* **339**, 451–458.

Halperin, M.L. & Kame, K.S. (1998) Potassium. *Lancet* **352**, 135–140.

Kumar, S. & Berl, T. (1998) Sodium. *Lancet* **352**, 220–228.

43 Acid-base disorders and arterial blood gases

Adrogue, H.J. & Madias, N.E. (1998) Medical progress: Management of life-threatening acid-base disorders. *New England Journal of Medicine* **338**, 26–34 and 107–111.

Gluck, S.L. (1998) Acid-base. *Lancet* **352**, 474–479.

44 Acute adrenal insufficiency

Oelkers, W. (1996) Current concepts: Adrenal insufficiency. *New England Journal of Medicine* **335**, 1206–1212.

45 Thyrotoxic crisis

Lazarus, J.H. (1997) Hyperthyroidism. *Lancet* **349**, 339–343.

46 Hypothermia and myxoedema coma

Danzl, D.F. & Pozos, R.S. (1994) Current concepts: Accidental hypothermia. *New England Journal of Medicine* **331**, 1756–1760.

Lindsay, R.S. & Toft, A.D. (1997) Hypothyroidism. *Lancet* **349**, 413–417.

Infectious diseases
47 Acute medical problems in the patient with HIV/AIDS

Cunningham, E.T. Jr & Margolis, T.P. (1998) Current concepts: Ocular manifestations of HIV infection. *New England Journal of Medicine* **339**, 236–244.

Monkemuller, K.E. & Wilcox, C.M. (1998) Diagnosis and treatment of colonic disease in AIDS. *Gastrointestinal Endoscopy Clinics of North America* **8**, 899–911.

Rosen, M.J. (1999) Intensive care of patients with HIV infection. *Seminars in Respiratory Infections* **14**, 366–371.

48 Septic arthritis

Goldenberg, D.L. (1998) Septic arthritis. *Lancet* **351**, 197–202.

49 Fever on return from abroad

Humar, A. & Keystone, J. (1996) Evaluating fever in travellers returning from tropical countries. *British Medical Journal* **312**, 953–956.

Haematological
50 Management of anticoagulation

Kearon, C. & Hirsh, J. (1997) Current concepts: Management of anticoagulation before and after elective surgery. *New England Journal of Medicine* **336**, 1506–1511.

Weitz, J.I. (1997) Low-molecular-weight heparins. *New England Journal of Medicine* **337**, 688–698.

51 Sickle cell disease

Davies, S.C. & Oni, L. (1997) Management of patients with sickle cell disease. *British Medical Journal* **315**, 656–660.

52 Anaphylaxis

Fisher, M. (1995) Treatment of acute anaphylaxis. *British Medical Journal* **311**, 731–733.

Project Team, Resuscitation Council (UK.). Emergency medical treatment of anaphylactic reactions. *Journal of Accident and Emergency Medicine*, 1999, **16**, 243–247.

Section 3: Procedures

53 Central vein cannulation

Mansfield, P.F., Hohn, D.C., Fornage, B.D., Gregurich, M.A. & Ota, D.M. (1994) Complications and failures of subclavian vein catheterization. *New England Journal of Medicine* **331**, 1735–1738.

Rosen, M., Latto, I.P. & Ng, W.S. (1993) Handbook of percutaneous central venous catheterisation (2nd edn). London: W.B. Saunders.

54 Pulmonary artery catheterization

Gomez, C.M.H. & Palazzo, M.G.A. (1998) Pulmonary artery catheterization in anaesthesia and intensive care. *British Journal of Anaesthesia* **81**, 945–956.

55 Temporary cardiac pacing

Fitzpatrick, A. & Sutton, R.A. (1992) A guide to temporary pacing. *British Medical Journal* **304**, 365–369.

Francis, G.S., Williams, S.V., Achord, J.L. *et al.* (1994) Clinical competence in insertion of a temporary transvenous ventricular pacemaker. *Circulation* **89**, 1913–1916.

Gammage, M.D. (2000) Temporary cardiac pacing. *Heart* **83**, 715–720.

56 Pericardial aspiration

Callahan, J.A., Seward, J.B., Nishimura, R.A. *et al.* (1985) Two-dimensional echocardiographically guided pericardiocentesis: experience in 117 consecutive patients. *American Journal of Cardiology* **55**, 476–479.

Krikorian, J.G. & Hancock, E.W. (1978) Pericardiocentesis. *American Journal of Medicine* **65**, 808–814.

57 DC cardioversion

Yurchak, P.M. (1993) AHA/ACC/ACP. Task Force Statement. Clinical competence in elective direct current cardioversion. *Circulation* **88**, 342–345.

58 Insertion of a chest drain

Hyde, J., Sykes, T. & Graham, T. (1997) Reducing morbidity from chest drains. *British Medical Journal* **314**, 914–915.

Miller, K.S. & Sahn, S.A. (1987) Chest tubes: indications, technique, management and complications. *Chest* **91**, 258–264.

59 Lumbar puncture
Petito, F. & Plum, F. (1974) The lumbar puncture. *New England Journal of Medicine* **290**, 225–227.
Practice parameters (1993) Lumbar puncture. *Neurology* **43**, 625–627.

60 Peritoneal dialysis
Ronco, C. & Bellomo, R. (1999) Renal replacement methods in acute renal failure. *Oxford Textbook of Nephrology*, Oxford. Oxford University Press (available on-line at www.doctors.net.uk).

61 Insertion of a Sengstaken-Blakemore tube
Haddock, G., Garden, O.J., McKee, R.F. *et al.* (1989) Esophageal tamponade in the management of acute variceal hemorrhage. *Digestive Diseases and Sciences* **34**, 913–918.

Index

abdomen, in critically ill patient 131
abdominal pain, acute 288–94
  causes 293
  examination 290
  investigation 291
  priorities 288–90
  site 289
acid-base disorders 353–63
  classification 356
  grading 357
  management 355–63
acid-base status 353, 354–5
acquired immunodeficiency syndrome 381–6 *see also* HIV/AIDS
activated charcoal 110–12, 125
active rewarming 34, 375
acute respiratory distress syndrome (ARDS) 165, 166
  causes 168
  diagnostic criteria 168
  management 170–1
adenosine 12, 15
adrenal insufficiency, acute 342, 364–8
  causes 366
  clinical features 365
  diagnosis 367–8
  investigation 366
  management 364–8
  priorities 364
  problems 368
adrenaline
  infusion 481–3
  in life support 7
adrenergic agonist dosage 480
alcohol
  abuse 86, 209
  withdrawal delirium 90–1
  withdrawal ('rum fits') 268–9
  withdrawal seizures 91
alteplase 228
amiodarone IV 42
anaemia, sickle-cell crisis 239
anaphylactic shock 414–16
anaphylaxis 37–8, 414–16
aneurysm
  abdominal aorta 36
  berry, rupture 242–5
  subarachnoid 243
angina, unstable 46, 52, 151–5
  drug therapy 154
  history taking 151
  management 152, 153–5
  priorities 151–5
  stratification of patients 152–3
anticoagulation 232–3, 403–8
antidotes to poisons 117
antithyroid therapy 371
aortic dissection 156–9, 160
  chest pain 51, 55
  classification 157
  hypotensive therapy 158
  priorities 156–9
aortic mural haematoma 159
ARDS *see* acute respiratory distress syndrome

arterial blood gases 353–3
   sampling 353–5
arterial puncture 427
arteritis 239
arthritis, septic 387–91
aspirin
   for ischaemic stroke 230
   poisoning 118–19
asterixis 86
asthma, acute 193–7
   bronchodilator infusions 195
   management 194, 196–7
   priorities 193–6
ataxia 88
atrial fibrillation 12, 15, 16, 23, 24–9
   drug doses 27
   management 33
   stroke and 232
atrial flutter 12, 19, 27
   drug doses 27
   management 29, 33
atrial tachycardia 21
   management 30–1
atrioventricular block
   first degree 31–2
   myocardial infarction and 145
   second degree 29, 30, 32–4
   third degree 34
atropine in life support 7
autonomic hyperactivity 90

bacterial meningitis 93, 247–53
   antibiotic therapy 248
   clinical features 248
   CSF formulae 250
   investigation 249
   management 249–51
   priorities 247–9
bacterial pericarditis 172–4, 447
berry aneurysm, rupture 242–5
beta-blockade 370
   reversal 32
biliary tract sepsis 89

bradyarrhythmias 17, 22
   myocardial infarction and 145
bradycardia, sinus or junctional
   31
breathlessness, acute 57–63
   diagnosis 60–2
   in HIV/AIDS 381–2
   investigation 59
   with normal chest X-ray 63
   priorities 57–9
   with raised JVP 62
bronchiectasis 209
brucellosis 395
bundle branch block 12

calcium, plasma 348
carbon monoxide poisoning 125–6
cardiac arrest 3–9
cardiac arrhythmias 10–35
   COPD and 203–5
   diagnosis 10–21
   priorities 10
cardiac pacing, temporary 438–46
   failure to capture and/or sense
      444, 445
   indications 443
   technique 443–5
   troubleshooting 445–6
   wire placement 438–41
cardiac syncope 74
cardiac tamponade 172, 175–7
   and pericardial tamponade 447
cardiogenic shock 36, 39–41
carotid artery dissection 92
carotid sinus
   hypersensitivity, testing 81
   massage 12
central vein cannulation 419–28
   choice of route 420
   complications 420
   indications 419
   right femoral vein puncture 425,
      426

right internal jugular vein
puncture 421–3
right subclavian vein puncture
424–5
technique 419–27
troubleshooting 427–8
central venous pressure
in hypotension 43, 45
interpreting CVP 421
method of measuring 422
charcoal, activated 110–12, 125
chest compression 4
chest drain
insertion of 455–60
technique 455–9
troubleshooting 459–60
chest pain, acute 46–56
causes 56
examination 52–3
further management 53–5
history taking 48–52
initial management 49
priorities 46–53
chronic obstructive pulmonary
disease (COPD) 63, 198–205,
209
breathlessness in 57
clinical assessment 199
investigations 200
management 201–3
priorities 198–200
ventilatory support 201
cigarette smoking 51
Clostridium difficile 281, 28
coma
causes
with focal neurological signs 70,
71
with hyperventilation 68
with neck stiffness 70
without signs 70, 71
eye signs 69
confusion in HIV/AIDS 382

confusional state, acute 84–91
clinical assessment 84–8
investigation 88
management 88–9, 91
mental state assessment 84
consciousness, clouding of 84
consciousness, transient loss 74–81
history taking 74–6
priorities 74–80
cor pulmonale 203
corticosteroids 367
critically ill patient 127–31
airway and breathing 127–8
causes 130
circulation 128–9
investigation 128
neurological status 129–31
priorities 127
cryptococcal meningitis 252
Cushing syndrome 164
cystic fibrosis 209
cytomegalovirus 397

DC cardioversion 42, 451–4
deep vein thrombosis 178–82
investigation 181
management 178–81
probability of 179
risk factors 180
stroke and 232
defibrillation 3, 4–7
delirium tremens 90, 91
causes 89–91
dementia, clinical features 87
diabetes 51, 319–27
blood glucose levels 321
management after myocardial
infarction 323–4
newly diagnosed, management
322–3
peri-operative assessment 324–7
treatment with oral hypoglycaemic
agents 326–7

diabetic ketoacidosis (DKA) 321,
        328–34
    causes 329
    fluid and electrolyte replacement
        330, 332
    infection and 333
    insulin infusion 331, 334
    investigation 329
    management 332–4
    priorities 328–32
diamorphine in sickle cell crisis 409
diarrhoea, acute 281–7
    causes 282–4
    examination 281–5
    investigations 285–6
    priorities 281–6
diazepam in status epilepticus 262
digoxin
    poisoning 125
    toxicity 17, 30–1
disorientation in time 84
disseminated intravascular
        coagulation 104–5
dobutamine infusion 484–5
dopamine infusion 484–5
Dressler (post–cardiotomy)
        syndrome 174
drug abuse, fever in 209
drug infusions 479–85

elderly, mental state examination 86
electrolyte disorders 336–52
embolism from the heart
    stroke and 235–6
    TIA and 238–9
emphysematous bulla 217
endocarditis 89
epilepsy 261–9
    causes 264
    diagnosis 266–8
    drug therapy 263
    investigation 262
    priorities 261–4

Epstein-Barr virus 397
exercise stress testing 149–50
eye signs in comatose patient 69

falciparum malaria 393–4, 397–9
fever
    drug abuse and 209
    headache and 53, 54
    after myocardial infarction 149
    on return from abroad 392–400
    stroke and 233
fibrillation, acute atrial
    hypotension and 42–4
fit *see* epilepsy; syncope
flecainide 28
flumazenil 66–7, 130
forced expiratory volume in 1 s 488,
        490
forced vital capacity 489, 490

gastric lavage 112–13
gastritis, erosive 279
gastrointestinal haemorrhage, upper,
        acute 273–80
    blood loss estimation 275
    investigation 275
    management 274, 277–8
    priorities 23–7
    problems 280
gentamicin 101
Glasgow Coma Scale 68, 72–3, 129
glaucoma, acute angle-closure 95
glycosuria 319–21
Guillain–Barré syndrome 256–60
    diagnostic criteria 257
    investigation 258
    management 258–9
    priorities 256–8
    problems 259

haematemesis 221, 273
haematoma, intracranial 70
haemoptysis 221–3

causes 222
  investigation 223
head injury 68
  signs of 68–70
headache 92–9
  clinical assessment 92–3
  with fever and no focal
      neurological signs 93, 94
  in HIV/AIDS 382
  with local signs 95
  with no abnormal signs 96–9
  with papilloedema but no focal
      neurological signs 94
  reduced conscious level/focal
      neurological signs 93
heparin
  low molecular weight 403
  unfractionated heparin (UFH) 403,
      404
hepatic encephalopathy, grading 297
hepatic foetor 86
hepatitis A and B 397
HIV/AIDS 209, 381–6
  breathlessness in 381–2, 383
  confusion 382
  impaired vision 386
  investigation 384
  neurological problems 382–6
  safety precautions 382
  spectrum of infection 385
  upper motor neurone signs 385–6
human immunodeficiency syndrome
    see HIV/AIDS
hydrocephalus, obstructive 70
hyperaldosteronism 164
hypercalcaemia 348–52
  causes 349
  drug therapy 351
  investigation 349
hyperglycaemia 227, 233
  management after myocardial
      infarction 323–4
hyperkalaemia 8, 344–6

diagnosis 345
  severe 302–4, 344–6
hyperlipidaemia 51
hypernatraemia 336–8
  diagnosis 337
  hypervolaemic 338
  hypovolaemic 336
  normovolaemic 338
hyperosmolar non-ketotic
      hyperglycaemia (HONK) 321,
      328, 335
hypertension 51, 160–4
  accelerated-phase 94
  examination 160–1
  history taking 160
  intravenous therapy 162
  investigations 161
  oral therapy 163
  subarachnoid haemorrhage and
      245
hypertensive encephalopathy 160,
      161
hyperviscosity syndrome 239
hypocalcaemia 352
  acute, with tetany 352
  causes 351
hypoglycaemia 19, 65, 107, 227, 319
  causes 320
hypokalaemia 14, 346–8
  diagnosis 347
hyponatraemia 338–42
  hypovolaemic 342
  management 338
  with neurological abnormalities
      338–40
  normovolaemic 342
  oedematous 342
  without severe neurological
      symptoms 341
hypotension 36–45
  causes 37
  correcting 308–9
  further management 41–5

haemorrhage and 36, 39
investigation 40
JVP in 129
myocardial infarction 142–5
priorities 36–41
pulmonary artery catheterization 429
hypothermia 373–7
investigation 374
priorities 373–4
hypothyroidism 342
hypovolaemia 36, 142
correcting 308–9
hypotension and 44–5
hypovolaemic shock
in gastrointestinal haemorrhage 274–6
hypoxia, hypovolaemia and 45

infection, acute confusional state and 89
influenza 209
inotropic/vasopressor therapy
dosages 42
hypotension and 41
myocardial infarction and 144
in refractory hypotension 45
insulin infusion
in diabetes 322
in diabetic ketoacidosis 331, 334
ischaemic stroke 230
isoprenaline infusion in bradycardia 11

jaundice 86, 397

left bundle branch block,
pulmonary artery catheterization and 437
Legionella pneumonia 395
leptospirosis 395, 397
life support
advanced 3–8, 6

basic 3, 5
liver disease
decompensation in 296
management 297–8
liver failure, acute 295–301
causes 300
complications 299
investigation 296
management 298–301
priorities 295–7
'liver flap' 86
lorazepam 262
low molecular weight heparin 403
lumbar puncture 461–6
anatomy of 464
in bacterial meningitis 247–9
contraindications 461
equipment 461
indications 461
problems 464–6
technique 462–4

malaria 70, 89, 94, 392–3
benign 399
falciparum 396, 398–9
Mallory-Weiss tear 273, 279–80
Marfan syndrome 51
melaena 273
memory, impaired short-term 84
meningitis 96, 100
CSF formulae in 465
see also bacterial meningitis;
tuberculous meningitis
mesenteric infarction 131
mesenteric vascular occlusion, causes 292
metabolic acidosis, causes 359
metabolic alkalosis, causes 360
methicillin-resistant *Staphylococcus aureus* (MRSA) 101
migraine 98–9
morphine in sickle cell crisis 409
multifocal atrial tachycardia 31

myocardial infarction, acute 137–50
    chest pain and 46, 52, 55
    drug therapy 147, 148
    ECG 50
    fever after 149
    investigation 140
    new murmur 147–9
    recurrent pain 147
    rehabilitation 19, 150
    sinus or junctional bradycardia
        related to 31
    thrombolytic therapy 141–3
myocardial necrosis 52
myxoedema coma, treatment of
    375–7

naloxone 66,107
nerve palsy VI 86
non-invasive positive pressure
        ventilation (NIPPV) 200
noradrenaline infusion 481–3
nystagmus 86

oesophageal rupture 51, 55
oesophageal ulcer 280
oesophagitis 280
oxygen delivery devices 361–2
oxygen therapy 363

pacemaker malfunction 34–5
pacing wire 438–46
pancreatitis 131
    causes 22
paracetamol poisoning 119–23
    liver failure and 295
paralysis, causes 260
passive rewarming 375
peak expiratory flow rate 487
peptic ulcer 278–9
pericardial aspiration 447–50
    complications 448
    equipment 447
    indications 447

technique 447–9
troubleshooting 45
pericardiocentesis 62, 173
pericarditis 52, 147, 172–4
    bacterial 172–4, 447
    causes 173
    ECG 50
    investigation 173
    viral ('idiopathic') 174
peripheral nervous system 491–5
peritoneal dialysis 467–71
    for acute renal failure 468–9
    antibiotic therapy and 470
    contraindications 467
    for core-rewarming in
        hypothermia 470
    indications 467
    technique 467–8
    troubleshooting 471
peritonitis
    causes 292
    generalized 131
    peritoneal dialysis in 471
pethidine in sickle cell crisis 409
phaeochromocytoma 164
phenobarbitone 265
phenytoin 265
Plasmodium ovale malaria 399
Plasmodium vivax malaria 399
pleurisy 52
Pneumocystis carinii pneumonia 381
    in HIV/AIDS 384
pneumonia 206–16
    antibiotic therapy 209–10, 211, 212
    aspiration (inhalation) 214–16
    breathlessness and 63
    chest X-ray 198
    community acquired 208
    differential diagnosis 208
    history 209
    investigation 207
    management 210
    priorities 206–10

Pneumocystis carinii 381, 384
sepsis and 100
pneumothorax 217–20
causes 220
central vein cannulation and 427
chest pain 51, 55
management 217–20
priorities 217
X-ray 198
poisoning 106–26
aspirin 116–17
carbon monoxide 125–6
conscious patient 106–9
digoxin 124, 125
elimination, increasing 113
management 110–16
paracetamol 117–23
plasma levels 110
poison, clues to 108–9
priorities 106–10
problems 115
psychiatric assessment 114–16
salicylate 118–19
supportive treatment 114
unconscious patient 109–10
Poisons Information Centres 116
polyneuropathy, acute idiopathic *see*
Guillain–Barré syndrome
potassium 343
priapism in sickle cell crisis 411
propofol 265
pseudoseizures 264
characteristics 265
psychosis, acute functional
clinical features 87
pulmonary artery catheterization
429–37
indications 429
technique 429–34
troubleshooting 434–7
wedge pressure measurement 433
pulmonary embolism 36, 46, 52, 55,
183–9

clinical presentation 184
priorities 183–6
thrombolytic therapy 187
pulmonary oedema 57, 63, 160, 165–71
blood pressure in 167–9
causes 166
hypotension and 36, 39–41
investigation 167
priorities 165–7
pulmonary artery catheterization
429
renal failure and 304

recovery position 66
renal artery stenosis, clinical features
163
renal failure, acute 302–15
causes 303, 304–7
clinical features 311–14
examination 306–7
investigation 305
management 309
priorities 302–9
ultrasound 307
urinalysis 308
renal replacement therapy
indications 310
respiratory acidosis, causes 358
respiratory alkalosis, causes 359
respiratory failure 200
in Guillain–Barré syndrome 259
type 204
respiratory function tests 486–90
resuscitation
stopping 8
successful 8–9
rewarming in hypothermia
active 374, 375
passive 375
rhinocerebral mucormycosis 333

salicylate poisoning 118–19
Seldinger technique 425–7

Sengstaken–Blakemore tube 472–6
  equipment 472
  indication 472
  technique 473–6
sepsis 36
  in ARDS 171
  in hypotension 45
sepsis syndrome 100–5
  antibiotic therapy 103
  investigation 102
  IV drug use and 104
  neutropenia and 102–4
  priorities 100–1
septic arthritis 387–91
  antibiotic therapy 390
  causes 388
  gonocccal cf non-gonococcal 389
  investigation 390
  management 388–91
  priorities 387
septic shock
  investigation 102
  malaria and 393–4
shock lung 165
'sick sinus syndrome' 31
sickle cell crisis 409–13
  indications for exchange
      transfusion 411
  investigation 410
  management 412
  priorities 409–12
  problems 413
sinoatrial disease ('sick sinus
      syndrome') 31
sinus (junctional) bradycardia 31
sinusitis, acute 95
sodium, plasma 336
sodium bicarbonate buffer in life
      support 7–8
spinal cord compression 254–5
status epilepticus 66
  generalized tonic-clonic 261–5
  non-convulsive 86

Stokes–Adams attack 74
stroke 70, 227–36
  cerebellar 235
  clinical features 229
  imaging 231
  investigation 228, 230
  management 230–3
  prevention 234–5
  priorities 227–30
  secondary prevention 234–5
subarachnoid haemorrhage 96, 242–6
  aneurysmal, clinical features 243
  causes 244
  clinical features 96, 97
  investigation 244
  priorities 242–5
  problems 245–6
subdural haematoma, chronic 235
suicide, poisoning and 116
supraventricular tachycardia
  drug doses 30
  management 34
SVT (AV nodal re-entrant
      tachycardia/AV re-entrant
      tachycardia) 29–30
syncope 74–83
  causes 76–7, 83
  diagnosis 77
  ECG 78–9
  investigation 82
  unexplained 81
syndrome of inappropriate ADH
      secretion (SIADH) 342, 343

tachyarrhythmia
  cardiac pacing and 445
  DC cardioversion and 451–4
  diagnosis 11–17
  myocardial infarction and 145–6
  ventricular (VT) 12–15
tachycardia
  diagnosis and management 13
  differential diagnosis 18

temporal arteritis 98
tension pneumothorax 37, 57
thiopentone 266
thyroid hormone replacement
in myxoedema coma 376
thyrotoxic crisis 369–72
antithyroid treatment 371
heart failure and 369
investigation 370
precipitants 370
priorities 369–72
thyrotoxicosis 25, 28
torsade de pointes 12, 24
transient ischaemic attack 237–41
diagnosis 238
investigation 239
neurological/visual symptoms,
causes 240
priorities 237–9
symptoms 241
tricyclic poisoning 8
tropical fever 393–9
incubation periods 394
investigation 397
management 393–7
meningism 395–7
priorities 392–3
septic shock 393–4
signs 395
troponin T and I 52
tuberculous meningitis 251–2, 395
tubular necrosis, acute 310–15
typhoid 94, 393–4
clinical features 396

unconscious patient 64–73
management 67–7
poisoning and 106–9

priorities 64–7
unfractionated heparin (UFH) 403,
404

Valsalva manoeuvre 12
variceal bleeding 276–7
vasovagal syncope 74
venepuncture 421–5
venous thrombo-embolism 51
ventilation 3–4
ventricular fibrillation (VF) 3, 4–6
DC cardioversion and 451
drug therapy 7–8
ventricular infarction, right 142, 144
ventricular septal rupture
pulmonary artery catheterization
437
ventricular tachycardia (VT) 3, 4–6
DC cardioversion 451
drug therapy 7–8
hypotension and 42
management 21–3
viral encephalitis 252–3
viral haemorrhagic fever 393

warfarin 234
clinical conditions affecting 406
indications 405
management of over-
anticoagulation 408
starting 407
Wernicke's encephalopathy 65, 86,
91, 107
wheeze 57
Wolff–Parkinson–White (WPW)
syndrome 12, 20, 30

xanthochromia 96